ALLEN COUNTY PUBLIC LIBRARY
P9-EEC-991

THE WOMAN'S GUIDE

TO HYSTERECTOMY

Expectations and Options

by Adelaide Haas, Ph.D.
Susan L. Puretz, Ed.D.

CELESTIAL ARTS
Berkeley, California

Celestial Arts Publishing
P.O. Box 7123
Berkeley, California 94707

Library of Congress Cataloging-in-Publication Data

Haas, Adelaide.
The woman's guide to hysterectomy: expectations and options /
by Adelaide Haas, Susan L. Puretz.
p. cm.
Includes bibliographical references and index.
ISBN 0-89087-743-2
1. Hysterectomy — Popular works. I. Puretz, Susan L. II. Title.
RG391.H33 1994 94-30362
618.1'453—dc20 CIP

Cover by Fifth Street Design
Text design and production by Star Type, Berkeley

First Printing, 1995

2 3 4 5 / 99 98 97 96 95

TABLE OF CONTENTS

ACKNOWLEDGMENTS

Every book is written and produced with assistance from many sources; ours is no exception. Our research would not have been possible without the support of Sieglinde Luskin, Robert and Virginia Nacamu, Lisa McKinney, Minna Haas, and Steve Sconfienza. Most importantly, the women who told us their stories provided the personal insights that introduce nearly all the chapters.

Our colleagues at the State University of New York at New Paltz aided us at every stage of this project: Associates in the Alumni Association; Rose Taft Waltzer; colleagues in the Sojourner Truth Library, especially Gerlinda Barley; Dr. Dudley Cahn, Donna Davis, and Gretchen Madoff, of the Department of Communication; Deana Groves, of the Department of Health and Physical Education; and Rhoda Nemerofsky, R.N., of the College Health Center. Their combined wisdom and efforts turned many awkward phrases into readable prose.

We received invaluable assistance from Mitchell Levine, M.D., and Carmella Parham, M.D.; Donna Meltzer, M.D.; Francoise Dunefsky, R.N.; and Sharon Cahn, R.N. All will find their contributions on the pages which follow.

William A. Smith, physical therapist, and Rose Mancuso, dietician at Kingston Hospital, gave thoughtful input regarding nutrition, diet, and exercise.

Ely Cohn, Ph.D., Ilka List, Dorothy Jessup, Merle London, and Louise Tricard gave helpful suggestions. Laurie Meltzer, Mary Phillips, and Gerald Silverman offered kind assistance. Ruth Haas, Hollise Carr, Aloysius Helminck, and Joseph Haas served as frequent reminders of the importance of our project.

Carole Brugnoni carefully prepared all the line-art in this work.

Deepest appreciation goes to the people at Celestial Arts. David Hinds saw the need for this book and agreed to publish our efforts. Veronica Randall, our dynamic editor, has been steadfast in her encouragement and enthusiasm. Linda Davis and the typesetting crew at Star Type were meticulous in their work.

Finally, we thank Kurt Haas and Phillip McDonald who have shared our commitment in writing this book. They understood the hours we needed to disappear into our studies and recognized that we had important messages for other women and their partners.

INTRODUCTION

Perhaps as a child you had your tonsils removed, or, as an adult, a fractured leg or arm was placed in a cast. These are ordinarily not perceived as very threatening experiences compared to the mere *thought* of hysterectomy. Hysterectomy not only evokes the anxiety associated with major surgery, but often also raises disturbing questions regarding youth, femininity, and sexuality.

For many women, hysterectomy is their first and only major surgery. One in three women has had this procedure by the time she reaches age 65. Hysterectomies are performed more than any other surgical procedure in the United States, with the exception of birth by Cesarean section. If hysterectomy has been recommended for you, it might help to know that you are not alone.

HOW THIS BOOK CAME TO BE WRITTEN

Addie's Experience

About ten years ago hysterectomy surgery was recommended for me, Addie Haas, because of enlarged fibroids. The gynecologist, Dr. K., at a routine annual checkup, commented, "those fibroids of yours are getting too big; we should plan to remove them."

Eager to avoid surgery, I sought several different medical opinions. I had read that the uterus decreases in size and that fibroids tend to shrink as women approach menopause. I was 43; maybe if I just stalled for a few years the problem would go away by itself. I checked with four different physicians — the gynecologist assigned by my insurance company, the family doctor, a female gynecologist at a large university medical center, and finally a male gynecologist who had performed the surgery on an acquaintance of mine. All agreed: "Take the uterus out! You've had your children, the fibroids have become too large to shrink, and they may impinge on your bladder or kidneys and cause serious problems."

I began to read as much as possible to prepare myself for what lay ahead. Poring over medical tomes and journals as well as popular magazines and books, I was dismayed at the limited amount of information available. Eventually I followed the professional advice, had the surgery, and recovered nicely. I was determined, however, to share what I learned with other women and to provide them with more complete and accurate information than I had.

Initially my intention in writing this book was to summarize medical information and make it available to women who were to have hysterectomies. As I read through the medical literature, however, I recognized that an important piece was missing. Women want to know more than technical facts. We also want to know how other women feel and react before, during, and after this surgery. In other words, we are interested in the patient's point of view.

I discussed it with my friend and colleague, Professor Susan Puretz. Recognizing the scope of this project, we decided to join forces and work together.

We felt that the best way to get women's perceptions and reactions to hysterectomy is to ask some direct questions. This was a large undertaking. The research for the book occupied us for almost three years .

Susan's Saga

In fall of 1990, I, Susan, was told I needed a hysterectomy. I ended up duplicating Addie's experience and feeling frustrated that there wasn't one source which answered all my myriad questions. All information had to be garnered piecemeal. I, of course, had one advantage that many women facing the prospect of hysterectomy don't have — I could use Addie as my quarterback, mentor, and advisor. I sought various medical opinions, and all doctors agreed that a hysterectomy was necessary. I was able to keep my ovaries, but my uterus was removed in a "bikini cut" procedure. I recovered easily, and my partner reports, and I believe, that today I am as fully vibrant, energetic, and sexy as before. This is reassuring information for women anticipating surgery.

THE RESEARCH PROJECT

The purpose of our investigation was to learn about hysterectomy from the patient's perspective. As a first step, we developed a questionnaire which asked numerous questions related to hysterectomy, health, sex, family, and relationships. We sent this pilot study to 22 women friends and acquaintances.

We were struck by two reactions: First, all 22 women filled out the questionnaire and returned it to us. Second, the responses were almost all detailed and lengthy. These women were eager to talk about their hysterectomy experiences. They also wanted to know more and to learn what our findings were.

Following their suggestions we improved the original questionnaire and then launched our major project — 1,200 questionnaires which were mailed to women who were in every fifth graduating class between 1945 and 1975 of a small public college. Two hundred and ninety (24 percent) responded. This is considered a good response rate for an unsolicited mail survey. Questionnaires were also distributed through four physicians' offices; 78 women participated in this way. All women were volunteers and assured of complete anonymity. The names you read in this book are not the real names of participants.

The respondents ranged in age from 21 to 84 years and the majority were from the northeastern states. Seventy-seven percent were college graduates. About 59 percent of the women who answered the survey had not yet reached menopause, 19 percent had experienced surgical menopause (had hysterectomies), and 22 percent were naturally past menopause.

THE QUESTIONNAIRE

The final questionnaire was eight pages long and consisted of both machine-codable items and open-ended questions. Quotations from women who responded are found at the beginning of many chapters. Further information regarding the questionnaire may be found in articles in the journals *Health Communication* and the *Journal of Women and Aging.*[1]

WHAT LIES AHEAD FOR YOU, THE READER

If you are the one in three women on whom a hysterectomy will be performed, you will read about other women's experiences. You will learn that the vast majority are glad they had the surgery and were generally well treated. You will learn answers to questions that are frequently asked to help you make decisions and act in an informed and assured manner. You also will become aware of options you have for avoiding surgery. You will learn how to become an active partner in your own health care.

ENDNOTES

1. Haas, A., & Puretz, S. L. Encouraging partnerships between health care providers and women recommended for gynecological surgery. *Health Communication,* 1992, *4* (1), 29 – 38.

Puretz, S. L., & Haas, A. Sexual desire and responsiveness following hysterectomy and menopause. *Journal of Women and Aging,* 1992, *5* (2), 3 – 15.

Chapter 1

PARTNERS

"Thank you for being interested in asking women about their health. I hope you will give the information to doctors." — Mary, age 39.

YOU'RE IN GOOD COMPANY

If you are reading this book because gynecological surgery has been prescribed for you, you're in good company. In the United States today, *one in three women has had a hysterectomy by the time she reaches age 65.*[1]

Mary Beth S., age 45, mentioned to her mother that her periods had become more uncomfortable than in the past. The parental response was, "well, you should probably have your uterus taken out. It's not doing you any good anymore. I had a hysterectomy when I was 43. Good-bye and good riddance is what I say." Mary Beth's husband echoed this sentiment more crudely. He told Mary Beth that when the wife of a friend from work had a hysterectomy at age 40, the colleague reported "they got rid of the nursery but kept the playpen." Mary Beth wondered whether any pleasure remained for the woman, since she had heard that the uterus is active in women's orgasm. (See Chapter Ten for a discussion of sex after hysterectomy.)

The more Mary Beth spoke with friends, the more she heard about women who had hysterectomies. She began to feel like a candidate for an elite club. A look at Table 1 – 1 confirms Mary Beth's observations.

EDUCATION MAY PROVIDE OPTIONS

Education and income level seem to be related to the likelihood of having a hysterctomy. According to a study of almost 12,500 women from 16 states, women with less education and lower incomes more often have hysterectomies than those from higher socioeconomic groups.[2]

TABLE 1 – 1

PERCENT OF U.S. WOMEN WHO HAVE HAD THEIR UTERUS REMOVED BY THE TIME THEY HAVE REACHED THE INDICATED AGES

Age	1970	1980	1990
20	.1	.1	.1
30	5.1	5.3	4.6
40	14.2	21.4	20.0
50	24.1	32.0	36.7
60	31.4	31.2	37.0
70	38.6	35.0	34.6
80	31.8	41.1	38.8

Adapted and interpolated from National Hospital Discharge Survey, unpublished data, National Center for Health Statistics, DCD.

This pattern holds true outside of the United States as well. Dr. R. Luoto and his associates at the University of Helsinki in Finland found that highly educated women had fewer hysterectomies compared to those with less schooling.[3] Possibly women with more education and better resources are less apt to accept one physician's recommendation. They may be better able to find alternatives to this major surgical procedure.

THE INSURANCE FACTOR

Women whose insurance is based on a fee-for-service to their physician are more likely to undergo hysterectomy than those who belong to a health maintenance organization (HMO). The obvious suspicion here, of course, is that a profit motive is in effect.[4]

While it appears that all women who belong to HMOs and require hysterectomies receive them, inappropriate *overuse* of the procedure in HMOs has been judged to be about 16%.[5] This is similar to the pattern found in HMOs for other procedures such as hernia surgery or appendectomy. Although it is reassuring to know that HMOs provide treatment when needed, excessive surgeries are of serious concern. Since HMOs schedule some unnecessary costly surgeries, one wonders if excesses occur when it is profitable to the physician.

Dr. Camilla Parham reports that currently most insurance companies compensate doctors for hysterectomy at a higher rate than myomectomies.[6] This can provide a not-so-subtle pressure for a gynecologist to perform the more traditional surgery to earn more money. It's almost the rule that the more you take out, the more you earn — regardless of the relative difficulty or time involved in the procedure. (Less tissue is removed in a myomectomy compared to a hysterectomy, but a myomectomy is generally considered to be a more difficult procedure.)

PHYSICIAN ORIENTATION

Hysterectomy is a procedure that has been around for a long time. Physicians, as most of us, often feel comfortable in a familiar routine. If hysterectomy was the approach to gynecological problems that was used by a doctor's teachers, there may be a tendency to stay with the "tried and true." A pattern of treatment develops which is hard to break.

Myomectomy and other options are newer and require special skills. Fortunately, medical doctors engage in "continuing education." As they develop competence and confidence in approaches which are less drastic than hysterectomy, alternatives will become more generally available.

TAKING CONTROL

"TELL ME WHAT TO DO." / "DON'T TELL ME WHAT TO DO."

In matters regarding our health, we often want to be taken care of — especially when we are ill and/or afraid. Despite this, more and more people today reject the traditional paternalism of many doctors. We don't want to be *told* what to do. Instead, we want to be *given information* so that we can make our own decisions.

But let's face it. Taking responsiblity is work. We need to ferret out the facts and learn how to interpret them. How can we even begin to make medical decisions, when physicians who have years of education and experience often disagree with one another?

Members of the medical community have considered this conflict. Linda and Ezekial Emanuel, a wife and husband team in which each holds both a Ph.D. and an M.D., write, "during the last two decades there has been a struggle over the patient's role in medical decision-making…there has been a movement to curtail physician dominance and [allow for] greater patient control."[7] The Emanuels' analysis leads them to pose the question, "What should be the ideal physician-patient relationship?" They recognize that no one style of interaction is suitable for all in every circumstance. However, they conclude that in general, a "deliberative model" in which clients come prepared to ask good questions, and physicians stand ready to relinquish some control and take time to discuss options, has much to commend it.

While information we learn from our doctor doesn't always lead to the right behavior (flossing, mammogram, pap smear, exercise), it gives us the option of informed choice. If we choose not to act on information, that is our decision. But when we act without knowledge, we really haven't chosen.

PARTNERS IN HEALTH CARE

A recent Gallup poll found that physician information to patients regarding both surgical (hysterectomy-induced) and natural menopause was often inadequate. Although about two-thirds of women reported that their doctors discussed physical symptoms such as hot flashes, night sweats, and osteoporosis, only about one-half talked about heart disease, hormone replacement therapy, cancer, or sex. In fact, most of the women reported that the information they had about menopause came primarily from magazines, books, television, and family and friends rather than their health care provider.

Dr. Wulf Utian, director of the North American Menopause Society, commenting on this survey, urged physicians to play a larger role in informing their patients on all aspects of menopause, including emotional, sexual, and physical concerns.[8]

While doctors must take responsibility for informing patients, we do not have to passively wait to be told. We can learn to ask the right questions and assume an active role in our health care.

This book is dedicated to helping women become better informed.

ENDNOTES

1. Graves, E. J. *1991 Summary: National Hospital Discharge Survey.* Advance data from vital and health statistics; no. 227. Hyattsville, MD: National Center for Health Statistics, 1993.

2. Kjerulff, K. H., Langenberg, P., & Guzinski, G. The socioeconomic correlates of hysterectomies in the United States. *American Journal of Public Health,* 1993(a), 83 (1), 106 – 108.

3. Luoto, R., Hemminki, E., Topo, P., et al. Hysterectomy among Finnish women: prevalence and women's own opinions. *Scandinavian Journal of Social Medicine,* 1992, 20 (4), 209 – 212.

4. Brody, J. E. Hysterectomy: the facts about the most common operation in the United States. *New York Times,* November 11, 1981.

Brody, J. E. A decline in hysterectomy surgery still falls short. *New York Times,* June 30, 1993, c14.

5. Bernstein, S. J., McGlynn, E. A., Siu, A. L., et al. The appropriateness of hysterectomy. A comparison of care in seven health plans. Health Maintenance Organization Quality of Care Consortium. *Journal of the American Medical Association,* 1993, 269 (18), 2398 – 2402.

6. Camilla Parham, M.D., personal communication.

7. Emanuel, E. J., & Emanuel, L. L. Four models of the physician-patient relationship. *Journal of the American Medical Association,* 1992, 267 (16), 2221 – 2226.

8. Randall, T. Women need more and better information on menopause from their physicians, says survey. *Journal of the American Medical Association,* October 13, 1993, 270 (4), 1664.

&

SUGGESTED READING

Adams, Patch, & Maureen Mylander. *Gesundheit!* Rochester, VT: Inner Traditions International, 1992.

Berczeller, Peter H. *Doctors & Patients: What We Feel about You.* New York: Macmillan, 1994.

Cornacchia, Harold J. *Consumer Health: A Guide to Intelligent Decisions,* 5th ed. St. Louis, MO: Mosby-Yearbook, 1992.

Heimlich, Jane. *What Your Doctor Won't Tell You.* New York: HarperCollins, 1990.

Inlander, Charles, B. *Your Medical Rights: How to Become an Empowered Consumer.* Boston: Little, Brown, 1990.

Inlander, Charles, B., & Karla Morales. *Getting the Most for Your Medical Dollar.* New York: Pantheon Books, 1991.

Jones, A., Kreps, G.L., & Phillips, G.M. *Communicating with Your Doctor: Getting the Most Out of Health Care.* Cresskill, NJ: Hampton Press, 1995.

Roter, Debra L., & Judith A. Hall. *Doctors Talking with Patients — Patients Talking with Doctors: Improving Communication in Medical Visits.* Westport, CT: Greenwood Publishing Group, 1992.

Walter, Douglas N. *Physician-Patient Decision-Making: A Study in Medical Ethics.* Westport, CT: Greenwood Publishing Group, 1985.

Chapter 2

A SHORT COURSE IN FEMALE BIOLOGY

"When I was growing up it was considered wrong to touch or look at your genitals. I was even afraid to wash myself properly. I'm glad those days are over." —Adrienne, age 62

"Most doctors don't understand that if you have any problems, even if you're fortunate and they're not serious, that you have legitimate concerns and want to understand what is happening with your body. Both male and female gynecologists have acted in ths way." — Merle, age 45

TAKING A LOOK: EXTERNAL FEMALE GENITALS

During the "flower-child" era in the 1960s when young men began to let their hair grow long for the first time since before the turn of the century, one would often hear the comment "from the back I can't tell if that's a boy or a girl." While the statement often was reflective of an anti-hippie political attitude, it was also true. Sometimes it is difficult to distinguish between males and females. Among *Homo sapiens,* the sexual dimorphism (difference) between sexes is far less marked than in other animal species. Additionally, few people possess the culturally ideal male or female form. Those who do often get photographed a lot or become models.

The external female genitals go by many terms, some technical and precise, and some more common and generally understood by scientists and nonscientists alike. Many words used for the female external genitals are considered crude, including pussy, snatch, cunt, and beaver. Others, such as "private parts," crotch, and groin, lack specificity. Betty Dodson notes that most terms tend to be negative.[1] She encourages women to be "cunt positive" and view their genitals as a "lotus flower unfolding."

Several words often incorrectly used interchangeably are pubic, pelvis, and vulva. **Vulva** is the accurate term for the visible female anatomical structures. **Pelvis,** which means "basin" in Latin, is the area that provides an attachment for the legs and supports the lower spine. It includes the **pelvic**

girdle — the two hip bones, and the **bony pelvis** — the bowl-like structure formed by the two hip bones and the bottom of the spinal column. **Pubic** refers to the anterior (front) portion of the hip bone.

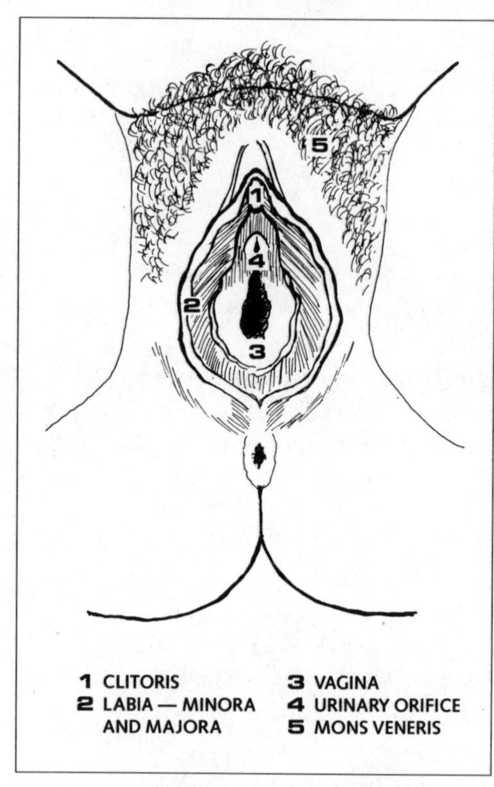

THE VULVA: EXTERNAL FEMALE GENITALS

The Vulva

ANATOMY

The vulva (or **pudendum**, Latin for "covering") includes the structures located in the space between the thighs — bounded in the front by the **mons veneris** and in the back by the **anus** (the external opening of the large intestine). The structures in the area encompassed by the vulva include the **mons veneris, labia majora, labia minora, clitoris,** and **vestibule.**

Mons Veneris · The mons veneris (or **mons pubis**) translates as "Mountain of Venus." Venus was the goddess of love, and the word **venereal** has the same linguistic root. The mons veneris, which is covered with hair from approximately age ten or twelve, consists of pads of fatty tissue lying below the skin and over the **pubic symphysis** (the joining place of the two pubic bones).

Labia Majora · The labia majora are two smaller longitudinal folds of skin that extend from the mons veneris and form the lateral (side) borders of the vulva. The labia majora (also known as the "major lips"), while hairy on the outside, contain only fat cells and sweat and oil glands on the inside. Under the skin are fibers of smooth muscle similar to the muscles of its homologue in the male, the **scrotum.** Like the male scrotum, the labia majora are temperature-sensitive — wrinkling in cold weather and appearing larger and softer in warm weather.

Labia Minora · The labia minora (or "minor lips") are two smaller longitudinal folds of skin located within the labia majora. They contain no hair or fat cells, but are rich in blood vessels, nerve endings, and oil glands. The minor lips form the side and lower borders of the vestibule and fuse at the top to form the clitoral prepuce which encloses the clitoris. The labia minora are highly erogenous and enlarge, during sexual excitement, flaring out to expose the vestibule.

Clitoris · Clitoris is a Greek word for "key." Thus, centuries before Masters and Johnson, the function of the clitoris was known! This small cylindrical erectile structure is situated at the top of the vestibule and at the lower border of the pubic symphysis. The clitoris consists of two leglike stalks, which fuse together to form the body or shaft and end in the glans — which projects outward. The entire clitoris, except for the glans, is underneath the upper part of the labia minora which, as mentioned earlier, form the clitoral prepuce.

The clitoris is homologous to the male's penis and, like the penis, contains two cylindrical, spongy erectile structures which may engorge with blood. This process causes the clitoris to increase in size and become erect. Like the penis, the entire area is replete with nerve endings and sensitive to stimulation. Direct rubbing or indirect stimulation by pulling or tugging can result in orgasm. Even removing the clitoris completely by circumcision will not completely destroy a woman's sensations and orgasmic capability. Because they are homologous organs, it should not be surprising that **smegma,** the white cheese-like substance produced by the glands in the penis, is also produced by the glands of the clitoris.

Vestibule · The vestibule, meaning "entry," describes the entire cleft enclosed by the labia minora. It houses the **hymen** and the openings of the **vagina, urethra, Bartholin's ducts,** and **Skene's ducts.**

Hymen · The term hymen (or "maidenhead") derives from Hymen, the Greek god of marriage. It is a thin, vascularized membrane that partially closes the external opening of the vagina. The spot of blood produced by the tearing of the intact hymen on the wedding night supposedly indicated that the bride was a virgin. The problem with this folk belief is that many women's hymens were ruptured before the first act of intercourse through participation in athletic endeavors such as horseback riding and gymnastics; conversely, a few hymens may remain intact even after intercourse.

Bartholin's Ducts · The Bartholin's ducts are situated on each side of the vestibule in the groove between the hymen and the labia minora. The ducts pass inward to the **Bartholin's glands,** which secrete a lubricating fluid during sexual excitement. According to Masters and Johnson, the lubrication from the gland is not of significant value.[2] The Bartholin's glands are homologous to the male's **Cowper's glands,** whose function is to provide pre-ejaculatory secretions which serve to cleanse the urethral canal.

Skene's Ducts · The opening of the Skene's ducts are located on either side of the urethral opening. The ducts serve as large collecting conduits for the **peri-urethral (Skene's) glands** — the homologues of the **prostatic gland**

(prostate) in men. Some anatomists think of the Skene's ducts (glands) and Bartholin's glands as vestigial remnants. Other sex researchers, however, claim that women experience ejaculation, and these ducts and glands are involved. Since the Skene's ducts (glands) are homologues of the prostate, the potential does exist for these tissues to produce an ejaculatory substance.[3]

SEXUAL FUNCTION OF THE VULVA

In many mammals, the vulva swells during their estrus, exposing the entrance way to the vagina. This serves as notice that they are ready and available.

In humans, the nature of the sexual advertisement is more subtle. Although the labia swell during **excitement,** the initial stage of the sexual response cycle described by Masters and Johnson,[4] it is only an overt signal if the genitals are exposed and not covered by clothing. Usually it is the thought of the "jewels" hidden under a woman's clothing that is the subtle attraction of the vulva.

While women can receive intense pleasure from stimulation of their labia, the major organ of the vulva which produces sexual arousal for the female is the clitoris.

The clitoris is generally acknowledged to be the primary source of a woman's orgasmic response. Whether it is the only stimulus or whether orgasm is produced by sexual intercourse, breast stimulation, or other stimulation, the physiological reflex response pattern is the same for all orgasms.[5]

While individuals may have preferences for intercourse or masturbatory orgasms and can describe why their particular preference is more satisfying, the old controversy that one type of orgasm is immature or inferior is considered ancient history.

REPRODUCTIVE FUNCTION OF THE VULVA

Technically, the vulva has no reproductive function. However, from a sociobiological perspective, since the vulva is a pleasure center, it may serve as a stimulus to encourage intercourse — thereby increasing the chances of an individual's reproductive success.

ON THE INSIDE: INTERNAL FEMALE ANATOMY

The Vagina

ANATOMY

The vagina, a muscular tube about three inches long, has walls made of three layers: a fibrous (elastic) outer coat, a muscular midsection, and a mucosal epithelial inner layer. The vagina is only potential space because its inner walls usually touch. It is normally quite acidic, with a pH of 3.5 to 5.5. That acidity, combined with the toughness of the inner epithelium, protects the vagina from infection. The acidity is a direct result of estrogen; the

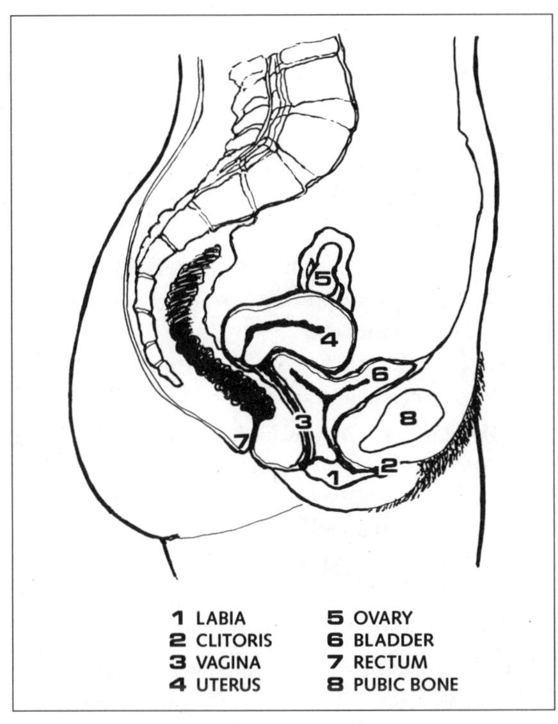

THE FEMALE SEXUAL/REPRODUCTIVE SYSTEM (SIDE VIEW)

lack of estrogen before puberty and after menopause causes the vagina to be more vulnerable to infection. Estrogen causes the basal cells of the vaginal epithelium to accumulate glycogen granules and proliferate. That extra glycogen provides the bacteria (**Doderlein's bacilli**) which are normal, healthy vaginal residents with a perfect environment. The bacteria break down the glycogen to form lactic acid which has a low pH. When women douche or use feminine deodorants, under the mistaken notion that their interior is "dirty," they in fact are destroying the "good guys" — the Doderlein's bacilli, which protect their vaginas.

SEXUAL FUNCTION

The role of the vagina in sexual satisfaction can be debated. The vagina has few nerve endings, and orgasm is often reached without vaginal entry. While the vagina may not be a very erogenous zone, the entire pelvic area's neural network (known as the pelvic plexus) contribute to the recognition of sensations within the vagina.

Vaginal Versus Clitoral Orgasm · Freud claimed that the sign of a mature woman was her achievement of a vaginal orgasm. He called the clitoral orgasm "immature," presumably because it is achievable through masturbation or other noncoital acts. According to Masters and Johnson, a vaginal orgasm is impossible, since their research has shown that it is the clitoris that is responsible for orgasm.[6] Anatomically that makes sense, since, as mentioned earlier, the clitoris is derived from the same embryonic tissue that becomes a penis in men. However, there are two possible anatomical explanations which support a vaginal orgasm model.

First, while the penis is made up of three spongy erectile bodies (two **corpora cavernosa** and a **corpus spongiosum** through which the urethra passes), the clitoris has only the corpora cavernosa. The female equivalent of the corpus spongiosum are the **vestibular bulbs.** Located internally and laterally alongside the vagina, they become engorged with blood during sexual excitement.

Second, the Skene's glands and ducts — the female tissue equivalent to the prostate gland — are located around the urethra. It is this "female prostate" that is suggested as the anatomical site of the **"G"-spot.** The G-(or **Grafenberg**) spot, named for the German physician who first described it in 1950, can be stimulated by pressing against the front wall of the vagina. If you are lying down on your back, the G-spot is on the upper vaginal wall, midway between the pubic bone and the cervix.

While some researchers[7] claim a central role for the G-spot in sexual excitement and ejaculation, Masters and Johnson take a cautious view. Masters and Johnson concede that some women may have a clearly erogenous area in their vagina, but these sexologists maintain that additional research is necessary to establish whether the G-spot exists as a distinct anatomic structure.[8]

Masters and Johnson take the same cautious view when discussing the possibility of female ejaculation. They report observing several cases of women who expelled a type of fluid that was not urine, but at the same time indicate that more research on the subject is required.

Vaginal Muscles and Sexual Pleasure · Surrounding the vagina are several muscular groups which hold it in place and also are active during coitus. As a result of childbirth and/or aging, these muscles sometimes lose their tone and don't grip the penis as tightly. This may be experienced by the woman and her partner as a loss of sensation. The condition is reversible, because the vaginal musculature is subject to the same type of conditioning or strength training as other muscles throughout the body. Dr. Arnold Kegel originally designed a series of exercises involving the muscles in the pelvic area to correct urinary incontinence without surgery. Women using these exercises reported increased sexual satisfaction as a beneficial side effect, and as a result, the exercises are now also used to treat certain sexual problems. For more information, see Chapter Ten.

Vaginal Lubrication and Sexual Pleasure · The source of vaginal lubrication was unknown until Masters and Johnson published the results of their scientific investigations.[9] Their research attributed the lubrication to **vasocongestion** (an increased amount of blood concentrated in the vessels and surrounding tissues) in the vaginal walls, which leads to moisture seeping through the vaginal lining. Lubrication starts within 10 to 30 seconds after the onset of sexual stimulation, but the quantity produced varies from one woman to another and also varies in the same woman from episode to episode. According to Masters and Johnson, the amount of vaginal lubrication produced is not necessarily an indication of the woman's level of sexual arousal; nor does it mean that a woman is "ready" for intercourse.[10]

REPRODUCTIVE FUNCTION

The vagina's role in reproduction is first to provide an entrance way from which sperm can begin their travels and later to act as a conduit through which the fetus passes on its way from the uterus to the outside world.

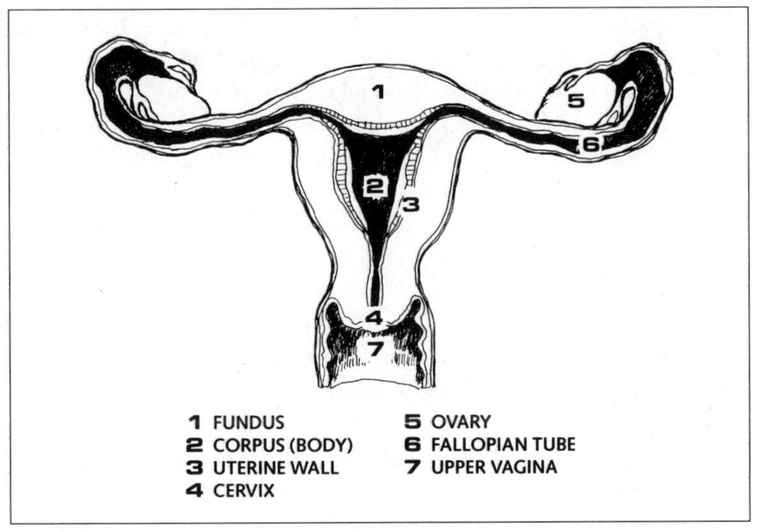

THE UTERUS

The Uterus

ANATOMY

The uterus is a hollow, thick-walled muscular organ that is about three inches long and pear-shaped. It is approximately two-and-a-half inches wide at the top and one inch across at the bottom. It has the ability to grow from a weight of two ounces to two pounds during pregnancy and then shrink back to its original size by six weeks after delivery. It is held in position by six ligaments which variously attach to the pelvic walls and the back (sacrum). When a woman stands erect with an empty bladder and rectum, the uterus lies almost horizontal, with its upper end (**fundus**) forward and at a right angle to the vagina. The interior of the uterus is divided into two parts by the **isthmus** — which is a slight constriction. The larger top portion is known as the **corpus** or body. The lower portion is known as the **cervix** (Latin for "neck"). About half of the cervix projects into the vagina. Many people erroneously think of the cervix as a separate organ when in fact it is part of the uterus.

The **external os** is the opening of the cervix into the vagina; the **internal os** is the opening in the other direction — into the corpus of the uterus. The openings to and from the cervix have diameters that are smaller than a straw, and the inner cavity of the corpus is flattened space — until pregnancy.

The wall of the corpus consists of three layers: the **perimetrium**, the outer layer of elastic fibrous tissue; the **myometrium**, the middle muscular layer which comprises most of the uterus; and the **endometrium**, the inner mucosal lining. The perimetrium and the myometrium allow the uterus to increase in size as the developing fetus matures, and then are responsible for the contractions and expulsion of the fetus. The endometrium is the tissue that thickens as first estrogen and then progesterone cause the uterus to prepare for a fertilized eggs's implantation. Endometrial tissue is sloughed off as the menstrual period when hormones subside — if no pregnancy has occurred.

In addition to this response to the ebb and flow of the hormones on a monthly basis, the uterus exhibits a lifelong curve of growth and development. At birth the newborn's cervix and corpus are about equal in size; however, in mature women the ratio of cervix to corpus is one to two. The infant's uterus enlarges prior to birth because of high maternal estrogen levels. Within days after delivery, it shrinks somewhat and its size then remains static until pubescence. At that time the ovaries start to produce hormones. The beginning of uterine growth is one of the earliest signs of approaching puberty, generally preceding the **menarche** (the onset of menstruation) by one to two years. The uterus has reached adult size by age 15 in approximately 60 percent of girls.

A woman who has been pregnant will have a larger uterus than a **nulliparous** (never pregnant) woman. However, after menopause, shrinking occurs, bringing the uterus back to its prepuberty size.

SEXUAL FUNCTION

The uterus is generally not thought of as a sexual organ; however, some sexologists have demonstrated that it plays a role in orgasm.

Masters and Johnson described in detail the physiological changes which occur throughout the body during the **sexual response cycle.**[11] The cycle consists of **excitement, plateau, orgasm,** and **resolution.** During the excitement stage the uterus pulls upward, while the inner two-thirds of the vagina expands. During the plateau stage there is further elevation and expansion of the uterus — known as "tenting." Muscular contractions of the uterus and vagina occur during orgasm.

While it is true that the uterus is involved during orgasm, it is also true that orgasm is a total body response. Brain wave patterns have distinct changes, and muscles in different body regions from the toes to the eyes contract during orgasm.[12] This entire body involvement is clearly good news if you anticipate hysterectomy and are worried that the surgical removal of your uterus might lead to a diminishment of sexual enjoyment.

REPRODUCTIVE FUNCTION

When we think of reproduction, it is the uterus which comes to mind. Although fertilization occurs in the fallopian tubes, it is in the corpus of the uterus that the developing embryo is nurtured and protected. An additional protection is provided by the cervix in the form of secretions, called a "**mucous plug.**" This plug separates the uterus from both the vagina and the outside environment, thereby lessening the possibility of infection.

The Fallopian Tubes

ANATOMY

The fallopian tubes arise from a pair of embryonic ducts known as **Mullerian ducts**. During early fetal development, if the embryo is to be a female, these ducts form the fallopian tubes, the uterus, and the top four-fifths of the vagina. Gabriello Fallopius, the 16th century anatomist for whom the tubes were named, thought they resembled curved trumpets, whereas more ancient anatomists thought of them as straight trumpets. In any case, the Greek word for trumpet or tube — **salpinx** — is also used for the fallopian tubes.

The major function of the fallopian tubes is to convey the egg from the ovary to the uterus. The tubes are approximately four inches long and are suspended by ligaments. Anatomists have divided the tube into three sections: the **intramural** portion, within the walls of the uterus; the **isthmus,** the narrow part adjoining the uterus; and the **ampulla,** nearest the ovary. The end which extends toward the ovary is called the **infundibulum,** and its small fingerlike extensions are known as **fimbria.**

SEXUAL FUNCTION

None.

REPRODUCTIVE FUNCTION

Cilia (hairlike projections) sweep the **ovum** (egg) from the ampulla, where fertilization usually occurs, to the uterus. At the ampulla-isthmic junction, transport of the ovum is delayed two to two-and-a-half days, a process called "tube locking" or isthmic block; however, by approximately three to four days after ovulation, the ovum has entered the uterus. While the egg is being propelled "downstream" to the uterus, if unprotected intercourse has occurred, sperm may be making their way "upstream" to meet it.

The Ovaries

ANATOMY

The ovaries are the female gonads and are homologous to the male testicles. The function of gonads is to produce seed and to manufacture hormones. However, while the male testes constantly create new seed, the ovaries serve as a storage facility for eggs which were developed in the first few weeks of fetal life. Another difference between the sexes' gonads is that hormonal production in males is constant with little variability, while in females it is cyclical.

The ovaries are roughly the size, shape, and weight of unshelled almonds. They are pinkish gray and present a dull exterior because they are not covered with a shiny **peritoneum** — the membrane that covers the inner organs. A peritoneal cover would not allow for the rupturing that occurs during ovulation. While the ovaries are smooth prior to puberty, the monthly scarring associated with the rupture and release of an ovum gives them a pitted surface. The ovaries are held in place by ligaments that connect with both the uterus and abdominal wall.

At birth the ovaries contain approximately 200,000 to 1,000,000 follicles, each housing an **oocyte** (an ovum in an early stage of development). The number decreases (for causes unknown) to about 10,000 to 50,000 by puberty. This is ample to permit several follicles to ripen each month for approximately 35 years.

SEXUAL FUNCTION

The main contribution of the ovaries to sex may be their production of the hormones estrogen and testosterone. While there is no doubt about estrogen's role in sex for other animal species and testosterone's role in human males, there is some question as to these hormones' sexual role in females. But we'll come to that later in this chapter.

REPRODUCTIVE FUNCTION

The reproductive function of the ovaries is both simple and complex. They are a holding chamber for the eggs necessary for reproduction, as well as the site for the production of the hormones which control reproduction. Each month a **graffian follicle**, housing an ovum, matures, ruptures the ovary, and sends an egg on its journey. The graffian follicle, which had also been producing estrogen, becomes the corpus luteum, producing progesterone and estrogen. If fertilization does not occur, the **corpus luteum** regresses, stops hormone production, and turns white — becoming the **corpus albicans** (white body). Several days later, menses starts and the ovarian cycle begins anew. (See the section "Puberty" later in this chapter for a more detailed description.)

THE BREASTS

ANATOMY

Anatomically the breasts are modified sweat glands. The 15 to 20 mammary glands within each breast are drained by a duct that opens into the nipple. Internally, mammary tissue is surrounded by varying amounts of fatty and fibrous tissue, which gives the breast its size and consistency. Externally, the nipple, located at the tip of the breast, is elevated and contains nerve endings. It is surrounded by wrinkled skin known as the **areola,** which extends outward in a circle for one to two centimeters. The areola contains many nerve and muscle fibers that serve to stiffen the nipple so the suckling infant can get a better grasp.

The breasts undergo changes in size and shape as a precursor to puberty, but reach their full physiological development only during pregnancy and lactation.

SEXUAL FUNCTION

The breasts have an erotic function and in many societies symbolize sexuality, femininity, and attractiveness. While there is no evidence to support the idea that breast size is related to a woman's sexuality — the bigger the sexier — this fallacy is still subscribed to by many men and women. This misconception has caused some women to seek to improve their sexual attractiveness through exercise or breast augmentation surgery. In reality, most women become sexually aroused when their breasts are stimulated, whether they are small- or big-breasted. The sexual sensitivity of the breast, areola, and nipples can vary and depends on such things as personal preference, situation, and habit.

REPRODUCTIVE FUNCTION

Although the breasts are not technically part of the reproductive organs, they may be involved in maintenance as milk suppliers once the act of reproduction has produced a baby.

BREAST SELF-EXAMINATION

In this age of mammography hype, one overlooked fact is that mammograms miss about 10 percent of breast lumps. All women, in addition to having periodic mammograms (on a schedule arrived at in consultation with a physician) should practice breast self-examination. The recommendation is to do this easy self-examination right after your menstrual period, because estrogen levels are low and as a result, breast tissue is less dense. After hysterectomy or natural menopause, breast self-examination may be done on the first day of each month as a helpful reminder.

The procedure is described in Chapter Three.

HORMONES

Females produce, primarily in the ovaries, two main groups of hormones: the **progestins** and the **estrogenic group. Testosterone,** the hormone associated with males, is also produced by the ovaries but in limited amounts. The adrenal glands also contribute small quantities of testosterone.

PROGESTERONE

Progestins are natural and synthetic compounds which produce changes in the uterus — after it has been previously prepared by estrogen. In humans, the naturally occurring progestin is **progesterone.** It accomplishes its function of preparing the uterus for implantation of a fertilized ovum and then maintaining it in several ways. It causes secretory changes in the uterine endometrium and affects other uterine tissue and vascular elements. Progesterone also inhibits uterine contractions and reduces motility of the fallopian tubes. This hormone causes the mucous secreted by the cells of the cervix to become more viscous, thereby creating the "cervical plug." It is responsible for a slight rise in basal body temperature, as well as an increase in excretion of water and sodium from the kidneys — both indications of the fertile time in the menstrual cycle.

ESTROGEN

The estrogenic group is comprised of several compounds, such as **estradiol, estrone,** and **estrol,** for which the term **estrogen** is generally used. The word estrogen comes from the Greek root *estro* — "to produce mad desire." In animals, estrogen, in addition to other things, is responsible for stimulating sexual urge during **estrus** — the female's receptive time. In humans, who do not experience estrus, estrogen's sphere of influence is nevertheless also large. Essentially a growth hormone with effects on the reproductive tract, fat distribution, and bone development, estrogen plays a critical role in the menstrual cycle.

Like progesterone, estrogen is produced cyclically and varies from approximately 40 picograms per milliliter of blood before menstruation to 250 to 300 picograms per milliliter at ovulation. After menopause, it hovers at below 20 picograms.

Estrogen's effects include the following:

1. Maintains the normal size and function of the uterus, fallopian tubes, and vagina. Estrogen causes the vaginal cells to accumulate glycogen, which is acted on by the Doderlein's bacilli to produce the acidic vaginal secretions mentioned earlier in our discussion of the vagina. Estrogen enhances the ability of the cilia in the fallopian tubes to move the ovum towards the uterus. At the same time, it causes the glands of the cervix to produce a clear, watery secretion, which facilitates sperm transport into

the uterus. Cyclically, it causes the uterine endometrium and the lining of the fallopian tubes to increase in size.

2. Controls production of gonadotropic hormones by its interaction with the pituitary and hypothalamus. This regulates the monthly menstrual cycle.
3. Influences growth, development, and maintenance of secondary sex characteristics.
4. Causes deposition of fat in all subcutaneous tissue, particularly in the buttocks, thighs, and breasts.
5. Causes the growth of duct tissue in the breast.
6. Causes an increase in bone formation. In girls, estrogen enhances the growth spurt at puberty, but it also has the opposite effect. It causes the closing of the epiphyseal cartilages at the ends of the long bones so that cessation of growth eventually occurs. This attribute led some parents in the 1960s and 70s to use estrogen as an antidote to their daughters' projected extremely tall stature. This use in prepubescent girls to arrest height was controversial, but was justified by some as important therapy for the psychological trauma that unusually tall girls may possibly experience.

   Because estrogen is involved in maintaining strong bones, after menopause, the lack of estrogen can lead to osteoporosis. For more information, see Chapters Eleven and Twelve.
7. Maintains the normal condition and function of mucous membranes and capillary walls of the mouth and nose. When estrogen levels are low, there may be a greater tendency to experience nosebleeds. In experiments on mice, the relationship of the olfactory bulb and their sense of smell has been connected to sexual events. For example, dense crowding in a cage will cause female mice to cease estrus cycles. That reaction can be prevented if the olfactory bulbs are removed. Also, the scent of a male will speed up a young female mouse's sexual maturity and make it cycle more regularly.

   The relationship in humans between estrogen and smell was documented in 1971, when Martha McClintock demonstrated that college roommates tended to have their menstrual period at the same time of the month.[13] Her research also showed that college women with boyfriends had shorter and more regular cycles than those that didn't. Another researcher, Michael Russel, demonstrated the same phenomena of menstrual synchronization among unrelated women who had a mixture of alcohol and underarm perspiration from a female donor dabbed on their upper lip.[14] All but one woman in the experimental group had a shift of their menstrual timing to that of the donor's cycle.

8. Provides protection against heart disease, possibly because it reduces blood cholesterol levels.
9. Promotes water and sodium retention. This is probably responsible for the bloating many women experience in the second half (after ovulation) of their menstrual cycle.
10. Possibly contributes to cognitive performance differences between the sexes; females in general are better at verbal expression, while males on the average have an advantage in certain quantitative and spatial abilities. Studies by Doreen Kimura support the controversial suggestion that high estrogen correlates with relatively higher performance of fine motor skills and relatively less success on spatial reasoning tasks. Her findings showed that postmenopausal women who receive estrogen therapy tended to perform fine motor tasks better on the days when they received the hormone than on the days when they did not.[15]

    Many question whether these differences are "real." Biologically oriented researchers support the physiological explanation for behavioral differences. Socially oriented researchers, on the other hand, claim that theories of sex differences in the brain have been constructed to account for differences in performance due to environmental conditioning.
11. Possibly connected to Alzheimer's disease. Dr. Toran-Allerand and her coworkers at Columbia University reported that receptors for estrogen and **nerve growth factor (NGF)** coexist in certain neurons in the basal forebrain.[16] The finding suggests that estrogen and NGF may act to influence the survival and health of those brain neurons. The implications for Alzheimer's disease revolve around the fact that this area of the brain contains cholinergic neurons which produce the neurotransmitter acetylcholine — vital for memory. In Alzheimer's, those nerve cells no longer produce acetylcholine — hence the loss of memory. Scientists are examining ways to treat cholinergic neurons with NGF — because in its presence, those neurons do not degenerate. The use of NGF suggested a similar role for estrogen. At the 1993 meeting of the Society for Neuroscience, Dr. Victor Henderson reported that taking estrogen replacement therapy appeared to both lower the risk of developing Alzheimer's, and made the symptoms milder if it did develop.[17]
12. Possibly involved in sexual functioning. In animals, the sex urge is tied to reproductive function. Large amounts of estrogen during estrus make female animals seek a partner, while at the same time making them more attractive to males.

    In humans, who have no estrus, sexual responsiveness is apparently influenced more by emotional and psychological factors than hormonal conditions. Studies support that the absence of estrogen does not change a woman's sexual desire (See Chapter Ten).

HOW HORMONES FUNCTION

Although estrogen and progesterone are produced in the ovaries, they are under the control of the brain. The direct impetus which causes them to be produced and secreted is the gonadotropic hormones produced by the **pituitary gland: follicle-stimulating hormone** (**FSH**) and **luteinizing hormone** (**LH**). At one time the pituitary gland was considered to be the master gland of the body — functioning independently. Now it is known that the brain, specifically the hypothalamus, controls the pituitary through releasing factors which travel from the hypothalamus directly to the pituitary. These releasing factors are sometimes grouped under the umbrella term **gonadotropin-releasing hormone (GnRH)**.

Positive and negative feedback mechanisms control the secretion of releasing factors. For example, in positive feedback — where an increase in one stimulates an increase in the other — a progesterone or estrogen increase causes LH releasing factor to be secreted by the hypothalamus. In negative feedback, a decrease in estrogen causes FSH releasing factor to be secreted. For more details, see "What Causes the Monthly Period?" later in this chapter.

FROM START TO FINISH

Puberty

Although we think of puberty as the start of our sexual being, it is actually the second time that our bodies are under the influence of our sexual hormones. The first time was during fetal development. Both males and females begin with the potential to become female. Testosterone in prenatal boys prompts the development of masculine organs. The lack of testosterone in females permits the structures to remain female. Not only were the reproductive organs affected in utero, but the hormones also acted on aspects of sexual differentiation in the developing brain. The principle was first demonstrated by studies with various species of lower mammals. While there is no disagreement that prenatal programming occurs in humans,[18] controversy exists regarding its extent.[19]

Puberty, then, is actually a reawakening for the hormones. Why the hormones become quiescent after their initial role in utero is not completely understood; however, the hypothesis is that the necessary neuronal connections are not in place until pubescence. While the terms puberty and pubescence are often used interchangeably, **pubescence** technically refers to the time period and the physical and biological changes leading to puberty. The term **puberty** is the point when the organism is actually able to reproduce; that is, to produce viable sperm or eggs. To be precise, then: pubescence culminates in puberty.

Whatever the term one uses, the events that occur are preordained.

Girls, at approximately 10 to 10½ years of age (which is about two years before boys), undergo a series of physiological and anatomical changes, including the obvious external ones of breast "budding"; broadening of the pelvic area; and hair growth in the vulvar and underarm regions. At approximately 12½ years of age, most American girls experience **menarche** — their first period. However, ovulation will not occur until about a year or so later. The production by the ovaries of that first egg heralds puberty. Growth and maturation will continue for the next several years. At the time of menarche the ovaries are one-third their adult size, reaching their maximum size and weight by the time a woman is 19 or 20. The average age for full reproductive capacity is approximately 23 — a good time to have a baby.

The average age for menarche has dropped in the United States from about 15 a century and a half ago to 12½ now, although the range is 9 to 17 years of age. The major factor theorized as contributing to an earlier age of menarche is better nutrition. Strenuous exercise seems to retard menarche. For every year of strenuous exercise — more than one hour daily — menarche may be delayed by approximately 5 months.

Menstruation

WHAT CAUSES THE MONTHLY PERIOD?

As mentioned earlier, although estrogen and progesterone are produced in the ovaries, they are under the control of the brain's hypothalamus. A woman's cycle is described as beginning on Day 1 of her menstrual flow. At that time, levels of estrogen and progesterone are at their lowest. The hypothalamus responds by secreting gonadotropin-releasing hormone (GnRH), which stimulates the pituitary gland to secrete follicle-stimulating hormone (FSH).

FSH does just that, and as a result, several follicles in the ovary start to mature. As they develop, they begin to secrete estrogen. The rising levels of estrogen register in the hypothalamus, and as a result of negative feedback, GnRH is withheld and FSH in the pituitary ceases to be released. Without this continued follicle stimulation, further growth of all but one follicle stops (why one follicle continues to grow is unknown). Estrogen levels briefly drop slightly as a result of the decrease from several to one follicle; however, that is soon more than compensated for as the one follicle continues to mature and secrete greater and greater quantities of estrogen. It also begins secreting progesterone.

These events have taken approximately 12 days (although it is the more variable part of the cycle). The effects of the increased quantities of estrogen have caused the endometrium of the uterus to start to proliferate. Changes

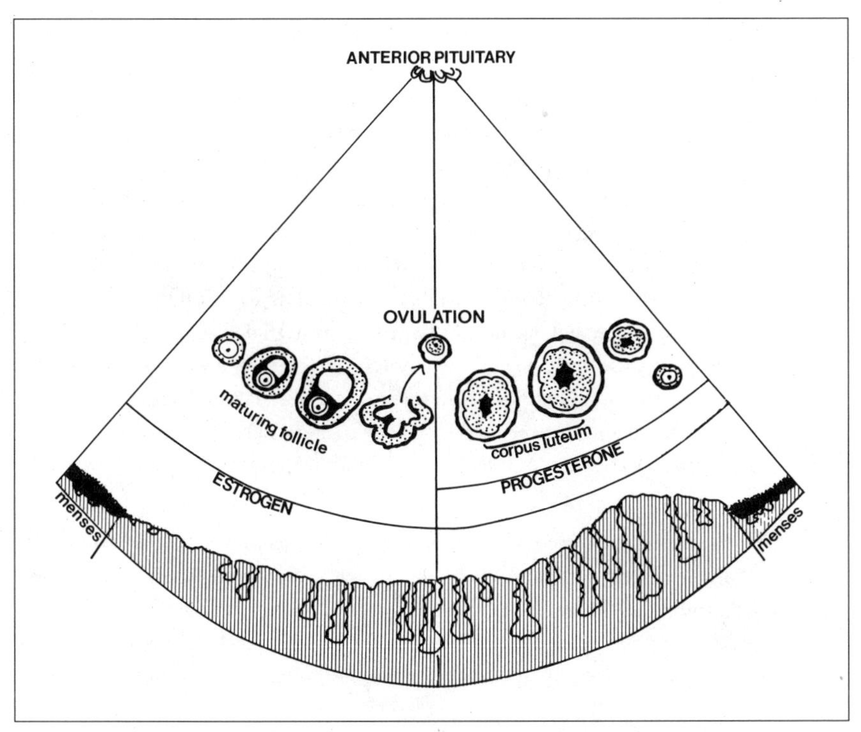

MONTHLY HORMONAL ACTIVITY

The pituitary gland releases follicle-stimulating hormone (FSH). As the follicle in the ovary matures in response to FSH, it secretes estrogen, which inhibits the production of FSH. As estrogen increases, it stimulates the pituitary to secrete luteinizing hormone (LH), which causes the follicle to ovulate (release an ovum). The corpus luteum is the body of cells left in the ovary after the ovum (egg) has been released; the corpus luteum produces large amounts of progesterone and estrogen, which enables the uterus to receive the fertilized egg. If the ovum is not fertilized, the inner lining (endometrium) of the uterus is shed and menstruation occurs.

in other reproductive organs are also noticeable as a result of increased levels of estrogen. For example, the cells of the vagina increase in size.

The rising amounts of estrogen and progesterone are detected by the hypothalamus, which causes GnRH to be secreted, which in turn stimulates the pituitary to release luteinizing hormone (LH). LH has a rapid effect on the ovaries, causing ovulation to occur within 16 to 24 hours. Ovulation involves the rupture of the ovarian wall by the graffian follicle — which has now grown so large that it takes up approximately one-third of the ovary. That rupture allows the ovum contained within the follicle to be released and begin its journey into and through the fallopian tubes.

Once ovulation has occurred, the cells of the graffian follicle (under the influence of LH) change and begin producing progesterone in large quantities. This transformed graffian follicle is now known as the **corpus luteum** (corpus for body and luteum for its yellow color). If fertilization occurs, then progesterone continues to be produced, the uterus lining is not shed, and the embryo has a place in which to develop.

If the egg is not fertilized, the corpus luteum starts to regress and ceases production of progesterone and estrogen approximately eight to ten days after ovulation. The corpus luteum becomes white and is then called the **corpus albicans.** The uterus responds to this hormonal deprivation by sloughing off its no-longer-needed, greatly enlarged endometrial lining. Approximately 28 days after the cycle began, the woman starts her menses (Latin for month — the approximate length of the cycle). The discharge is a combination of uterine blood and dead tissues and is the equivalent of approximately two to four ounces. The start of the bleeding is the start of the new cycle.

THE OVARIAN AND ENDOMETRIAL CYCLE

This process, viewed another way, can be seen as involving two cycles which are occurring simultaneously — the ovarian and endometrial cycles. Each mirrors and correlates with the other, as shown in Table 2 – 1. The purpose of the ovarian cycle is to produce an ovum, and the purpose of the endometrial cycle is to prepare a haven to nourish and maintain the fertilized ovum.

TABLE 2 – 1
THE REPRODUCTIVE CYCLE

Ovarian Cycle (prepares the egg)	**Endometrial Cycle** (prepares the haven)
No equivalent	Menstrual
Follicular phase	Proliferative phase
Ovulation	No equivalent
Luteal phase	Secretory phase

Ovarian Cycle · *Follicular phase.* During this phase there is initial follicle growth under the stimulation of FSH. FSH has been secreted because of a drop in estrogen during the prior luteal phase. Follicle maturation occurs with a concomitant rise in the estrogen level, so that by the 12th day the increase is sufficient to start a precipitous LH increase.

Ovulation. The surge of LH leads to the final steps of follicle maturation, causing it to rupture. Some women can tell when they are ovulating because they suffer from **mittelschmerz,** a German term for pain in the middle (of the month). The pain is in the abdominal region and the ovaries are very tender to touch. Some women experience some breakthrough bleeding, while others can judge when they're ovulating by the consistency of their vaginal mucosal discharge. It becomes very thick, viscous, and sticks together somewhat like rubber cement. This condition of elasticity is known as **spinbarkeit,** and under the microscope the mucosa exhibits a branching pattern known as **ferning.** Finally, women who have been monitoring their temperatures with a basal body thermometer know when they have ovulated because their temperature rises at least 0.4 degrees fahrenheit.

Luteal phase. There is an increase in production of progesterone and estrogen. The corpus luteum reaches full maturity and then starts to regress if fertilization has not occurred. Estrogen and progesterone decrease.

Endometrial Cycle · *Proliferative phase.* The endometrial wall is very thin, but under the stimulation of estrogen, begins to grow.

Secretory phase. The glands of the endometrium become swollen and fill up with secretions of fat and glycogen in preparation for pregnancy. If the egg is not fertilized, progesterone diminishes and the lining of the uterus breaks down.

Menstrual phase. The superficial two-thirds of the endometrium is almost all sloughed off as part of the menstrual flow.

THERE'S MORE TO THE CYCLE THAN BLOOD

As recently as 1981 and despite the increasing frankness with which Americans discuss sexuality, a survey conducted for the manufacturer of Tampax™ tampons found that many people are still uncomfortable about the topic of menstruation.[20]

In this study of attitudes toward menstruation, only 35 percent of the respondents said that it was appropriate to talk about it at the office, and a similar 33 percent thought it fitting to mention in social situations. More than one-third of the respondents said that even at home, women should conceal the fact that they are menstruating.

Fifty-six percent of the women in the survey agreed that women should abstain from intercourse during menstruation, while 8 percent believed that women should avoid contact with others during this time. Those beliefs are based on religious convictions and old myths.

While these attitudes are personal opinion, it is well substantiated that women experience physical and emotional changes during the cycle. The perceptions of these alterations are very individual and even vary within the same person. The range of symptoms include: breast tenderness, abdominal cramping or discomfort, fatigue, moodiness, edema (swelling of some body parts), lower back pain, tension, general joint achiness, shoulder or knee pains, headache, nausea, irritability, and depression. They may occur before the period — that is, premenstrually — or during the time of menstrual flow.

Because of estrogen's wide-ranging nongenital effects, it should not be surprising that women experience such a variety of premenstrual and menstrual physical and emotional symptoms. That this is not just an American female phenomenon was confirmed recently by researchers at State University of New York, Buffalo who found that women in Italy and Bahrain experienced similar symptoms.[21] These biologically based changes are entirely normal, although the whys and wherefores are still a biomedical mystery. For women who find the discomfort disconcerting, **anti-prostaglandin** medication — aspirin or ibuprofen — has been shown to be very effective in relieving many menstrual symptoms.

While almost all women experience some premenstrual symptoms, a small proportion of women experience them severely enough so that it disrupts their lives. Those women are said to be suffering from **premenstrual syndrome (PMS).**

Some scientists believe the syndrome is caused by hormonal changes, but they have been unable to document any differences in quality and types of hormones between women with severe and those with only a few symptoms. Although many theories and remedies have been advanced for treating PMS, at this time no one therapy has proven effective in treating the constellation of symptoms. Probably awareness that a PMS problem exists is the single most helpful measure. Trying to keep this time as stress-free as possible, as well as treating some of the more annoying symptoms, may be other ways of dealing with PMS.

Menopause

As menarche signals the beginning of reproductive life, so menopause heralds its end. The term **menopause** refers to the final cessation of menstruation either as a normal part of aging or as a result of surgery. In a broader sense, as the term is commonly used, it denotes a one- to several-year period during which a woman adjusts to a diminishing and then absent menstrual flow and the physiologic changes that may be associated. Technically, this lead-up time is known as the **climacteric.**

Whether we look at menarche and menopause as simply physiological changes which are age-dependent milestones in our reproductive lives, or we view them as diseases in the medical sense, our perceptions will dictate how we handle these stages.

Increasingly, more research is being conducted and information is becoming available on the formerly taboo topic of menopause. Some credit this interest to the aging of the "baby boomers" — the large number of women who were born in the decade following World War II and who are now approaching their menopause. It is estimated that in the next two decades, approximately 40 million Americans will pass through menopause and have to deal with questions of menopausal symptoms, hormone replacement therapy, and sexuality. More reliable data on those concerns should start to become available from well-controlled prospective studies that are now in process. Experts predict a mother lode of information from a federally funded project called the Women's Health Initiative, which is monitoring the health of approximately 140,000 females nationwide who are 50 years or older.

Some good news for women whose menopause was surgically induced comes from a study which looked at whether differences in onset of menopause — it currently ranges from age 38 to age 58 — are indicators of health and aging.[22] The findings have lead the researchers to suggest that early natural menopause is associated with a shorter life span, but in the surgically postmenopausal woman, the age of menopause is unrelated to mortality.

Menopause is characterized by increasing irregularity of menstruation and cessation of ovulation. To what extent the onset of menopause is determined by exhaustion of the egg supply in the ovaries, by failure of hormone production by the ovaries, or by changes in the overall mechanism controlling reproductive function is uncertain. Research reported in the *New England Journal of Medicine* indicated that with donated eggs, four of seven postmenopausal women 40 to 44 years old became pregnant and gave birth to healthy babies.[23] More recently, the media reported one woman age 62 who was pregnant and one 59 who had just delivered a baby — after implantation of a donated fertilized egg.[24] These cases may prompt a redefinition of the term menopause.

What is certain about menopause is that estrogen and progesterone levels decrease. Eventually estrogen levels drop so low that they no longer cause the uterus to prepare for an embryo. As a result, menstruation ceases. Usually the stoppage is gradual, with menstrual cycle irregularities occurring over a period of years. Other symptoms women experience include the common ones of **hot flashes** (or **flushes**), night sweats, and vaginal dryness or soreness with sexual intercourse, as well as irritability, insomnia, headaches, **incontinence,** weight gain, fatigue, depression, and backaches.

Some changes can be directly attributed to decreasing estrogen levels, such as thinning and drying of vaginal and urinary tissues and aging skin. Painful intercourse arises as a result of these changes to the vagina.

Some women require no treatment at menopause, as the problems are or are perceived as minor. Most complaints pass by themselves in a few weeks or months, or at the most two or three years. However, the fact that studies are still being done on whether menopause causes stress or depression indicates the pervasiveness of the beliefs concerning menopause's negative effects.

Dr. Karen Matthews and her colleagues at Pittsburgh and Duke Universities recently tested 541 randomly selected menstruating women from the ages of 42 to 50. Three years later, they reexamined 102 of those women who had ceased menstruating. The women's physical and psychological health was tested before and after their menopause. This research was unique because past studies on menopause and mental health tended to rely on women's recollections rather than on objective tests. Older studies also used as subjects groups of women who sought psychological treatment rather than a more representative group. Matthews' findings were that, contrary to popular beliefs, menopause does not cause stress or depression in most healthy women, and it may even improve mental health for some.[25]

Because we live in an era when "medicine cures all," we believe that we have to "cure" the manifestations of menopause. The issue of hormone replacement therapy to make up for the diminution of estrogen has become a lightening rod for the women's health movement. In Chapter Eleven we discuss the pros and cons of its use.

In 1973, the appearance of *Our Bodies, Ourselves,*[26] written by a group of Boston women, heralded a new era. Women realized that they were really capable of understanding their bodies and that evolved into wanting to gain control of them. For those Boston women, "body education is core education. Our bodies are the physical bases from which we move out into the world; ignorance, uncertainty — even, at worst, shame — about our physical selves create in us an alienation from ourselves that keeps us from being the whole people that we could be."[27]

Learning and knowledge empower.

ENDNOTES

1. Dodson, B. *Selflove and Orgasm.* New York: Privately Printed, 1983.

2. Masters, W. H., & Johnson, V. E. *Human Sexual Response.* Boston: Little, Brown, 1966.

3. Sevely, J. L., & Bennett, J. W. Concerning female ejaculation and the female prostate. *The Journal of Sex Research,* 1978, 14(1), 1 – 20.

4. Masters, W. H., & Johnson, V. E. *Human Sexual Response.* Boston: Little, Brown, 1966.

5. Masters, W. H., & Johnson, V. E. *Human Sexual Response.* Boston: Little, Brown, 1966.

6. Masters, W. H., & Johnson, V. E. *Human Sexual Response.* Boston: Little, Brown, 1966.

7. Ladas, A. K., Whipple, B., & Perry, J. D. *The G-Spot and Other Recent Discoveries About Human Sexuality.* New York: Holt, Rinehart and Winston, 1982.

8. Masters, W. H., Johnson, V. E., & Kolodny, R. C. *Masters and Johnson on Sex and Human Loving.* Boston: Little, Brown, 1986.

9. Masters, W. H., & Johnson, V. E. *Human Sexual Response.* Boston: Little, Brown, 1966.

10. Masters, W. H., & Johnson, V. E. *Human Sexual Response.* Boston: Little, Brown, 1966.

11. Masters, W. H., & Johnson, V. E. *Human Sexual Response.* Boston: Little, Brown, 1966.

12. Cohen, H., Rosen, R.C., & Goldstein, L. Electroencephalographic laterality changes during human sexual orgasm. *Archives of Sexual Behavior,* 1976, 5, 189 – 199.

13. McClintock, M. Menstrual synchrony and suppression. *Nature,* 1971, 229, 244 – 245.

14. Russell, M. J., Switz, G. M., & Thompson, K. Olfactory influences on the human menstrual cycle. *Pharmacology, Biochemistry, and Behavior,* 1980, 13, 737 – 738.

15. Kimura, D. Sex differences in the brain. *Scientific American,* 1992, 267(3), 118 – 125.

16. Toran-Allerand, C. D., Miranda, R. C., Bentham, W. D., et al. Estrogen receptors colocalize with low-affinity nerve growth factor receptors in cholinergic neurons of the basal forebrain. *Proceedings of the National Academy of Sciences of the United States of America,* 1992, 89(10), 4668 – 4672.

17. Angier, N. How estrogen may work to protect against Alzheimer's. *New York Times,* March 8, 1994, c3.

Hilts, P.J. Studies suggest estrogen lowers Alzheimer's risk. *New York Times,* November 10, 1993, a23.

18. Diamond, M. Human sexual development. In Beach, F., ed. *Human Sexuality in Four Perspectives,* pp. 22 – 61. Baltimore: John Hopkins University Press, 1972.

Money, J., & Ehrhardt, A. A. *Man & Woman, Boy & Girl.* Baltimore: John Hopkins University Press, 1972.

19. Ehrhardt, A. A., & Meyer-Bahlburg, H.F.L. Effects of prenatal sex hormones on gender-related behavior. *Science,* 1981(March 20), 211, 1312 – 1318.

20. Brozan, N. Menstruation: Survey finds it's still uneasy subject. *New York Times,* June 22, 1981, c8.

21. Brody, J. PMS is a worldwide phenomenon. *New York Times,* November 11, 1992, c10.

22. Snowdon, D. A., Kane, R. L., Beeson, W. L., et al. Is early natural menopause a biologic marker of health and aging? *American Journal of Public Health,* 1989, 79(6), 709 – 714.

23. Sauer, M. V., Paulson, R. J., Lobo, R. A., A preliminary report on oocyte donation extending reproductive potential to women over 40. *New England Journal of Medicine,* 1990, 323(17), 1157.

24. Schmidt, W. E. Birth to 59-year-old raises British ethical storm. *New York Times,* December 29, 1993, a1 & a6.

25. Matthews, K. A., Wing, R. R., Kuller, L. H., et al. Influences of natural

menopause on psychological characteristics and symptoms of middle-aged healthy women. *Journal of Counseling and Clinical Psychology,* 1990, 58(3), 345 – 351.

26. Boston Women's Health Collective. *Our Bodies, Ourselves.* New York: Simon and Schuster, 1973.

27. Boston Women's Health Collective. *Our Bodies, Ourselves.* New York: Simon and Schuster, 1973, p. xix.

SUGGESTED READING

Ayalah, D., & I. Weinstock. *Breasts: Women Speak About Their Breasts and Their Lives.* New York: Summit Books, 1979.

Bly, Robert. *Menopause Workbook.* New York: HarperCollins, 1994.

Boston Women's Health Book Collective. *The New Our Bodies, Ourselves. Updated and Expanded for the '90s.* New York: Simon & Schuster, 1992.

Callahan, Joan C., ed. *Menopause: A Midlife Passage.* Bloomington, Ind.: Indiana University Press, 1993.

Cutler, Winnifred, & Delso-Ramon Garcia. *Menopause: A Medical Guide for Women.* New York: Norton & Co., 1993.

Golub, S. *Periods: From Menarche to Menopause.* Newbury Park, CA: Sage Publications, 1992.

Hall, Judy, & Robert Jacobs. *Menopause Matters: A Practical Approach to Midlife Change.* Rockport, MA: Element Books, 1994.

Lark, Susan M. *Menopause Self Help Book.* Berkeley, CA: Celestial Arts Publishing, 1990.

Madaras, L., & J. Patterson. *Womancare: A Gynecological Guide to Your Body.* New York: Avon Books, 1981.

Murray, Michael T. *Menopause: Getting Well Naturally.* Roseville, CA: Prima Publishing, 1994.

Notelovitz, Morris, & Diana Tonnessen. *Menopause and Midlife Health.* New York: St. Martin's Press, 1993.

Chapter 3

NORMAL GYNECOLOGICAL MAINTENANCE

"I feel that it is my right as a responsible consumer of my own health care to shop around for talented and able medical treatment. I am currently cared for by an adult male who, although board certified in the most sophisticated laser procedures and having graduated with honors from respected schools, has all the interpersonal skills that one might expect from a bowling ball. You can be sure I won't stay with him long." — Miriam, age 58

GETTING STARTED

The Odds Are Against Women

Millions of women regularly visit our doctors even when we believe we are perfectly healthy. We go for many reasons, but particularly for checkups and assistance with regard to our gynecological — sexual and reproductive — health. As a result, our interactions with the doctor who provides gynecological care are likely to be the most important medical encounters of our adult lives.

As women, we are at a disadvantage in our medical care. Women undergo more exams, laboratory tests, and blood pressure checks than men, but are less likely to receive major diagnostic or therapeutic interventions. Also, women receive fewer preventable services than recommended, including cancer screening tests.[1] This may be partly due to financial barriers to health care caused by lower income and/or less insurance. Interestingly, the gender of your health care provider can make a difference. A 1993 study indicated that women who visit a female physician for their usual health care are more likely to have had a Pap test within the past three years and to have previously had a mammogram than women whose primary physician is male.[2]

Health issues affecting women, like osteoporosis or the menstrual cycle, have been the subject of surprisingly little research. In diseases affecting both sexes, such as Alzheimer's and heart disease, only men have been generally studied. Instruments used in heart surgery were designed for men's larger arteries — because heart disease was traditionally viewed as a man's disease. Furthermore, heart disease is usually treated less aggressively in women.[3] Women, until recently, have been left out of clinical trials of new drugs under the assumption that chemicals act the same in men and women.

What You Can Do to Even Your Odds

Since you may be starting at a disadvantage, it is up to you to equalize your chances of getting the best medical care possible. That process begins with selecting your gynecologist. If possible, you should begin your search for a suitable doctor when you are well. Don't wait until you are ill, because you may be hurried, anxious, or confused, and as a result the doctor you choose may not be the most qualified and compatible. The discussion and guidelines that follow, while directed specifically at helping you choose a gynecologist, are useful for choosing any physician.

IDENTIFYING PROSPECTIVE GYNECOLOGISTS

Information from friends, neighbors, relatives, family physicians, county medical societies, local health departments, and telephone directories can be the source for identifying prospective gynecologists. Most people pick a physician based on personal recommendations from friends and family. These recommendations will probably provide you with a sense of the doctor's interpersonal skills ("he has a great bedside manner," "she feels for her patients," "she listens"); however, you will likely learn little about other important critical criteria such as medical training, board certification, and affiliations.

So, how do you find out about their qualifications? To proceed knowledgeably you first need to know what attributes make a good doctor.

Qualifications / Training · Medical training, normally a four-year program, usually begins after completion of a college education. At medical school graduation, students take the Hippocratic oath and are pronounced Doctors of Medicine (M.D.). To begin to practice medicine as a general practitioner (G.P.) they also need to complete a one-year internship and pass licensing examinations, administered by the State or National Board of Medical Examiners. Most do not become general practitioners. Nowadays, more than 70 percent of doctors become specialists, which requires additional training. The primary care physician that you see is most likely a specialist in family practice or internal medicine. To become a specialist, doctors must complete residency training in their chosen area.

A residency of from one to six or seven years, depending upon the specialty, provides doctors with intensive training in a particular branch of medicine. Only physicians who have passed speciality examinations following their residency are termed **board certified** and are able to say that they are specialists. Some physicians, who have *not* passed board exams, say that they "limit their practice to (for example) ob/gyn" — thus avoiding erroneously labeling themselves as gynecologists while at the same time giving the public the impression that they are certified specialists.

Affiliations. At a minimum, the physician you choose should be board certified. When there are complicated medical problems and you need to choose a specialist, you will improve your chances of getting the best doctor possible if you choose one who is on the faculty of a medical school and is affiliated with and has admitting privileges at a teaching hospital.[4] It makes sense, in these cases, to turn to doctors who teach, do research, and practice in teaching hospitals. They will be on the "cutting edge" of the discipline, will be involved in transmitting information to the next generation of physicians, and will be current and conversant with the field.

Getting in the Know · Guidance in helping you select a competent physician can be obtained from several sources.

Local medical societies. Call the local medical society. County medical societies maintain up-to-date information about their members, including their specialties and hospital affiliations.

Call 1-800-776-CERT to confirm your doctor's certification. This is a service provided by the American Board of Medical Specialties.

Consumer organizations. Many special interest groups maintain lists of doctors around the country whom they would recommend for particular problems. See the Appendix for some groups that maintain lists of obstetricians and gynecologists.

Reference books available in your library. A book published by the American Board of Medical Specialties, *The ABMS Compendium of Certified Medical Specialists,* will tell you whether your doctor is board certified. The listings in this book are not complete. First of all, some physicians choose not to be included. Second, although the directory offers physician-provided information on medical school attended, residencies, fellowships, and so on, only the facts about board certification are verified. Finally, there is a lag time in the publication, so some material is outdated.

The *American Medical Directory* or state medical directories list all licensed physicians in the country or specific state. While they include all kinds of biographical information on medical backgrounds, the data is not rigorously checked.

A 1,100-page tome, *6,892 Questionable Doctors* lists doctors, dentists, chiropractors, and podiatrists in 40 states who have been found to be medically negligent and have been disciplined by their state licensing agency. Discipline can take a variety of forms from probation to license removal. If your library does not have the book, you can get it from the publisher: Public Citizens Health Research Group, Department QD, 2000 P Street NW, Washington, D.C. 20036.

POPULAR BOOKS AND MAGAZINES AVAILABLE IN BOOKSTORES

Examples of these are: Robert Arnot's *The Best Medicine: How to Choose the Top Doctors, the Top Hospitals and the Top Treatment*, and Donald Vickery and James Fries' *Take Care of Yourself: The Complete Guide to Medical Self Care.* Another good source is *U.S. News and World Report,* which for the last several years has conducted a survey of leading physicians and has published an "honor roll of the best of the best."

Summary: the doctor you choose as your physician should be:

1. A graduate of an accredited medical school
2. Board certified in the specialty you need
3. Someone you are comfortable with

And if there is a serious problem,

4. Appointed to the faculty of a medical school, and
5. Affiliated and have privileges at a teaching hospital.

SELECTING YOUR MEDICAL CARE PROVIDER

Compatibility · The information about the doctor which you have carefully researched does not tell you whether you are going to get along. Compatibility is somewhat like a marriage — there are no objective criteria that predict success.

Part of compatibility involves communication skills and part involves style. Studies have shown that many doctors and patients could benefit if their discussions were somewhat more friendly and less businesslike. Although some physicians naturally listen to their patients with empathy, data suggest that too often many are abrupt, apparently uninterested in patients' distress and prone to controlling the medical interview. A study in 1984 found that three-quarters of the patients studied were interrupted by their physicians within the first 18 seconds of beginning to describe their symptoms.[5] While some doctors may believe this is efficient, researchers find that it unduly limits the physician's ability to obtain crucial information from the patient.[6] A recent study suggests that doctors would do well to listen more and talk less. While many physicians assume the first complaint is the most important, there is usually no relationship between the order in which patients bring up their concerns and their medical significance.[7] When doctors dominate, patients don't medically do as well as when the patients exert more control.[8]

As for style, in one study of more than 1,000 letters from dissatisfied patients at a large Michigan HMO, the most common complaints had to do with a lack of compassion on the physicians' part. Patients' complaints included that their physicians never looked at them, made them feel humiliated, or used medical or technical jargon that left them confused.[9]

Male Versus Female · A considerable number of women, who have lost patience with the gruff imperiousness displayed by some gynecologists, are beginning to suspect that the best guarantee against insufferable behavior and paternalism is to make sure the doctor is a woman.

One of this idea's loudest advocates is a man. In his book *Women and Doctors,* Dr. John M. Smith argues that men have no business being gynecologists, and that women have been mistreated and abused by their male physicians.[10] A growing body of data shows that female physicians spend more time with their patients and interrupt them less often than men do.[11] While there have been predictions that female doctors would be less interventionist and more "natural," studies of the number of surgical procedures performed or drugs prescribed have shown no significant sex difference.[12] On the other hand, an informal survey of doctors in several Boston hospitals reported that female doctors were 20 times more likely than males to prescribe estrogen replacement therapy for menopausal patients.[13] Whether it's because female physicians have a greater understanding of the female body in transition or are just empathic is not clear.

The problem with choosing a female physician is finding one. Only 20 percent of gynecologists now in practice are women. However, 40 to 51 percent of the current medical school student body are female; therefore, in not too many years, women should be readily available as physicians. The option will then be yours to choose a male or female physician.

Nontraditional Medicine · Alternative medicine has been around for years, but the scientific community has tended to have a hands-off attitude. However, in 1992, the National Institutes of Health established an Office for the Study of Unconventional Medical Practices. Alternative medicine had come of age. Under their aegis, the merits of therapies outside mainstream healing will be studied. In the meantime, what constitutes "alternative medicine" as opposed to quackery needs further investigation.

THE FIRST VISIT

Your first visit should include an interview in order for you to get a sense of the doctor. That initial interview also allows you the opportunity to establish a relationship with the doctor when you are not in the middle of a crisis. When you call to schedule your first office visit with either a medical doctor or osteopathic physician, explain that you do not have an urgent problem, but that you would like to consult the doctor, and that an appointment within the month is acceptable. While on the telephone you might also ask about fees if you are not in an HMO or managed care program.

When you visit the office, note the general atmosphere. One patient has been quoted as saying, "Never go to a doctor whose office plants have died." More importantly, is it hospitable or cold, efficient or slovenly; are the aides courteous or abrupt? Both the staff and the office atmosphere often reflect a doctor's basic attitudes.

It is a good idea, when seeing a physician for the first time, to have obtained your medical records from your previous doctor. The file belongs to you and should be provided free of charge.

Don't be embarrassed about asking the doctor questions during this interview. This is the time to find out about his or her philosophy of health care, when he or she is available, how he or she responds to calls. The answers and the way they are communicated are good indications of whether a good doctor-patient relationship is possible.

Below is a checklist which you might want to answer after your first visit.

1. Are you comfortable around the doctor?
2. Are you allowed to talk or does the doctor do most of the talking?
3. Is the doctor a good listener or are you constantly interrupted?
4. Do you feel hurried or pressured by the doctor?
5. Does the doctor take notes of what you said?
6. Is the doctor willing to answer questions? One of those questions should be "Is the doctor available for emergencies?"
7. Does the doctor explain what she or he is doing during the various phases of the examination?
8. Is the exam you receive thorough?
9. Do you have to wait "too long" to see the doctor? (Unless you are informed of an emergency situation, you should not usually spend more than 15 to 30 minutes in the waiting room.)
10. Does the doctor treat you with courtesy and respect?
11. How long do you have to wait to get a follow-up appointment?
12. What type of hospital privileges does the doctor have?
13. What type of insurance will the doctor accept? If you are not covered by a plan, what are the billing and payment procedures?

You have carefully chosen your medical care provider based on recommendations and research into the person's qualifications. Your first visit will confirm whether you should continue with this individual or whether you need to search again. If after your first visit you are not satisfied — shop around. The more experience you have with medical providers, the easier it becomes to evaluate them.

PARTICIPATORY GYNECOLOGICAL HEALTH CARE

Your Doctor's Role

Your doctor's obligation is to provide you with a thorough examination. It begins with an interview during which your entire medical history is taken. The interview should include discussing in some detail: the diseases or conditions that run in your family; your medical history, including past illnesses, allergies, current medications, disabilities, vaccinations, operations, and medical problems; and details of your current lifestyle, which could include the nature of your work, your level of satisfaction in it, and your recreational pursuits. Finally, the interview should include discussion of any current symptoms or problems. See the Appendix for items to be included in a history.

After the history is taken, you will be asked to undress and put on a gown. Before the physical examination begins you may be asked to provide a urine sample. This serves two purposes — first, it allows a check for signs of infection and excess sugar, protein, and so on; and second, the empty bladder will make the examination more comfortable. Usually prior to the doctor's examination, the nurse will take your weight, pulse, and blood pressure. If you have not had your blood tested recently, a blood sample may be taken to screen for anemia and other ailments.

THE PHYSICAL EXAMINATION

When your examination begins, if your doctor is male, another woman — either a nurse or an assistant — is likely to be present during the exam. This is for both your comfort and the doctor's legal protection.

While you are sitting, the doctor will check:

1. your face for acne or unusual hairiness — signs of hormone excess
2. your neck for thyroid gland enlargement, and
3. your breasts for lumpiness or growths.

This might be the time that the doctor discusses breast self-examination and shows you how and when to do your self-exam (preferably right after your period or, if you are postmenopausal, at the same time each month). The doctor should also discuss mammography with you.

You will then probably be asked to lie on your back, knees bent and feet in the stirrups — the **lithotomy position**. This position is the only way a doctor can properly do a gynecological examination. Your abdomen and breasts will be checked both visually and with **palpation** (touch) as the doctor looks for abnormal growths or signs of infection.

Breast Examination · The doctor will reexamine your breasts after you move from a sitting to lying position. You will probably be asked to place one of your hands behind your neck. This helps flatten and spread out the breast over the chest wall.

In this position, the doctor will palpate with flat fingers gently in small circular motions, moving around the entire breast as if it were an imaginary clock face. The procedure is repeated after the fingers are moved approximately an inch in towards the nipple. It make take three or more circles to palpate every part of the breast, including the nipple. The nipple will also be gently "milked" to detect any discharge. The entire process is repeated on the other breast. Your underarms will be examined for enlarged lymph nodes, since breast tissue extends into that area.

The purpose of the palpation is to discover any lumps or masses, areas of nodularity, thickening, or tenderness.

Breast Self-Examination · You should be looking for these same things when you examine your own breasts using the *same technique* as just described. A good time to begin practicing is after the doctor's visit. You are not as likely to be as concerned about the dismaying variations in consistency that you may find, since the professional exam probably reassured you that all of those possible little irregularities are normal. In ensuing months, as long as the nodules and thickenings remain the same size and are diffusely scattered, there is usually nothing to worry about.

One other part of breast self-examination involves visual inspection. Before beginning the palpation, you should stand in front of a mirror with good lighting and look at your breasts. Turn from side to side, looking at your breasts with your arms relaxed at your sides. Look for any change in the size or shape of the breast, puckering or dimpling of the skin, changes in the nipple such as scaling, changes in the direction of the nipple, or drainage. Lift your arms over your head and check to see whether your breasts move up and down together. Lift your breasts to look for sores or dimpling. Bend forward and check for any abnormality in the shape of the breasts.

NOTE: While recommendations have been made for years for women to practice breast self-examination, the reality is that most women do not. For the estimated 60 percent or more of women who do not practice breast self-exam, many claim they have tried at some point in their lives; almost all believe that it should be done. Studies have shown that women who learn the routine usually discontinue it after a few months, although those who were instructed by a doctor or other medical provider are more likely to continue than those acquiring the technique from another source.

Internal Examination · The internal examination of the vagina and cervix necessitates the use of a **speculum,** a metal or plastic instrument that opens like a duck's bill to spread the vaginal walls. Years ago, one common complaint made by women against their gynecologists was that they "shoved in a cold speculum." In response to those mounting criticisms, some physicians are

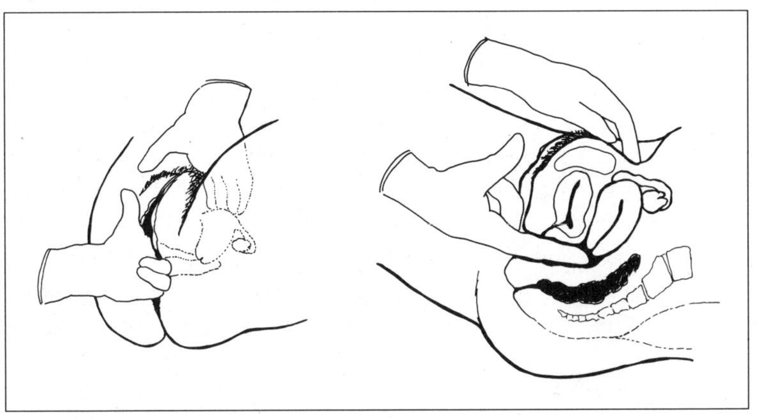

PELVIC EXAM

The physician uses a bimanual (two-handed) method to check the position and size of the ovaries and uterus.

now more sensitive and use a warm speculum or the disposable plastic type. If you follow the direction to relax and concentrate on not tensing up, you should experience a mild pressure that is neither uncomfortable nor painful.

Once the speculum is in place, the doctor will usually take a swab of cervical tissue for a Pap smear. The doctor may also take a sample of some vaginal tissue or discharge to test for infection if that is indicated.

After the speculum is removed, the doctor will don sterile gloves and insert one or two lubricated fingers into your vaginal opening while pressing on your abdomen with the other hand. This manual examination allows the physician to check your uterus and ovaries for abnormal size or growths.

The doctor will then insert one gloved finger into your rectum and the other into your vagina to continue manual observations. By remaining relaxed, these procedures should not be painful. If they are, inform the doctor.

During all of the above procedures, the doctor should be communicating with you and describing what is being done and why. That will aid immeasurably in allowing you to be relaxed.

That last procedure typically ends the physical examination. After you have dressed, you will see the doctor in the office to review all findings and recommendations. A reminder — do not be intimidated. Ask questions. For a list of possible questions, see pages 44 and 45.

The office visit often concludes with a reminder of when to return for another checkup, and a follow-up suggestion for you to schedule a mammogram.

Mammogram · A three-step early breast cancer detection program includes: (1) examining your breasts monthly, (2) seeing your doctor regularly, and (3) making an informed decision on when to have a **mammogram** — which is an X-ray of the breast.

With any cancer, chances of survival increase the earlier it is detected. Early detection of breast cancer occurs usually through mammography and results in a cure rate that is greater than 90 percent.

Mammography, routinely used since the late 1950s, involves placing a woman's breasts, one at a time, on a metal plate. Two X-rays of each breast, one from the top and one from the side, are taken and developed on photographic film. Mammography is currently recommended as a screening technique on an annual basis for women over 50 and women in high-risk groups.

Breast cancer risk factors include:

Age over 50
Personal history of breast cancer
Family history of breast cancer
Never giving birth, or birth after age 30
Long menstrual history (periods started early and ended late in life)
Obesity

Mammograms, in addition to acting as a screening tool to detect some cancers before they are felt, can verify a doubtful diagnosis when a mass is discovered by palpation. Diagnostic mammograms also can determine exact locations for biopsy or for surgery. They also serve as a "baseline" against which future mammograms can be compared to see if there have been recent changes.

The procedure is not 100 percent accurate, and much depends on the skill and experience of the interpreter of the films; that is, a radiologist. There have been cases of **false positives** (mistaken diagnoses of cancer) and **false negatives** (missed cases). False positives tend to foster biopsies as the physician tries to ascertain the nature of the suspicious lesions. However, not every finding on a mammogram needs to be handled as a major medical intervention. Rather, depending on the nature of the lesion found by the X-ray, the area might be examined by a sonogram, by a needle aspiration biopsy (which does not involve surgery and can be done in a physician's office), or by another mammogram in three to four months. That follow-up mammogram can serve to confirm or negate the original diagnosis.

False negatives may prompt some women to ignore the symptoms of a possible cancer that appear between mammograms. If a lump is discovered, even within weeks of a negative mammogram, it should be treated as suspicious and looked at by a doctor. In spite of these problems, the majority of medical care researchers find the cost-risk benefit to be in favor of using mammograms as a screening tool for women over 50 and those in the previously defined high-risk groups.[14]

Despite the fact that nearly 85 percent of breast cancer cases occur in women over 50 years of age,[15] and the fact that there is a confirmed clear benefit (at least a 30 percent reduction in deaths for women over 50 who were screened every year or two),[16] vast numbers of women in this age group have not been taking advantage of this screening tool. In 1990, it was estimated that 40 percent of women over 50 had never had a mammogram.[17] Worse yet, a recent study reported that, between 1985 and 1992,[18] the proportion of women over 50 years of age seeking mammograms fell. This low mammogram usage by women over age 50 is of major concern to health professionals, as evidenced by the January 1994 issue of the *American Journal of Public Health,* which was primarily devoted to strategies directly related to raising the awareness and prevention of breast cancer.

While there is no question about the benefits of mammography for women over age 50, the big focus of debate concerns at what age and at what intervals mammograms should be taken regularly. According to an editorial in the *Journal of the American Medical Association,* the United States since 1987 has been the only developed nation encouraging mammography screening for asymptomatic women under 50 years of age.[19] In December of 1993, the National Cancer Institute stopped recommending that women in their 40s have mammograms every one to two years.

The debate concerning the age to begin mass routine screening with mammography centers on these issues. Less than 20 percent of all breast cancers occur in women under age 50. Additionally, "false positive" results on mammograms in this age group prompted approximately two-and-a-half times as many unwarranted biopsies and three times as many unnecessary diagnostic procedures as for women over age 50.[20] The Canadian National Breast Cancer Study[21] and a statistical analysis of relevant studies on mammography screening[22] concluded that there is no basis for the promotion of screening in women under age 50.

However, the issue is not as clear-cut as it seems. To demonstrate the volatility of the debate, it is worth noting that the National Cancer Institute, by changing its policy, had overruled the advice it received from its general advisory body, the National Cancer Advisory Board.[23] Further, The American Cancer Society and the American College of Radiology still recommend that women 40 to 50 years of age undergo routine mammography screening.

Mammography critics claim that younger women's denser breasts can make it more difficult to pick up tumors; however, supporters of early breast X-rays state that mammography has been vastly improved, making it easier to find tiny tumors.

Because of the controversy regarding mammograms for women 40 to 49, an informed decision at age 40 is important. You need to know the drawbacks (for example, unnecessary biopsies and diagnostic procedures, and psychological trauma) as well as the benefits (early detection, less invasive surgery, and better survival rates).

When you look at the information arguing against a mammogram for women 40 to 49 years of age, realize that the statistics used relate to the value of mass screening in health care cost dollars (cost/benefit). While health care costs are important, you should not necessarily let societal economic considerations influence your individual decision.

NOTE: On October 1, 1994, a new law took effect which mandates that mammography centers must provide demonstrably high-quality X-ray pictures, and their staffs must be adequately trained. Unfortunately, as of 1993 only 6,384 of the approximately 11,000 – 12,000 mammography units in the United States were accredited by the American College of Radiology. The American Cancer Society (1-800-ACS-2345) and the National Cancer Institute in Bethesda, Maryland (1-800-4-CANCER) can tell you which centers in your area are accredited.

Whatever your decision, when you start to have mammograms, choose an accredited facility. Double reading of mammograms (that is, having your X-ray read by two board certified radiologists) is likely to be especially valuable for younger women.

Preparing for a mammogram. Dress comfortably in a two-piece outfit such as slacks or a skirt and a blouse. Do not use deodorant, powder, ointment or perfume on your breasts or underarms before your mammogram. These substances leave a residue which can be detected by X-rays, distorting the mammogram. Be aware that breast compression is not dangerous and does no damage to the breast tissue. Remember, any discomfort you may feel is only temporary.

Your Obligation

Gynecological care, even at its best, can be awkward and sometimes embarrassing. As a result of criticism from participants in the feminist movement, many gynecologists have been trying to modify their attitudes and behavior. However, you too have responsibility toward the quality of the doctor-patient relationship.

KEEPING A RECORD

Because a thorough medical history will be taken during the initial exam, you should be prepared. Keeping a record book or file of important medical milestones such as major illnesses, operations, and vaccinations is helpful and should be brought with you on your first visit. You should also be ready to answer questions about your family's medical history. If possible, you should jot down a family tree listing major illnesses such as cancer, diabetes, stroke, or heart disease that have affected parents, siblings, aunts, and uncles.

If you are among the 24 percent of women who report seeing no other doctor besides a gynecologist, it's important to tell your gynecologist that he/she is your only physician. Routine additional tests might then be included, such as those for cholesterol or blood sugar. These wouldn't ordinarily be assessed, because your gynecologist may assume that you've already received these tests elsewhere.

Your first obligation for being prepared for the visit begins weeks or months before your scheduled visit. You need to be as good a detective about your own body as possible. One way of doing this is to keep a health diary which documents any illnesses, bodily changes, and persistent or unusual symptoms. Because of the cyclicity of women's hormones, you can expect bodily changes in response to the rising and falling levels of estrogen and progesterone. For example, your temperature can vary by as much as 1.6 degrees (from 97.2 prior to ovulation to 98.6 – 98.8 afterwards) during your monthly cycle, which is why you should have a baseline of those normal temperature fluctuations.

Women have been known to exhibit a variety of bodily changes throughout their monthly cycle, which include nosebleeds, headaches, listlessness, depression, aching joints, constipation, and bloat because of hormonal fluctuations. Note carefully your pattern over several months. In addition, you should be able to describe to the doctor how long your periods last, when your last one began, and how heavily you bleed (i.e., the number of tampons or pads you use daily). Keeping a written record will help in recognizing symptoms which are part of your normal cycle and others which might indicate problems.

COMMUNICATING WITH THE DOCTOR

Some women are uncomfortable discussing family or sexual matters with a physician. Others view their doctor as an authority figure too busy or knowledgeable to be questioned. In either case these women leave the office with unanswered questions, uncertain of the diagnosis or how to follow the recommended treatment.

Many women hold back information, waiting for the doctor to ask everything — figuring the doctor will ask if she or he needs to know.

Honest, open communication with your doctor is vital to your health. The more information you provide, the more likely it is that the physician will make the correct diagnosis.

A national health survey indicated that the typical gynecological visit lasts only 13 minutes, which is possibly why most of us feel pressured and don't ask questions. You should not worry about the length of the visit. You are paying for the doctor's care and attention, and your health is at stake. So, ask questions and do not be embarrassed no matter how they sound.

Take Control of Your Health — Ask Questions · Medicine is a business as well as a science and an art. If you recognize this, you will be better able to negotiate for the purchase of the very specialized services that doctors and hospitals are selling.

In dealing with the medical profession, you should not regress to the behavior of an anxious child and allow yourself to be led passively through your medical experience. The medical care business thrives on this passivity. But this can be harmful to you. You should not be distracted from using your critical faculties in dealing with doctors. At the very least, choosing medical care should be given the same consideration that applies to the process of selecting a new car, house, or appliance.

One way to increase the effectiveness of the visit is to write down your questions before the visit. Writing down "difficult" questions sometimes makes it easier to address them in person. You might even want to rehearse — talking about them with a friend or relative or in front of the mirror. By doing this you will be able to ask the questions with confidence in the doctor's office. Remember, you are the one in control — it's your health, your time, and your money.

In addition to your prepared questions, if a procedure is performed or the doctor says something which you don't understand, ask about it. You need to understand what is happening in order to make intelligent decisions about your medical care in the future. While you are being examined, if a procedure is performed or the doctor says something which you don't understand, continue to question the doctor.

The People's Medical Society, a consumer health advocacy organization, says that there are three broad categories of questions which should be asked. They are:

1. Which tests are being given, what are the alternatives (if any), and what can be done if the tests disclose a problem?
2. On what basis was the diagnosis made: tests, symptoms, or an educated guess?
3. Why is a particular therapy being suggested, and what is the doctor's experience with the treatment?

A list of more specific questions to ask your doctor can be found in Chapter 6, page 100.

Two questions to ask your physician's office staff are:

1. What type of insurance will the doctor accept?
2. Does the doctor use an in-house laboratory for tests? If so, will my insurance cover those costs? If not, will I be referred to a facility or hospital where the costs will be covered by my insurance?

Take notes during the visit. Jot down highlights of what the doctor says, particularly if there are important instructions you might forget. Consider bringing a family member or close friend with you. While this person may not be able to stay with you during the physical examination, she or he can provide moral support and help you recall details of the doctor's explanations during the post-examination discussion.

INSURANCE

The U.S. health care system was built primarily on a lucrative partnership of fee-for-service medicine and private insurance. Modern health insurance in the United States began as hospital insurance in 1929. During the 1930s it expanded to cover hospital, surgical, and medical services and was purchased on an individual basis.

Now health insurance has more varieties than almost any other type of insurance, although, in general, it can be classified as either private or public. The public health insurance plans include Medicare and Medicaid. Private sector plans include traditional prepaid **fee-for-service insurance** and **group prepaid insurance** which, since 1973, are known as **Health Maintenance Organizations (HMOs).**

Until recently, doctors and hospitals had a free hand to set their own fees and pass the cost of their services on to private insurance carriers — or their patients, if the individual had no insurance. Costly procedures and their accompanying bills were rarely questioned. This was a major contributing factor to burgeoning health care expenses.

The high cost of medical care, coupled with the fact that more than 37 million Americans were either uninsured or underinsured, prompted President Clinton's attempt to correct the U. S. health delivery system. He is the latest American president since Teddy Roosevelt to advocate a system of national health insurance for the United States. Harry S. Truman presented legislation during his administration, but it was defeated by the specter of "socialized" medicine raised by the American Medical Association and insurance companies.

September 22, 1993 marked another attempt. President Clinton's health care reform proposal was generated because the issue of rising health care costs had become the second most important concern (after the economy) of the American public in the 1992 election. That there would be a change in the system was a given; the form it would take was still up for grabs when we went to press in 1995.

In the 1980s the cost of medical care increased so astronomically that insurance companies began complaining. The result was the beginning of "**managed care**" programs, which allow insurance companies to monitor the quality of treatment and determine its appropriateness for the patient's condition. Managed care programs require policyholders to seek **second opinions** before undergoing most surgery, to use outpatient facilities for specified procedures, to use participating doctors and hospitals, and to obtain insurance company approval before starting a proposed course of treatment for certain illnesses.

Although the term managed care is now used to specify a new system, in actuality the oldest managed care providers are the group prepaid practice plans. The oldest is Kaiser Permanente which was started in the 1940s. At one time the distinctions between fee-for-service, traditional insurance, and group prepaid (HMO) policies were great. Nowadays, the differences have blurred. Many insurers have adopted the HMO label — providing health care for their members for a fixed monthly premium. They range from restrictive arrangements found in the original prepaid group practices to loose confederations of doctors whose practices are mirror-images of the old-fashioned, fee-for-service medicine. The proliferation of many different types of HMOs makes it confusing to select coverage and requires much time and effort to make an informed decision.

ENDNOTES

1. Clancy, C. M., & Massion, C. T. American women's health care: a patchwork quilt with gaps. *Journal of the American Medical Association,* 1992, 268(14), 1918 – 1920.
2. Clancy, C. M., & Franks, P. Physician gender bias in clinical decision-making: screening for cancer in primary care. *Medical Care,* 1993, 31(3), 213 – 218.
3. Clancy, C. M., & Franks, P. Physician gender bias in clinical decision-making: screening for cancer in primary care. *Medical Care,* 1993, 31(3), 213 – 218.
4. Arnot, R. *The Best Medicine: How to Choose the Top Doctors, the Top Hospitals and the Top Treatment.* Reading, Mass.: Addison-Wesley, 1992.
5. Beckman, H. B., & Frankel, R. M. The effect of physician behavior on the collection of data. *Annals of Internal Medicine,* 1984, 101(5), 692 – 696.
6. Roter, D., & Frankel, R. M. Quantitative and qualitative approaches to the evaluation of the medical dialogue. *Social Science and Medicine,* 1992, 34(10), 1097 – 2103.

7. Roter, D., Lipkin, M. Jr., & Korsgaard, A. Sex differences in patients' and physicians' communication during primary care medical visits. *Medical Care,* 1991, 29(11), 1083 – 1093.

8. Greenfield, S., Kaplan, S. H., Ware, J. E. Jr., et al. Patients' participation in medical care: effects on blood sugar control and quality of life in diabetics. *Journal of General Internal Medicine*, 1988, 3(5), 448 – 457.

9. Beckman, H. B., Frankel, R. M., Kihm, J., et al. Measurement and improvement of humanistic skills in first-year trainees. *Journal of General Internal Medicine,* 1990, 5(1), 42 – 45.

10. Smith, J. M. *Women & Doctors: A Physician's Explosive Account of Women's Treatment — & Mistreatment — in America Today.* New York: Grove/Atlantic, 1992.

11. Angier, N. Bedside manners improve as more women enter medicine. *New York Times,* June 21, 1992.

12. Angier, N. Bedside manners improve as more women enter medicine. *New York Times,* June 21, 1992.

13. Angier, N. Bedside manners improve as more women enter medicine. *New York Times,* June 21, 1992.

14. Fletcher, S. W., Black, W., Harris, R., et al. Report of the International Workshop on Screening for Breast Cancer. *Journal of the National Cancer Institute,* 1993, 85, 1644 – 1656.

15. Davis, D. L., & Love, S. M. Mammographic screening. *Journal of the American Medical Association,* 1994, 271, 152 – 153.

16. Shapiro, S. The call for change in breast cancer screening guidelines. *American Journal of Public Health,* 1994, 84(1), 10 – 11.

17. U.S. Department of Health and Human Services, Public Health Service. Mammography and clinical breast examinations among women aged 50 years and older — behavioral risk factor surveillance system. *Morbidity and Mortality Weekly Report,* 1992, 42, 737 – 741.

18. Kerlikowske, K., Grady, D., Barclay, J., et al. Positive predictive value of screening mammography by age and family history of breast cancer. *Journal of the American Medical Association,* 1993, 270, 2444 – 2450.

19. Davis, D. L., & Love, S. M. Mammographic screening. *Journal of the American Medical Association,* 1994, 271, 152 – 153.

20. Kerlikowske, K., Grady, D., Barclay, J., et al. Positive predictive value of screening mammography by age and family history of breast cancer. *Journal of the American Medical Association,* 1993, 270, 2444 – 2450.

21. Miller, A. B., Baines, C. J., To, T., et al. Canadian National Breast Screening Study: 2. Breast cancer detection and death rates among women aged 50 to 59 years. *Canadian Medical Association Journal,* 1992, 147(10), 1477 – 1488.

Russell, C. Doubts about mammograms (Canadian Study questions guidelines for women under 50). *Washington Post,* November 14, 1992, A1.

22. Elwood, J. M., Cox, B., & Richardson, A. K. The effectiveness of breast cancer screening by mammography in younger women. *Online Journal of Current Clinical Trials,* February 25, 1993, Document 32.

23. Marwick, C. NCI changes its stance on mammography. *Journal of the American Medical Association,* 1994, 271, 96.

SUGGESTED READING

Aldrich, C. Knight. *The Medical Interview: Guide to the Doctor-Patient Relationship.* Pearl River, NY: Parthenon Publishing Group, 1993.

Arnot, Robert. *The Best Medicine: How to Choose the Top Doctors, the Top Hospitals and the Top Treatment.* Reading, Mass.: Addison-Wesley,1992.

Consumer Reports. "Alternative Medicine: The Facts." A three-part series in January, March, and May of 1994.

Ellig, David H. *Never Get Naked on Your First Visit: A Patient's Survival Guide.* Mesa, AZ: Med Ed AZ, 1992.

Jones, J. A., Gary L. Krebs, & Gerald M. Phillips. *Communicating With Your Doctor: Getting the Most Out of Health Care.* Cresskill, NJ: Hampton Press, 1995.

Lobanov, Igor, & Silvia Shepard-Lobanov. *Key to Choosing a Doctor.* Woodbury, NY: Barron's Educational Series, 1991.

Navarro, Vicente D. *Dangerous to Your Health: The Crisis of Medical Care in the United States.* Holmes, PA: Cornerstone Books, 1993.

Pell, Arthur R. *Diagnosing Your Doctor: A Straightforward Guide to Asking the Right Questions and Getting the Health Care You Deserve.* Minnetonka, MN: Chronimed Publishing, 1991.

Porter, Sylvia. *Sylvia Porter's Guide to Your Health Care: How You Can Have the Best Health Care for Less.* New York: Avon Books, 1990.

Raffel, Marshall W., & Norma K. Raffel. *The U. S. Health System: Origins and Functions.* Albany, NY: Delmar Publishers, 1994.

Roberts, Marc J., & Alexandra T. Clyde. *Your Money or Your Life: The Health Care Crisis Explained.* Garden City, NY: Doubleday & Co., 1993.

Shulman, Neil, & Letitia Sweitzer. *Better Health Care for Less.* New York: Hippocrene Books, 1993.

Smith, John M. *Women & Doctors: A Physician's Explosive Account of Women's Medical Treatment — & Mistreatment — in America Today.* New York: Grove/Atlantic, 1992.

Vickery, Donald, and James Fries. *Take Care of Yourself: The Complete Guide to Medical Self Care.* Reading, Mass.: Addison-Wesley, 1993.

Wekesser, Carol. (Ed.) *Health Care in America: Opposing Viewpoints.* San Diego, CA: Greenhaven Press, 1994.

Chapter 4

SYMPTOMS, TESTS AND DIAGNOSES

"I kept putting off my gyn test and Pap smear. I was so busy — new husband, new job — I didn't know when I could schedule it. When I finally went, I was diagnosed with low-grade cervical cancer. Thank goodness it had not had time to spread." — Sally, age 35

In this chapter some common gynecological concerns will be discussed, including those that may possibly merit hysterectomy. We begin our discussion with symptoms and their possible causes. In some cases a single disorder may be heralded by more than one symptom. On the other hand, a problem such as abdominal discomfort may occur in several conditions. For this reason, you may need to consult medical personnel to schedule appropriate tests to arrive at an accurate diagnosis. These procedures are described in the second section of this chapter.

SYMPTOMS THAT RAISE QUESTIONS

A good look at the human body, and particularly some understanding of the female and male physiology, almost always stimulates awe and admiration. Our many organs normally function ceaselessly and healthfully. Occasionally, however, problems arise.

Heavy or Abnormal Periods

For most women the menstrual period lasts about three to five days, and the amount of blood and other substances expelled is roughly two to four ounces (a quarter to half of a cup). Since we don't normally collect our menstrual flow in a measuring cup, it may be difficult to accurately determine how much is lost. Furthermore, the number of days of bleeding, the length of the cycle, and even the amount of flow varies considerably from woman to woman. Concern is appropriate when there is a marked change from your previous pattern.[1]

One way to document the amount of flow is to keep a record of the number of tampons and/or sanitary napkins you use over the course of your period. Recognize, of course, that many women routinely change these after using the toilet and/or taking a shower, while others do not. Often, therefore, it does not help to compare your use with that of others unless you account for these specifics. It is *your* pattern that is of concern.

Excessive bleeding is naturally scary. A truly heavy flow, especially one with many clots, may cause worry about hemorrhaging. At the least, we wonder whether we will become weak or anemic. Very heavy periods may also cause embarrassment.

News About Heavy Bleeding · Heavy bleeding alone, including clots, is rarely a sign of cancer or infection of the uterus or ovaries. It is far more likely that your heavy bleeding is due to the benign uterine tumors commonly called **fibroids**, a troublesome IUD, or other causes.

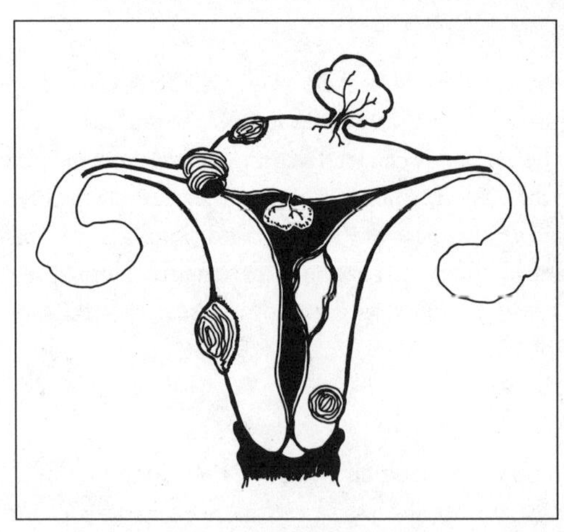

FIBROIDS OR MYOMATA

These benign growths of uterine tissue may occur above, below, on the outside or the inside of the uterus.

UTERINE FIBROIDS

Benign growths of uterine tissue are known as fibroids. The medical term **myomata** or **myomas** (**myoma** for just one) or **leiomyomata** is used for these growths which are derived from the smooth muscle or connective tissue of the middle of the three uterine layers. Fibroid-like growths from the endometrium into the uterine muscle are **adenomyomata**; the term **adenomyosis** is used to describe the condition.

Fibroids may make themselves known to you through heavy or irregular menstrual bleeding and cramps. If they are of sufficient size, you might feel them as firm rounded lumps in your abdomen. Myomata may cause the need to urinate frequently, if they press on your bladder. Your medical caregiver can feel them when doing an internal examination. Further confirmation of the presence of enlarged fibroids is available through the use of the X-ray and ultrasound procedures described later in this chapter.

The development of fibroids is influenced in part by the hormone estrogen. While fibroids may be present in the uterus at birth, they do not start to grow until hormonally triggered after puberty. Stimulated by estrogen, they often enlarge during pregnancy, and then withdraw following delivery. They may also grow while you are using birth control pills. Once you begin menopause, the normal reduction in estrogen production causes fibroids to shrink unless you are on hormone replacement therapy.

Although it is possible to have a single fibroid or myoma, they mostly manifest themselves in multiple numbers. Their size is usually stated in terms of how far advanced in pregnancy their growth makes your uterus appear. Dr. Vicki Hufnagel[2] describes a 12-week (three-month) uterus as "relatively small — less than 3½ inches in diameter." She notes, but disagrees with, the rule of thumb among gynecologists that a 12-week sized uterus or larger warrants a hysterectomy. While there is no consensus on what is meant by "small" and "large," Hufnagel's observations suggest that a less than 12-week size might be considered small; a greater than 12-week size would be large. Occasionally a medical practitioner may use fruit terms to describe size, such as "grapefruit-sized," or "like a watermelon."

Experts are agreed that if the fibroids are relatively small and do not cause significant discomfort or other symptoms, it is best to leave them alone. If you are in your 40s and even if they are fairly large, you can expect them to diminish in size with menopause if you do not use hormone replacement therapy. You should recognize this as an option. If you are younger and expect to have children, however, fibroids that measure to the size of a six-month pregnancy may interfere with your ability to carry the fetus. Even smaller ones may cause problems, depending on their location in the uterus. In this case, a **myomectomy**, removal of just the fibroids, may be the procedure of choice.[3] (See Chapter Six: Treatment Options.)

Physicians may attempt to rush you into a hysterectomy by using the term fibroid **tumor**. Because myomata are benign and do not spread like malignant cancer cells, the word tumor, although accurate, is unnecessarily frightening when referring to these growths. In no case do fibroids warrant an emergency hysterectomy unless you are hemorrhaging. If you decide to consider hysterectomy, take time to get more than one medical opinion and to make your decision thoughtfully. Enlarged fibroids in the uterus are the most common cause for hysterectomy.

Additional Causes of Abnormal Menstrual Bleeding · **Intrauterine Devices (IUDs)** used for contraception may cause unusually long and/or heavy menstrual discharge or cramping. Prompt removal of the offending device should correct the problem.

If you have not been practicing contraception, excessive or irregular bleeding may be due to an **ectopic** (out of place or tubal) **pregnancy**. The fertilized egg may be developing in a fallopian tube or other area unable to sustain an embryo; it needs to be removed. If such a pregnancy results in hemorrhage, emergency medical attention and possibly surgery would be required.

Hormonal, endocrine, and related factors may cause abnormal bleeding. Ovarian dysfunction and inadequate progesterone production can result in periods with extra heavy flow. Similarly, either an over- or under-productive thyroid gland could contribute to abnormally heavy periods. Accurate diagnosis and medication should relieve the condition.

The hormones in oral contraceptives may result in **breakthrough bleeding** (spotting) — irregularly spaced small endometrial discharges. A change in contraception or even switching to another brand of birth control pill may provide a remedy. Alternatively, you may simply live with the inconvenience.[4]

Abnormally heavy bleeding must not be ignored. Let your medical practitioner be the one to determine the cause. Blood tests to measure hemoglobin and determine whether you need iron supplements are recommended.

TABLE 4 – 1

POSSIBLE REASONS AND REMEDIES FOR HEAVY VAGINAL BLEEDING

Reason	Possible remedy
Uterine fibroids	Myomectomy or hysterectomy
Intrauterine devices (IUDs)	Removal of device
Ectopic pregnancy	Surgery
Ovarian dysfunction	Variable
Low progesterone	Progesterone pills
Oral contraceptive hormones	Change pills
Uterine polyps	Surgical removal of polyps
Hypo- or hyperthyroidism	Thyroid medication

Note: Each of the above requires careful medical evaluation and treatment related to individual findings.
Sources: Benson & Pernoll, 1993; Berkow, 1992.

POSTMENOPAUSAL BLEEDING OR DISCHARGE

During the years prior to menopause, loosely from about age 40 to 50, the menstrual period *normally* is *more irregular* than it had been in the past. This is with the exception of the teen years, when irregularity is commonplace because the menses are just beginning. Women going through menopause, whose menstrual cycles have seemingly stopped, may have a brief resumption of flow after several quiet months. This is ordinarily an entirely normal event. *Bleeding is not considered pathological unless other revealing symptoms accompany it or it has resumed six months or more after menstruation had apparently stopped. In these cases, medical attention is definitely warranted.*

If you have not had a menstrual period in six months or more, and then notice bleeding, you should see a physician. This may be symptomatic of endometrial cancer or complex hyperplasia. A clinical examination and office biopsy may be necessary to evaluate the condition. A D&C may be recommended, if the initial examination and biopsy indicate that this is warranted.[5] The following chapter discusses cancer — its diagnosis and treatment.

Abdominal Pain or Discomfort

PRIMARY DYSMENORRHEA

The vast majority of women have experienced some cramping and/or pelvic or back pain associated with menstrual periods. This is called **primary dysmenorrhea** when it is simply the result of uterine contractions, and there is no pathological cause. Primary dysmenorrhea is most common among younger women, especially those who have not given birth.

SECONDARY DYSMENORRHEA

Secondary dysmenorrhea, painful menstruation caused by physical problems, is more likely to occur in women over age 30. It may be due to IUD use, polyps, fibroids, or endometriosis. Abdominal pain may also be caused by infection and inflammation within the fallopian tubes, ovaries, and/or uterus.

PELVIC INFLAMMATORY DISEASE (PID)

Inflammation of the fallopian tubes is called **salpingitis.** Since other major organs within the pelvis such as the cervix (**cervicitis**), uterus (**endometriosis**), or ovaries (**oophoritis**), are also often infected, many physicians and patients refer to any of these four conditions as **pelvic inflammatory disease** or **PID.**

Symptoms of this infection are lower abdominal pain, menstrual-like cramping, and possibly abnormal vaginal discharge and fever. The diagnosis is not always obvious, since PID sometimes mimics the signs of ectopic pregnancy, ovarian cysts, or appendicitis. The difficulty in diagnosis prompted one cynic to suggest that PID actually stands for "physician in doubt."

Occasionally an IUD or cervical cap used for contraception prompts the inflammation, but most often a sexually transmitted disease (STD) is the cause. Any number of STD microorganisms may be responsible for PID, particularly those causing gonorrhea and chlamydia. Other pathogens, not sexually transmitted, such as the streptococcus and the tubercular bacteria, have also been found to cause PID. Occasionally injury during childbirth or gynecological surgery may result in PID.

PID may become chronic, so once you have it, you may have repeated episodes. These may result in damage to the reproductive organs, pain during intercourse, and impaired fertility.[6]

You may be able to avoid chronic PID by taking precautions against STDs, such as always using a condom, and undergoing a regimen of antibiotic treatment. Infrequently, in advanced cases or if the cause was injury during previous gynecological treatment, surgery, such as hysterectomy, may be required.[7]

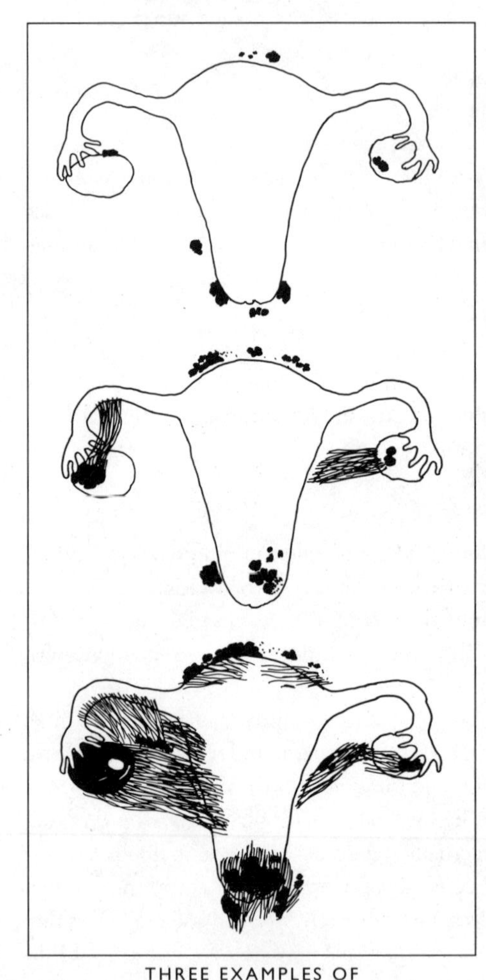

THREE EXAMPLES OF ENDOMETRIOSIS

Endometrial tissue, seen as dark splotches in this diagram, may be found in places other than the endometrium.

ENDOMETRIOSIS

Pelvic pain may be due to **endometriosis,** which is the presence of endometrial tissue in abnormal places. While many women with endometriosis suffer only mild discomfort, others experience severe pain.

The endometrium, the inner lining of the uterus, normally thickens and grows during each menstrual cycle and is subsequently sloughed off during menstruation. Sometimes, however, endometrial tissue migrates and may attach and develop in places other than the uterus. Endometrial tissue may end up in the ovaries, vagina, fallopian tubes, cervix, and even the intestines. Why and how migration occurs is unknown, but when endometrial tissue adheres to inappropriate organs, these structures are likely to become painfully engorged with blood during the menstrual cycle.

Laparoscopic examination is usually required to confirm the diagnosis of endometriosis. Mild cases may be helped by diet modification including the avoidance of dairy products, fat, sugar, alcohol, and caffeine. Hormonal drugs, including birth control pills, or Danazol, a synthetic steroid, are sometimes prescribed and may be helpful, but could have side effects which should be explored. Laser surgery utilizing a laparoscope is effective in eliminating the offending tissue. Hysterectomy accomplishes the objective of removal of the uterus, the original source of endometrial tissue.[8] See Chapter Six for a fuller discussion of treatment options.

More Causes of Pelvic Pain · If you are postmenopausal, pain in your lower abdomen together with fever may indicate an abscess in your fallopian tubes and/or ovaries, appendicitis, or an infected gall bladder. The pain and fever may or may not be accompanied by bleeding or discharge. Any of these problems would likely require surgical treatment.[9]

If you experience pain in the lower abdomen and have had your uterus and/or ovaries removed, your body may be signalling an **adhesion** resulting from the previous surgery. Adhesions are tissue growths that attach to, and may cause constriction of, the intestines or other organs. Pain, particularly if severe, *must not be ignored.*

A medical consultation should rule out obstructions, abnormal growths, adhesions, infections, and nongynecological problems. If you are confident that these are not causes of your pain, and that your discomfort is primary dysmenorrhea, treatment with over-the-counter antiprostaglandin medication such as aspirin and ibuprofen should be helpful. Exercise and diet recommendations are discussed in Chapter Thirteen.

Severe Unusual Pain

Whether you are pre- or postmenopausal, and have a uterus or do not, severe, unusual pain is the way your body signals a potentially serious problem. Do not be a heroine (or hero) and bite your lower lip, take it on the chin, or demonstrate your courage. Severe abdominal pain must receive medical attention.

> Rose, aged 55, had had her uterus and one ovary removed eight years earlier, when she was 47. One morning, following a delicious restaurant meal the night before, she experienced stomach cramps. Convinced that she had probably eaten too much or possibly that in spite of its tastiness the dinner had given her food poisoning, Rose patiently waited for a bowel movement, vomiting, or simply time to ease the situation. As the days passed, her stools were normal and she felt no need to vomit. On the other hand, the abdominal pain persisted.
>
> Two weeks went by and Rose became concerned about her pain. It was intermittent rather than constant. In some ways she felt as she did when she had been ready to give birth. The cramps were increasing in frequency and intensity. She sensed the need to "pass this thing" out of her system but did not know what to do.
>
> Finally, at the insistence of her husband, Rose consulted a physician, who rushed her to the emergency room of the local hospital. Following evaluation, it was concluded that the restaurant meal had noth-

ing to do with the present problem. (Food poisoning tends to resolve itself within a couple of days.) Unable to diagnose this abdominal distress by either routine clinical examination or more elaborate tests such as colonoscopy and CAT scans, a laparatomy (exploratory abdominal surgery) was performed. This operation revealed adhesions from the hysterectomy, eight years before, which were obstructing the bowel and had to be removed. Were the situation allowed to persist, it could have resulted in gangrene, a potentially critical condition.

TABLE 4 – 2
SOME CAUSES AND TREATMENTS FOR ABDOMINAL PAIN

Cause	Possible Treatment
Primary dysmenorrhea	Aspirin, antiprostaglandin medication; or anti-inflammatory drugs such as ibuprofen
Endometriosis	Elimination of dairy products, caffeine, alcohol; hormone therapy; surgical removal of tissue or hysterectomy
Pelvic inflammatory disease	Varies, depending on cause
Intrauterine device	Removal of device
Uterine fibroids	Surgical myomectomy or hysterectomy
Uterine polyps	Surgical removal of polyps
Abscess in fallopian tubes or ovaries	Antibiotics
Gall bladder infection	Antibiotics; stop oral contraception; surgery
Appendicitis	Antibiotics; surgery
Adhesions from earlier surgeries	Surgery

Note: Each of the above requires careful medical evaluation and treatment related to individual findings.
Sources: Benson & Pernoll, 1993; Berkow, 1992.

PAIN DURING INTERCOURSE

Persistent pain in the genital area during sexual intercourse is called **dyspareunia.** It may sometimes be the result of emotions like guilt, fear, lack of desire, or inhibitions that block pleasure. While pain may be due to psychological, relationship, or sexual technique problems, dyspareunia just as often has a physical cause. Occasionally hymenal tissue may be left, even in a sexually experienced woman, which can cause discomfort. In other cases, insufficient lubrication, growths, lesions, or infections in the genital tract may be the culprit. The causes of pain during intercourse require careful inquiry, enabling appropriate treatment.[10]

Vaginismus is characterized by painful involuntary contractions of the outer third of the vagina, leaving the organ tightly closed and impenetrable. It is possible, but extremely rare, for a penis, finger, or other object to be in the vagina when the spasmodic contraction occurs. In such cases, the object is expelled. (Some men, having heard of this condition, erroneously fear having their penis "caught" in a vagina.) Like dyspareunia, vaginismus may have a psychological/emotional or a physical origin, or some combination of these. Mostly the vaginal closing seems to be a defensive response largely outside the woman's control. Typically the woman who has had pain with intercourse, for whatever reason, is more likely to experience vaginismus. She is, in effect, reflexively sparing herself intercourse leading to pain. Vaginismus and dyspareunia often require treatment directed both at physical problems and the sexual attitudes and interactions of the couple.[11]

URINARY INCONTINENCE

Stress incontinence, leaking urine when there is increased abdominal pressure such as while sneezing, laughing, running, or straining, is quite common and is found at all ages. In younger women who have given birth, this problem may be due to an injury that occurred during delivery. Among women who have had abdominal surgery, including hysterectomy, an adhesion left from the operation may interfere with the normal functioning of the bladder. In women past menopause, estrogen deficiency may lead to relaxation of the pelvic floor, resulting in poor bladder control. Additional causes of urinary incontinence include nerve pathology, growths in the abdominal region, urinary tract infection, or possibly a tumor in the bladder. In all cases, marked changes in bladder control must not go unexamined. While treatments vary, most women find successful resolution of this problem.[12]

VAGINAL HERNIAS

Cystoceles, enteroceles, and rectoceles. A hernia is a protrusion of an organ or mass of tissue through an abnormal opening. Vaginal hernias may involve intrusion or bulging of the bladder (**cystocele**), the rectum (**rectocele**), or, less commonly, small intestine (**enterocele**) into the vagina.

Most vaginal hernias do not result in clear symptoms. When the hernias do make themselves known, signs may include a feeling of fullness in the vagina, lower abdomen, and bladder; urinary frequency, and constipation. In cases of cystocele, the bladder may not be able to empty fully and this can result in urinary infection. Similarly, the lack of adequate bowel movement associated with rectocele may result in fecal impaction.

The cause is not always clear, but obesity and tissue weakened by injury or surgery are frequent correlates. Childbirth, however, is the most common contributor. About half of all women who have given birth develop some herniation, but usually not until they reach their 50s or even later.

Vaginal hernias which are mild may be managed by losing some weight (sounds easier than it is!), and avoiding heavy lifting and straining. Kegel exercises, discussed in Chapter Ten, may also be helpful. Some physicians recommend the use of a **pessary** for cystoceles, enteroceles, and rectoceles. This rubber or plastic ball or ring inserted high into the vagina may provide some temporary relief. Laxatives and enemas may be recommended in the case of rectocele. In severe conditions of some duration, corrective surgery will probably be recommended. However, since the hernias recur in about one out of ten surgical cases, you should attempt noninvasive treatments first.[13]

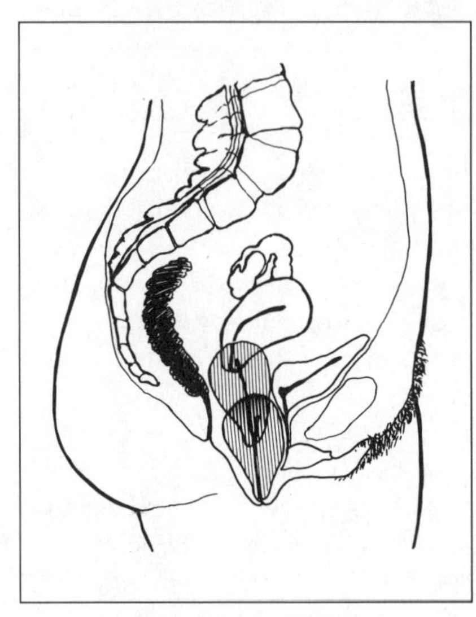

PROLAPSED UTERUS

Top example shows the uterus in normal position. Shaded examples show prolapsed positions.

UTERINE PROLAPSE

A prolapsed uterus is the abnormal protrusion of the uterus through the pelvic floor. The herniation may be minimal, the uterus descending only partway down the vagina. Or the prolapse may be more marked, the uterus descending so deeply into the vagina that the cervix is present at the vaginal entrance. It is often also associated with cystocele and rectocele.

Symptoms may be slight and resemble those found in vaginal hernias. Often these are accompanied by a sense of heaviness in the pelvic region and frequent low back pain. Standing for considerable periods may aggravate these problems.

Uterine prolapse is fairly common, especially among older women who gave birth many years earlier. It may be due to naturally caused damage or (less likely today when Cesarean sections are so frequently performed) forceps used during a difficult vaginal delivery. During the time of childbirth, the muscles which support the uterus may be injured. Over the years they become progressively weaker, finally resulting in prolapse.

As with the other vaginal hernias, the simplest treatment for uterine prolapse is to avoid behaviors, such as straining, heavy lifting, and prolonged standing, which bring on the symptoms. The next focus of treatment might be the use of a pessary. Finally, if you feel a more definitive solution is needed, surgery can be beneficial.[14] Treatment options are described in Chapter Six.

TESTS THAT ANSWER QUESTIONS

Office Procedures

PAP SMEAR

In 1928, Dr. George Papanicolaou developed a simple procedure that now is used routinely on healthy women as a screening for cervical cancer.

Primarily used to identify abnormal cervical cells, the **Pap smear** also often can disclose vaginal cancer as well as suggest infections including monilia (a yeast infection), condyloma (vaginal warts), and possibly chlamydia, prior to the appearance of any symptoms. Physicians agree that the Pap test is one of the most valuable, inexpensive screening procedures available.

Scheduling the Test · Both the National Cancer Institute and the American College of Obstetricians and Gynecologists recommend a first Pap smear at age 18, or earlier for those who are sexually active at a younger age. The test should be given annually for at least three consecutive years. If these three exams show normal results, the interval between tests may be extended to not more than three years. But women who are at "high risk" for cervical cancer should have the test once a year. You are considered high risk if you have had cervical or uterine cancer, previous abnormal Pap smears, genital herpes or warts, or multiple sexual partners; if you smoke or take birth control pills; or if your mother took DES (diethylstilbestrol) while pregnant with you.[15]

TABLE 4 – 3

WOMEN WHO ARE AT HIGH RISK FOR CERVICAL CANCER

You are considered to be high risk for cervical cancer if:

1. Your mother took DES while pregnant with you
2. You have had cervical or uterine cancer
3. You have had previous abnormal Pap smears
4. You have genital herpes or warts
5. You take birth control pills, or
6. You smoke.

Sources: Benson & Pernoll, 1993; Berkow, 1992.

Most American gynecologists believe that limiting the annual screening to women who are "at risk" is inadequate. They recommend that *all women have a Pap smear once a year throughout life.* They maintain that this procedure should be continued *even following hysterectomy*, since the Pap smear is effective in detecting vaginal cancer and may also reveal various gynecological infections.[16]

Procedure · You should make an appointment to have the Pap test midway in your menstrual cycle, when you do not have your period. To get ready for the examination, do not douche, or use vaginal medication or tampons for 24 hours prior to the test. It is most comfortable to have an empty bladder, so try to urinate after you arrive at the doctor's office. You might ask the nurse or receptionist if they will be requiring a urine sample, in which case one visit to the bathroom will serve two purposes.

The Pap test is often part of the routine gynecological examination. You lie on your back on the examining table with your feet in stirrups. The physician or nurse practitioner places a speculum into your vagina to open the passageway. A swab or wooden spatula is inserted, and samples of cells are taken from the upper vaginal walls, the opening of the cervix, and the cervix itself. The procedure takes only a few minutes. You may feel some discomfort, but there should be no pain, and the procedure is considered free of risks. **Negative,** meaning normal, results are usually telephoned or mailed to you within one to two weeks. Although not all physicians extend this courtesy. For a more complete description of the findings, you should ask for a copy of the laboratory report.

CLASSIFICATION OF CERVICAL TISSUE

Tissue cells taken in a Pap smear are classified by three different labeling methods: **"Class," WHO,** and **Bethesda.** The class system, devised by Papanicolaou, is the traditional method of categorizing tissue taken during a Pap smear, although this system has largely been supplanted by two other modes of classification. The World Health Organization (WHO) introduced the **CIN system** in 1973. The letters stand for **cervical intraepithelia neoplasia,** which refers to new tissue growth among the epithelial cells of the cervix. In 1988, the National Institutes of Health devised nomenclature, known as the **Bethesda system.** A major feature of this system is the identification of **squamous intraepithelial lesions**, or **SIL**, which is considered to be a more accurate diagnostic term.

Classes I and II are **benign**, noncancerous cells; these have no CIN or SIL categorization. Class III suggests atypical cells called **dysplasia;** the cells may be precancerous. Class IV results indicate a **malignant** or cancerous condition. Class V is indicative of **invasive** cancer.[17]

The WHO method identifies three categories of atypical cells. CIN I and CIN II are mild and moderate dysplasia respectively. CIN III is severe dysplasia or **carcinoma in situ,** which means that cancer cells have been found in the top layer of tissue.

The Bethesda system identifies two classes of SIL: low-grade and high-grade. The distinction is that low-grade SIL may not require medical treatment, while high-grade SIL indicates moderate to severe dysplasia and carcinoma in situ which must be treated. This system also reports on the adequacy of the smear. Table 4 – 4 shows the relationship between the Pap, WHO, and Bethesda systems.

CAUTIONS!

The Pap smear is a good but not perfect screening test. If your test results show that you have CIN, there is a strong possibility that you actually do not have cancer. First of all, CIN I is mild dysplasia and not cancer. Second, the nature of the testing procedure is such that cells are often hard to "read," and cancer cells are suspected where they do not exist. Of course, you must not disregard a "positive" (problem) Pap result. It is a signal to you and your physician that further testing is necessary. Colposcopy and cervical biopsy, to be described later in this chapter, may also be used when Pap results are unclear or point to a possible cancer.[18]

TABLE 4 – 4

SYSTEMS USED TO CATEGORIZE CELLS FROM A PAP TEST

Description	Class	WHO*	Bethesda**
Normal smear; no abnormal cells	1	Benign	Benign
Inflammation is present, but no cancer	2	Benign with inflammation	Benign
Abnormal cells are present in the lower third of the epithelial tissue; mild dysplasia; may not require treatment	3	CIN I	Low-grade SIL
Abnormal cells occur in lower 2/3 of epithelial tissue; moderate dysplasia; will require medical treatment	3	CIN II	Low-grade or high-grade SIL
Abnormal cells occupy the entire epithelial tissue; severe dysplasia	3	CIN III	High-grade SIL
Carcinoma in situ	4	CIN III	High-grade SIL
Invasive carcinoma	5	Invasive cancer	Invasive cancer

* WHO, the World Health Organization, utilizes the term **cervical intraepithelial neoplasia** (CIN).

** The National Institutes of Health devised the Bethesda system which identifies **squamous intraepithelial lesions** (SIL).

Adapted from Rose, 1993; Tierney, et al., 1994.

The opposite situation also exists. A "negative" or no problem result on the Pap smear is not a guarantee that you do not have abnormal cells. Depending on your doctor's techniques and the skill of the laboratory, an "all clear" report may actually mean that for roughly 8 in 10 women no dysplasia or precancerous cells are present. However, this leaves the other 2 in 10 who do in fact have a problem. Fortunately, both laboratory and office procedures involving Pap screening are constantly being improved. But given the current situation, repeated — at least annual — tests are generally recommended.

While the Pap test is a safe, inexpensive, and generally reliable screening test for cervical cancer and may suggest various genital infections, it should be recognized that the Pap test does not screen for either endometrial or ovarian cancer. If these are suspected on the basis of other evidence, surgery will almost surely be required.[19]

"PRECANCEROUS" TISSUES AND MALIGNANCIES

Dysplasia · Dysplasia is the medical term used for any abnormality in the size or shape of an adult cell. Dysplasias can involve any tissue in the body. They can range in severity from a **benign**, relatively harmless condition to **invasive** cancer, meaning the tumors have spread beyond the surface layer of tissue.

It is essential to recognize that it has not been established that a benign dysplasia will eventually develop into cancer if left unchecked. Nevertheless, many physicians use the term "precancerous" for benign dysplasia, which prompts most women into quick compliance with any surgical recommendation. This may not be necessary, as you will see in Chapter Five: Cancer.

The importance of routine Pap smears must be stressed since both benign cervical dysplasia and early cervical cancer tend to be symptom-free. Should you be notified that you have "mild dysplasia" or CIN I (cervical intraepithelial neoplasia, category I), you need not panic that you will develop cancer. You must, however, have further investigation. This normally involves sending tissue taken during office colposcopic examination and endocervical curettage to a laboratory for microscopic evaluation. If you have been diagnosed with dysplasia, you will be considered to be at higher risk for cervical cancer and therefore may require treatment and medical follow-up.[20]

While the causes for mild dysplasia and cervical cancers are not really known, these abnormal cells are more likely to occur in women who smoke, have multiple sexual partners, use oral contraception, or have genital warts. Although no cause-effect relationship has been documented, it can't hurt to engage in possible preventive measures. These include giving up smoking, limiting the number of sexual partners, switching to a diaphragm or condom, and obtaining treatment for vaginal warts.[21]

Cancerous cells in the uterus may let themselves be known by abnormal uterine bleeding and discharge. If cervical cancer is diagnosed, treatment is essential. If the cancer cells are limited to the cervical area, cryotherapy (freezing), a loop excision (LEEP), or laser treatment which removes all involved cells may be adequate. If there is evidence that the cancer has gone beyond the cervix, a total hysterectomy (uterus, ovaries, and fallopian tubes removed) with follow-up radiation may be required. Almost 100 percent of women with carcinoma in situ (CIN II or CIN III) and about 90 percent of those with early invasive cancer (cancer which has gone beyond the site of origin) can be cured.[22] (For further discussion of cancer, see Chapter Five.)

COLPOSCOPIC EXAMINATION AND CERVICAL BIOPSY

A **colposcope** is an instrument which looks like a microscope and is placed at the opening of the vagina to provide a 10 to 40 times magnification of the vagina and cervix.

Colposcopic examination is recommended if Pap results are suspicious or a lesion was noted in your vagina or cervix. Women who have had pain or bleeding during intercourse may also be advised to undergo this procedure. It is used to check for possible cancer or to monitor a precancerous condition.

A colposcopic examination can be administered at any time, but heavy menstrual bleeding may interfere with the procedure. You should also not douche prior to the procedure. As with the Pap smear, an empty bladder helps to make the procedure more comfortable.

The examination is performed with you on your back, feet in stirrups. The speculum opens the entrance to the vagina where the scope is then placed. The physician looks through the eyepieces and may take pictures of the vaginal walls and cervix. Cotton swabs may be used to "paint" the area with acetic acid (vinegar) and then iodine to allow better visualization. If suspicious areas in the vagina are spotted, a **biopsy** may be conducted. A biopsy means removal of tissue which can then be microscopically examined and analyzed. A **curette,** a small spoon-shaped instrument, may be used to scrape tissue from the inside of the cervix. The removed cells are sent to a lab for evaluation for malignancy.

Usually colposcopy and biopsy take a few minutes or somewhat longer if adequate time is taken to thoroughly examine the area and talk with the patient. The procedure may be uncomfortable but should not be overly painful. The colposcopy itself poses no risks, but the scraping of tissue for biopsy usually results in a small amount of vaginal bleeding and very rarely pelvic infection. You will be advised to avoid sexual intercourse, douching, and the use of tampons for about one week following a biopsy so that the cervix has time to heal. An antiprostaglandin such as *Motrin* may be used prior to or following the procedure to prevent cramping.

The results of colposcopic examination, cervical biopsy, and Pap smears are generally compared. Together they can confirm or rule out a diagnosis of cervical cancer. If they show conflicting results, you may need to repeat some of the tests or be asked to undergo **loop excision.**[23]

LOOP EXCISION

The **loop electrosurgical excisional procedure** (LEEP) is a relatively new procedure which is sometimes used instead of cervical cone biopsy, described later in this chapter. LEEP is also known as **loop excision of the transformation zone** (LETZ) and **large loop excision of the transformation zone** (LLETZ).

The loop excision is performed quickly in a doctor's office with local anesthesia. A low-current, high-frequency electrical generator and thin wire loops are used to remove suspicious cells or a cone of tissue as in cervical cone biopsy. This tissue is then microscopically evaluated or biopsied.

Loop excision is a relatively inexpensive and effective testing procedure which is free from short-term or long-term complications.[24] Cryotherapy and laser procedures are described in Chapter Six.

Sonograms and Magnetic Resonance Imaging

ULTRASOUND

Ultrasound is a way of creating pictures (**sonograms**) of internal organs by using sound waves. A **transducer**, a small, hand-held wandlike instrument, sends sound waves to the organs which reflect the waves in varying ways depending on the organs' density. These reflected waves are converted by computer and transmitted to a monitor, making the organs visible. Ultrasound can identify enlargement of the uterus or ovaries, which may suggest a likelihood of internal infection, cysts, or growths. If you are pregnant, it can provide information about the health of a developing fetus. Ultrasound cannot determine whether cancer is present.

Ultrasound tests are generally performed on an outpatient basis in a hospital or doctor's office. This means that you go to the hospital but will not spend the night. Either of two preparation methods are used that require drinking a great deal of water. (1) You may be told to arrive at the hospital about an hour before the test, at which time you must drink about four glasses of water. (2) Alternatively, you may be asked to drink eight glasses of water prior to your appointment. In either case, you will not be permitted to urinate until after the test is over. You will probably experience discomfort from your water-filled bladder, but hang in there — the test takes just 15 to 30 minutes. The purpose of the full bladder is to force the intestines out of the pelvis so as to improve the visualization of the uterus and ovaries.

After removing your lower garments and putting on a hospital gown, you lie on your back on an examining table. A surgical gel is applied to your belly. This helps in the transmission of the sound waves. It also serves as a lubricant so that the transducer can glide more easily. A technician moves the transducer back and forth over the lubricated area. You may be asked to roll onto your side from time to time. Throughout the procedure, sound wave pictures of your organs, or fetus, can be seen on the TV-like screen called an oscilloscope. These images are saved for later study.

Ultrasound techniques are considered safe, with no known risks. They do not involve pain, radiation, or body penetration. These procedures have been used without mishap for more than 20 years.[25]

MAGNETIC RESONANCE IMAGING (MRI)

Magnetic resonance imaging (**MRI**), also called **nuclear magnetic resonance** (**NMR**), is a sophisticated technique for studying the body. It is quite reliable in diagnosing benign diseases of the uterus and ovaries such as fibroids or other abnormalities. It can help the physician define areas requiring corrective surgery. However, since it is quite expensive, it is not usually the first method of examination.

MRI is based on the fact that the hydrogen atoms within our bodies respond to a magnetic pull, and the electrical resonance produced by this movement can be translated into a picture of our internal organs. For this reason, you will need to wear a hospital gown and remove any metal objects on your body. You will probably be disqualified for testing if you have a pacemaker, artificial limb, or even an IUD.

MRI takes place while you lie on a special table which is electronically guided inside a large magnetic tube. You will be asked not to move during the examination, which lasts about half an hour. About one-third of the people receiving this test experience some anxiety or claustrophobia. Some report that the sensation is like being "in a coffin."[26] However, no physical side- or after-effects have been reported. To date it is considered a safe and valuable diagnostic tool.[27]

X-ray Techniques Using Contrast Dyes

The next three techniques involve the use of contrast dyes to enhance X-ray visibility. If you have a history of allergic reactions, specifically to iodine or other contrast materials, discuss this with your doctor before you schedule X-rays. If you do not know whether you have these allergies, insist on being tested for them. You should also be sure to inform the radiologist or technician of your allergies before you begin any of these procedures.

INTRAVENOUS PYELOGRAM (IVP)

An IVP is a special form of X-ray in which dyes are injected to evaluate the kidneys. If fibroid tumors have caused significant enlargement of the uterus, the function of the kidneys may be affected. An IVP can detect kidney stones, cancer in the kidney, and other kidney problems. Normal X-rays are generally not adequate for assessing the kidneys because these organs cannot be readily distinguished from other abdominal tissue.

The IVP should NOT be administered if there is a chance that you are pregnant, since X-rays can damage the developing baby. If you are diabetic, there is a risk that the dye will damage your kidneys.

To prepare for an IVP, you will be told not to eat or drink for the preceding 12 hours. You also will be instructed to take a laxative and enema the evening before the test since the presence of stool in the large intestine can interfere with test interpretation. The IVP is generally performed on an outpatient basis in a hospital.

After emptying your bladder, you will lie on your back on an X-ray table, and an initial picture will be taken of your abdomen. A contrast dye will be injected into a vein inside your elbow. This substance will be transmitted through the bloodstream to the kidneys, ureter, and bladder. Several X-ray pictures will be taken as the dye travels. You will then be asked to urinate, and a final X-ray picture will be taken when you return.

Since the test takes about one hour, you might want to bring something to read during the time you are left alone between X-rays. Also, since the room may be cool, you might want to wear knee socks. If you don't come prepared and begin to feel chilly, do not be embarrassed to ask for a blanket. You will not have had anything to eat or drink for several hours, so you may want to bring a snack and some fruit juice for after the procedure. It is good to drink plenty of fluids after the test to help further wash the dye out of your system.

During testing, if you have breathing difficulties, nausea, excessive sweating, or other abnormalities, report these problems immediately so that you can receive appropriate attention. If you feel fine for the first ten minutes, the chances are excellent that you can safely tolerate the IVP. Only about 1 percent of the people tested experience a mild allergic reaction, and even fewer have serious problems.

In view of the risks involved, you will probably be asked to sign a consent form prior to examination. You should not consent to this test unless your doctor gave you a good reason for its use and you are not likely to develop adverse reactions as noted in the paragraphs above.[28]

HYSTEROSALPINGOGRAM

The hysterosalpingogram is an X-ray procedure used in examining the uterus for fibroid tumors and other abnormalities. It can also detect fallopian tube blockage and in some cases even correct this by forcing a tube open.

The test requires the use of a dye which is injected through the cervix. If you might be pregnant or have allergies to X-ray contrast materials, you should not undergo this examination. The procedure is normally administered within seven days after the start of your menstrual period to rule out the likelihood of pregnancy.

To prepare, you will probably be asked to fast for several hours. You may also be given a sedative prior to the test. You will lie on your back on the examining table with your feet in stirrups. The physician will swab the exterior of the vagina, then insert a speculum. Contrast material is placed in the cervix through a tube called a **cannula.** X-ray pictures are taken, and you should be able to view your abdomen on a fluoroscope, which looks like a television screen, as the dye moves through your body.

You may feel some cramping during this procedure. If your fallopian tubes are blocked, the contrast material may cause a fairly sharp pain.

You should be off the table in less than half an hour. Since you will be uncomfortable following the test and possibly unsteady, you should be sure to arrange for someone to drive you home.

You may continue to feel slightly dizzy, and have abdominal discomfort and a bloody vaginal discharge for a few days. If you have severe pain, a heavy discharge, a fever, or a discharge which continues for more than four days, you should report it to your medical caregiver.

A number of risks are associated with hysterosalpingogram, although these occur in fewer than 1 percent of women undergoing the procedure. Infections may occur, which are usually treatable with antibiotics. More seriously, the uterus or fallopian tubes can be injured by the pressure of the dye. Also, a remote possibility exists that the contrast medium might enter the bloodstream, causing dangerous side effects. This test should only be used when there is a strong justification, such as to determine the cause of infertility.[29]

COMPUTERIZED AXIAL TOMOGRAPHY (CAT or CT SCAN)

The CT, or CAT, scan has been in use since the 1970s and has replaced many more invasive tests. The pelvic CT scan is used to directly study the uterus or ovaries; an abdominal CT scan, which is aimed higher on the body, can be helpful in diagnosing cysts, tumors, and abscesses of organs such as the liver, pancreas, and kidneys.

Basically, CT works by scanning the area to be studied and taking X-ray photos of various cross-sections of tissue. A computer processes and retains the X-ray information. With this technique, body organs and changes over time can be examined in great detail.

You are not to eat for four hours or to drink for one hour prior to this test. You may have to take an enema to cleanse your bowels. Occasionally sedatives are given to relax you.

As with some of the other X-ray procedures described, a contrast material (dye) may be injected into a vein, which might induce a feeling of general bodily warmth. Sometimes the dye is administered by mouth, and you will need to drink several glasses of a lemony-tasting thick liquid.

The CT scan uses high-tech equipment, and you may be struck by this when you go to the room for the procedure. Wearing a hospital gown, you lie on a table that electronically moves you into a large circular-shaped scanner which makes buzzing or clicking sounds as it takes X-rays from various angles. A technician in another room will instruct you when to take a breath and when to hold still.

A CT scan may require anywhere from ten minutes to about one hour. There is no pain involved, although, as with MRI, some women report that they feel a little claustrophobic while inside the scanning ring. Potential risks relate to the use of the dye and X-ray exposure. In both cases these are negligible.

Again, if you are allergic to various substances, especially iodine used in the dye, be sure to talk to your physician and/or technician beforehand. Sometimes medications can be used to counteract the possibility of an allergic reaction.

The levels of radiation from the X-rays are very low and should pose no problems except possibly to the developing fetus in pregnant women. So try to avoid a CT scan if you may be pregnant.[30]

Procedures Requiring Anesthesia and/or Surgery

DILATION AND CURETTAGE (D&C)

More commonly known as **D&C**, dilation and curettage describe the dilation or opening of the cervix and the scraping of the inner lining of the uterus, the **endometrium,** with an instrument called a **curette.** This procedure has been widely used for a number of purposes.

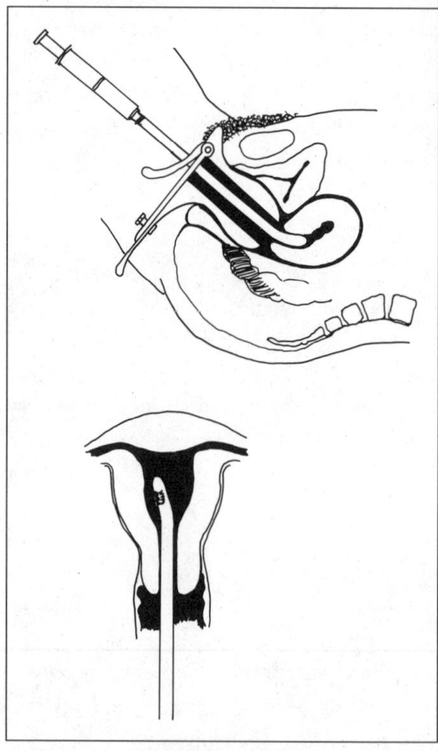

ENDOMETRIAL BIOPSY

Tissue is removed from the inner lining of the uterus for microscopic analysis.

The D&C was once a common way to abort a pregnancy by removing the embedded fetus between the second and fourth months. On the other hand, a D&C may be used to help determine the cause of infertility, by studying the scraped endometrial tissue and assessing its receptivity to housing a fertilized egg. A D&C can help diagnose menstrual problems such as those caused by uterine polyps or fibroids, and can be used as effective treatment for some menstrual disorders. It is also a screening procedure for endometrial cancer.

The D&C is performed either in a physician's office or in the hospital, generally on an outpatient basis. No matter what location, you will probably be told to arrive an hour or two early and to avoid food and drink for about 12 hours before the procedure. You will be relaxed by a mild sedative such as Valium; then local, spinal, or possibly general anesthesia will be administered.

For the D&C, you will lie on your back with your feet in the usual gynecological stirrups. Your cervical opening will be enlarged by the physician inserting rods of successively increasing diameter through your vagina into your cervix. When the opening is of sufficient size, the curette is inserted and samples of endometrial tissue are removed from the inside of your uterus. If you have general anesthesia, you sleep through all of this and feel nothing. If you have local or spinal anesthesia, you should not feel pain, but you may notice some mild cramping.

A D&C is usually accomplished within half an hour. Risk of damaging the cervix or uterus is very low. However, all anesthesia carries a very small risk of complications, especially if general is used. At the extreme, general anesthesia may, very rarely, result in death. If you are a relatively healthy person, this probability is significantly diminished. It is well to bear in mind that in the use of anesthesia there is a progression of risks. A local carries the least likelihood of serious complications, a regional or spinal has slightly more risk, and a general is the most hazardous. You need to weigh this information against your own and your physician's preferences for you to be asleep and unaware of what is going on.[31]

No matter which type of anesthesia is used, be sure to have someone drive you home, since you will feel fatigued and achy. You should plan extra rest for several days following a D&C, and avoid vigorous exercise, heavy physical work, and lifting. You should not engage in sexual intercourse or douche for a week or so. You will need to use a menstrual pad for several days. Notify your health care provider if the bleeding is excessive or you have a fever.[32]

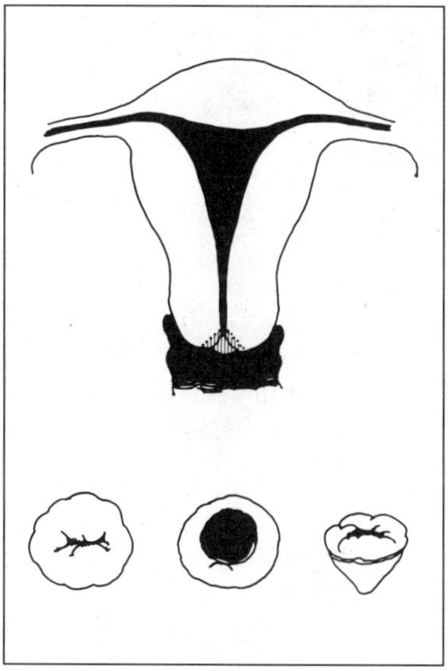

CERVICAL CONE BIOPSY
A cone of tissue is surgically removed from the cervix.

CERVICAL CONE BIOPSY

Cone biopsy may be used to confirm surgically a diagnosis of cervical cancer. It may also be treatment, if all abnormal cells are removed during the procedure. The term comes from the "cone" of tissue which is removed from the cervix and then examined microscopically for cancerous changes. Cervical cone biopsy is performed less frequently today than it was a decade ago.[33] LEEP, an office procedure described earlier in this chapter, is often used instead.

For cervical cone biopsy, you may be admitted to a hospital, probably as an outpatient. You will be told to avoid food and drink for 12 hours prior to admission. Since general anesthesia is normally used, you will not be conscious for the half hour or so of surgery. Entry to the cervix is gained through the vagina.

Cervical cone biopsy carries the risks inherent in the use of anesthesia as well as of complications such as infection, significant bleeding, and interference with later pregnancies.

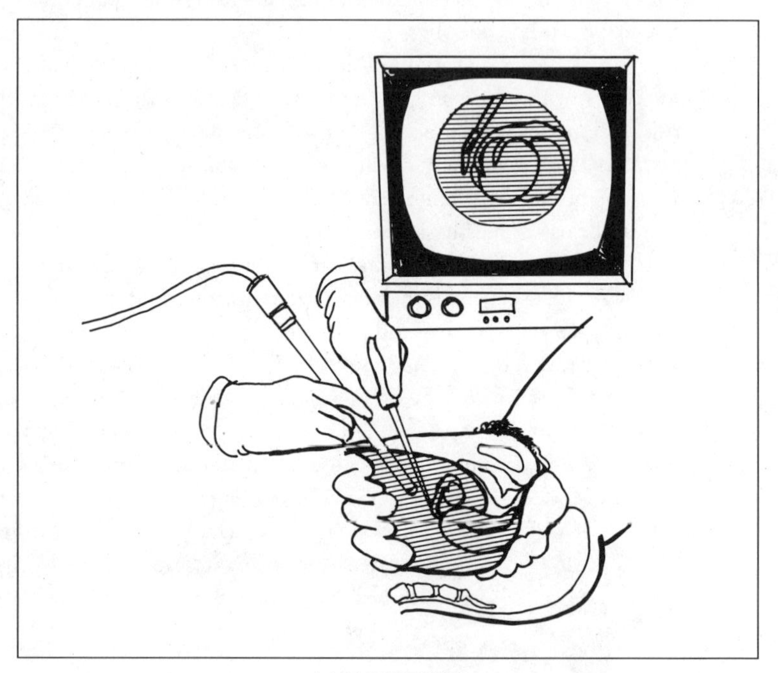

LAPAROSCOPY

Through the use of a laparoscope, surgical incisions may be kept relatively small.

LAPAROSCOPY

Also known as **peritoneoscopy**, and **pelvic** or **abdominal endoscopy**, this procedure views the abdominal organs by means of a special lighted scope (a **laparoscope**) which is inserted through a very small cut made in the abdominal wall. The image is then transmitted to a video monitor.

Laparoscopy often is used when a physical exam, ultrasound, and X-ray studies are inconclusive. It can provide information regarding the shape and health of the uterus, ovaries, fallopian tubes, appendix, gallbladder, liver, intestines, bladder, and other organs. It is useful in the diagnosis of cancer, endometriosis, ovarian cysts, ectopic pregnancy, fibroid tumors, and other causes of abdominal pain or heavy bleeding.

Although laparoscopy may be done on an outpatient basis, you should have someone drive you home from the hospital. Be prepared to feel tired and achy for several days. Some women report feeling pretty well immediately following the procedure, probably due to the various relaxant drugs, but quite uncomfortable a day to a week or so later.

Since general anesthesia will probably be used, you will be told not to eat or drink for about 12 hours prior to the test. You may take a prescribed sedative the night before to help you relax. If local or spinal anesthesia is used, you may be awake but not feel the procedure. The portion of your pubic hair just below your abdomen may be shaved.

As you lie on the operating table with your feet raised slightly, your belly will be cleansed with an antiseptic. A **catheter** will probably be inserted through your urethra in order to keep your bladder empty. Another long slender tube, a **cannula,** may be placed into your vagina in order to move your uterus for better viewing.

Carbon dioxide or nitrous oxide will be injected into your abdomen through a small cut below or in your navel. This gas gently forces up the abdominal walls, something like a balloon, and permits better visualization of your organs. The tip of the laparoscope is then placed into the incision, and your organs are examined.

Sometimes laparoscopic techniques are used for sterilization by tubal ligation ("tubes tied through 'band-aid' surgery"), removing suspicious tissue for biopsy, draining cysts, and even hysterectomy (as covered in Chapter Six). In these cases, a second small horizontal cut is made at the pubic hairline and the treatment instruments are inserted through this while viewing takes place through the laparoscope. A third cut may be made to remove an organ.

Laparoscopic examination, even with treatment, generally does not take more than one hour. If you had general anesthesia you should be fully awake in a few hours, ready to walk and return home. However, some people feel nauseous and tired for a few days. You should not engage in heavy lifting or exercise for about one week.

Laparoscopy is an invasive procedure and therefore carries risks. It is very rare but laparoscopy may result in damage to an internal organ with resultant bleeding and possible need for transfusion. Again, the odds are in your favor that you will have no problems.[34]

LAPAROTOMY

Laparotomy is an extensive surgical procedure in which a fairly large incision is made in the abdomen. It is recommended in cases when the patient is unable to have laparoscopy because of scarring, or when laparoscopy would not allow for adequate visualization. Compared to laparoscopy, laparotomy involves greater risk, cost, and recovery time.[35]

ENDNOTES

1. Benson, R. C., & Pernoll, M. L. *Benson & Pernoll's Handbook of Obstetrics and Gynecology*, 9th ed. New York: McGraw Hill, 1993.
2. Hufnagel, V. with Golant, S. K. *No More Hysterectomies*. New York: New American Library, 1988.
3. Benson, R. C., & Pernoll, M. L. *Benson & Pernoll's Handbook of Obstetrics and Gynecology*, 9th ed. New York: McGraw Hill, 1993.
4. Benson, R. C., & Pernoll, M. L. *Benson & Pernoll's Handbook of Obstetrics and Gynecology*, 9th ed. New York: McGraw Hill, 1993.
5. Feldman, S., Berkowitz, R. S., & Tosteson, A. N. A. Cost-effectiveness of strategies to evaluate postmenopausal bleeding. *Obstetrics and Gynecology*, June 1993, 81 (6), 968 – 975.
6. Buchan, H., Vessey, M., Goldacre, M., et al. Morbidity following pelvic inflammatory disease. *British Journal of Obstetrics and Gynaecology*, June 1993, 100 (6), 558 – 562.
7. Benson, R. C., & Pernoll, M. L. *Benson & Pernoll's Handbook of Obstetrics and Gynecology*, 9th ed. New York: McGraw Hill, 1993.

   Branch, Jr., W. T. *Office Practice of Medicine*, 3rd ed. Philadelphia: W. B. Saunders, 1994.
8. Benson, R. C., & Pernoll, M. L. *Benson & Pernoll's Handbook of Obstetrics and Gynecology*, 9th ed. New York: McGraw Hill, 1993.

   Branch, Jr., W. T. *Office Practice of Medicine*, 3rd ed. Philadelphia: W. B. Saunders, 1994.

   Lark, S. M. *Fibroid Tumors and Endometriosis*. St. Louis, MO: Mosby Publishers, 1993.
9. Berkow, R., ed. *Merck Manual of Diagnosis & Therapy*, 16th ed. Rahway, NJ: Merck Sharp & Dohme Research Laboratories, 1992.
10. Haas, K., & Haas, A. *Understanding Sexuality*. 3rd ed. St. Louis, MO: Mosby-Yearbook, 1993.
11. Haas, K., & Haas, A. *Understanding Sexuality*. 3rd ed. St. Louis, MO: Mosby-Yearbook, 1993.
12. Branch, Jr., W. T. *Office Practice of Medicine*, 3rd ed. Philadelphia: W. B. Saunders, 1994.
13. Benson, R. C., & Pernoll, M. L. *Benson & Pernoll's Handbook of Obstetrics and Gynecology*, 9th ed. New York: McGraw Hill, 1993.

Branch, Jr., W. T. *Office Practice of Medicine,* 3rd ed. Philadelphia: W. B. Saunders, 1994.

14. Benson, R. C., & Pernoll, M. L. *Benson & Pernoll's Handbook of Obstetrics and Gynecology,* 9th ed. New York: McGraw Hill, 1993.

Branch, Jr., W. T. *Office Practice of Medicine,* 3rd ed. Philadelphia: W. B. Saunders, 1994.

15. Branch, Jr., W. T. *Office Practice of Medicine,* 3rd ed. Philadelphia: W. B. Saunders, 1994.

16. Freund, K., & Buttlar, C. A. The use of cervical cytology to identify women at risk for chlamydial infection. *American Journal of Preventive Medicine,* 1992, 8 (5), 292 – 297.

Benson, R. C., & Pernoll, M. L. *Benson & Pernoll's Handbook of Obstetrics and Gynecology*, 9th ed. New York: McGraw Hill, 1993.

Arroyo, G., Linnemann, C., Wessler, T. Role of the Papanicolaou smear in diagnosis of chlamydial infections. *Sexually Transmitted Diseases,* 1989, 16 (1) 11 – 14.

17. Rose, P. G. Cervical cancer. *Emergency Medicine,* March 1993, 25 (4), 133 – 140.

18. Jones, D. E., Creasman, W. I., Dombroski, R. A., et al. Evaluation of the atypical Pap smear. *American Journal of Obstetrics and Gynecology,* September 1987, 157 (3), 544 – 549.

McKinnon, K. J., Ford, R. M., & Hunter, J. C. Comparison of cytology and cervicography in screening a high-risk Australian population for cervical human papillomavirus and cervical intraepithelial neoplasia. *Australian and New Zealand Journal of Obstetrics and Gynaecology,* May 1993, 33 (2), 176 –179.

Mann, W., Lonky, N., Massad, S., et al. Papanicolaou smear screening augmented by a magnified chemiluminescent exam. *International Journal of Gynaecology and Obstetrics,* December 1993, 43 (3), 289 – 296.

Toffler, W. L., Pluedeman, C. K., Sinclair, A. E., et al. Comparative cytologic yield and quality of three Pap smear instruments. *Family Medicine,* 1993, 25 (6), 403 – 407.

19. Benson, R. C., & Pernoll, M. L. *Benson & Pernoll's Handbook of Obstetrics and Gynecology*, 9th ed. New York: McGraw Hill, 1993.

Berkow, R., ed. *Merck Manual of Diagnosis & Therapy*, 16th ed. Rahway, NJ: Merck Sharp & Dohme Research Laboratories, 1992.

20. Benson, R. C., & Pernoll, M. L. *Benson & Pernoll's Handbook of Obstetrics and Gynecology*, 9th ed. New York: McGraw Hill, 1993.

21. Benson, R. C., & Pernoll, M. L. *Benson & Pernoll's Handbook of Obstetrics and Gynecology*, 9th ed. New York: McGraw Hill, 1993.

22. Benson, R. C., & Pernoll, M. L. *Benson & Pernoll's Handbook of Obstetrics and Gynecology*, 9th ed. New York: McGraw Hill, 1993.

23. Benson, R. C., & Pernoll, M. L. *Benson & Pernoll's Handbook of Obstetrics and Gynecology*, 9th ed. New York: McGraw Hill, 1993.

Berkow, R., ed. *Merck Manual of Diagnosis & Therapy*, 16th ed. Rahway, NJ: Merck Sharp & Dohme Research Laboratories, 1992.

24. Apgar, B. S., Wright, T. C. Jr., & Pfenninger, J. L. Loop electrosurgical excision procedure for CIN: see comments. *American Family Physician,* August 1992, 46 (2), 505 – 520.

Mayeaux, E. J. Jr., & Harper, M. B. Loop electrosurgical excisional procedure: see comments. *Journal of Family Practice,* February 1993, 36 (2), 214 – 219.

25. Tierney, Jr., L. M., McPhee, S. J., & Papadakis, M. A., eds. *Current Medical Diagnosis & Treatment 1994.* Los Altos, CA: Appleton & Lange, 1994.

26. Shuchman, M. When a 'noninvasive' scan causes pain. *New York Times,* November 3, 1994.

27. Mitchell, D. G. Benign disease of the uterus and ovaries: applications of magnetic resonance imaging. *The Radiologic Clinics of North America,* July 1992, 30 (4), 777.

28. Tierney, Jr., L. M., McPhee, S. J., & Papadakis, M. A., eds. *Current Medical Diagnosis & Treatment 1994.* Los Altos, CA: Appleton & Lange, 1994.

29. Tierney, Jr., L. M., McPhee, S. J., & Papadakis, M. A., eds. *Current Medical Diagnosis & Treatment 1994.* Los Altos, CA: Appleton & Lange, 1994.

30. Benson, R. C., & Pernoll, M. L. *Benson & Pernoll's Handbook of Obstetrics and Gynecology*, 9th ed. New York: McGraw Hill, 1993.

31. Tierney, Jr., L. M., McPhee, S. J., & Papadakis, M. A., eds. *Current Medical Diagnosis & Treatment 1994.* Los Altos, CA: Appleton & Lange, 1994.

32. Benson, R. C., & Pernoll, M. L. *Benson & Pernoll's Handbook of Obstetrics and Gynecology*, 9th ed. New York: McGraw Hill, 1993.

33. Benson, R. C., & Pernoll, M. L. *Benson & Pernoll's Handbook of Obstetrics and Gynecology*, 9th ed. New York: McGraw Hill, 1993.

34. Benson, R. C., & Pernoll, M. L. *Benson & Pernoll's Handbook of Obstetrics and Gynecology*, 9th ed. New York: McGraw Hill, 1993.

35. Benson, R. C., & Pernoll, M. L. *Benson & Pernoll's Handbook of Obstetrics and Gynecology*, 9th ed. New York: McGraw Hill, 1993.

SUGGESTED READING

Dusek, Dot, & Daniel Girdano. *The Body as Teacher: Symptom Metaphors for Health.* Winter Park, CO: Paradox Publishers, 1992.

Inlander, Charles B., & Jim Punkre. *The People's Medical Society Healthy Body Book: Test Yourself for Maximum Health.* New York: Viking Penguin, 1991.

Moskowitz, Mark, A., & Michael E. Osband. *The Complete Book of Medical Tests.* New York: Ballantine Books, 1984.

Sobel, David S., & Tom Ferguson. *The People's Book of Medical Tests.* New York: Summit Books, 1985.

Chapter 5

CANCER

"When I heard that it might be cancer, I was sure that I was going to die. Well, it's been eight years, and I'm still here. I think that scary time in my life made me recognize that every day is a gift to be treasured." — Barbara, age 50

WHAT IS CANCER?

The human body is composed of millions of cells which follow their own life cycles. They form, develop, die, and are sloughed off in orderly and predictable ways. Cells have special shapes and generally names that reflect their appearance. For example, "cuboidal" cells line the inside of the uterus, and they are somewhat cubelike.

Cells in various parts of the body are also **differentiated,** so that, for example, cells of the uterine lining look different from those found in the clitoris, and so on. Well-differentiated cells are what are expected and normal for a particular type of tissue.

Tumor is the general term used to describe abnormal cell growth, and a **malignant tumor** is called a **cancer**. Cancer cells appear undifferentiated; they do not look like the normal cells for that part of the body. They also are potentially **invasive;** that is, they may grow beyond the tissue in which they originated. Cancer cells may metastasize, meaning break off and start growing in a relatively distant part of the body. In both instances, they may seriously, even fatally, damage body organs.

We must stress that not all unwanted cell growth is cancerous. For example, enlarged uterine fibroid tumors (clusters of myometrial cells) are growths which are not normal and may interfere with the body's healthy function. Yet, fibroids and many other tumors are benign; they remain confined and do not invade healthy cells. In short, unlike malignant cells, they are not potentially fatal.

TYPES OF CANCER

Cancers are categorized according to where they are located. They may occur in the vulva, vagina, uterine cervix, uterine corpus, ovaries, and breasts,

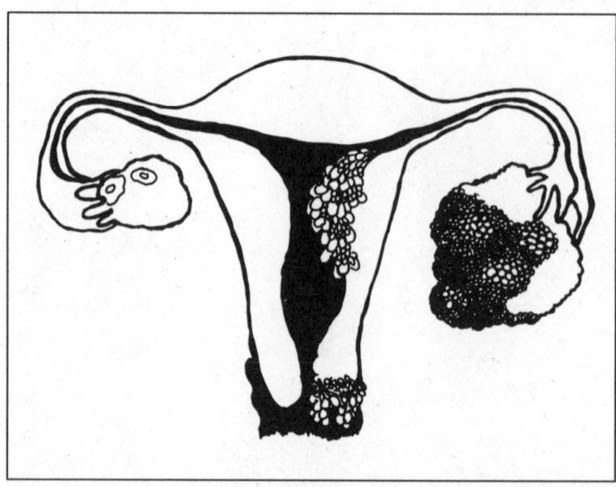

UTERINE AND OVARIAN CANCER

Cancer cells tend to be irregular in size and shape, and are categorized according to where they are located.

as well as in other parts of the body. Cancers are also labeled according to **histology**, or cell characteristics and type of cell.

Carcinoma, the most common kind, starts in the epithelium, the layer of cells that cover the body's surface or line internal organs and glands. The majority of pelvic malignancies are carcinomas — either **squamous cell, epidermoid,** or **adenocarcinoma** (originating in gland-forming tissue). Each type of tumor has its own cell growth pattern; therefore, histological information as well as cancer location may influence treatment and prognosis.[1]

CLASSIFICATION

Three methods of classifying cervical tissue were described in Chapter Four. You might want to refer to pages 60 – 61.

In brief, cells are categorized by Class, CIN (cervical intraepithelial neoplasia), and SIL (squamous intraepithelial lesion).

Class 1 cells are normal, with no CIN or SIL rating. Class 2 cells are somewhat atypical, but not cancer, and also have no CIN or SIL equivalent. Class 3 cells may be CIN I, II, or III — low-grade or high-grade SIL. For this reason the class number is not sufficiently informative. A Class 3 Pap report may indicate anything from a mild to severe dysplasia. If abnormal cells are found in the lower third of the epithelial tissue it would be described as mild dysplasia and may require no treatment. Class 3 also encompasses CIN II and high-grade SIL indicating that abnormal cells are clearly present in the lower two-thirds of the epithelial tissue. The condition is moderate dysplasia, and medical treatment will be needed.

Class 4 cells are the equivalent of CIN III or high-grade SIL. Abnormal cells are throughout the entire epithelial tissue. This is carcinoma in situ (pronounced "in sigh too"). It must be treated.

Class 5 refers to invasive carcinoma. Cancer cells have spread below the first layer of tissue. Appropriate medical and surgical attention are critical.[2]

CANCER ODDS

The chances of getting cancer of the female genital-reproductive system are relatively low. However, the odds of breast cancer are significant. Table 5 – 1 shows the overall lifetime probability of an American woman developing various cancers.

Cancer of the Vulva and Vagina

Malignancies of the external female genital organs are fairly uncommon. Vaginal cancer is frequently the result of metastasis from another location such as the uterus, ovaries, colon, or breasts. Maternal use of DES has also been implicated. Lifestyle behaviors may sometimes be a factor in both vulvar and vaginal cancer.[3]

TABLE 5 – 1
PERCENTAGE OF AMERICAN WOMEN DEVELOPING PARTICULAR CANCERS IN THEIR LIFETIME

Cancer Location	Percentage
Breast	11.0
Uterine body	2.4
Ovaries	1.4
Uterine cervix	0.6
Vagina/Vulva	.3

Sources: American Cancer Society; U.S. National Institutes of Health, National Cancer Institute, *Cancer Statistics Review,* 1973 –1987, 1990; U.S. National Center for Health Statistics, *Vital Statistics of the United States,* annual.

RISKS

DES-Related Cancer · The drug **diethylstilbestrol (DES)** is a synthetic estrogen that was used from 1945 to 1971 to treat a variety of pregnancy and childbirth problems. It allegedly improved the probability of conceiving a child and reduced the likelihood of miscarriage and premature birth. In fact, DES was not very effective in assuring a healthy birth, but has had serious effects on the DES children years later.[4]

Signs of DES exposure. Since DES was sold under a number of names and people typically do not recall what medications they took 20 or more years ago, it is often difficult to document DES exposure, but clues exist. If any of these apply to you, it is a good idea to discuss the possibility of DES exposure with your gynecologist.

1. You were born in the United States between 1945 and 1971.
2. Your mother had difficulty conceiving or carrying a baby to term during those years.
3. You were born during the critical years and have had fertility problems, miscarriage, or premature births.
4. Your gynecologist reports that you have vaginal or cervical malformations or other anatomical signs that may indicate DES exposure.[5]

Lifestyle and Vulvar or Vaginal Carcinoma · Although cancer of the vagina is often the result of metastasis from another part of the body, both vulvar and vaginal cancer may be related to number of sexual partners.

This has led to the suspicion that a microorganism, transmitting an infection during intercourse, may play a causative role. The human papillomavirus (HPV), the virus associated with genital warts, has been specifically implicated. Other factors have been found to correlate with genital cancer. These include cigarette smoking as well as having a weakened immune system such as from HIV infection or treatment with steroids or chemotherapy.

Cervical Cancer

Cancer of the uterine cervix is generally believed to warrant hysterectomy. While definitive causes have not been found, a number of contributing factors have been documented.

RISKS

Lifestyle may play a role in the chances of cervical cancer as well as in malignancies of the external genitals as noted earlier. This linkage has been suspected for more than a century, when Dr. Rigoni-Stern first observed in 1842 that cervical malignancies in women were almost never found among nuns.[6]

Interestingly, the strongest contributor to cervical cancer may be having sexual intercourse within a year of puberty. This may be because at this time, the cervix is undergoing considerable change and may be more vulnerable.

Other associations with cancer of the cervix are cigarette smoking, a relatively large number of sexual partners, a partner who has multiple partners, use of oral contraception, or a history of sexually transmitted disease including genital warts. As with vulvar cancer, it has been theorized that cervical cancer may be due partly to infectious microorganisms. However, the linkage is far from definitive. For example, although 95 percent of cervical cancers contain the human papillomavirus (HPV), only 3 – 4 percent of women with HPV develop cervical cancer. This is analogous to the hypothetical observation that 95 percent of people who broke bones at a winter resort were skiing, but only 3 – 4 percent of skiers broke bones.[7]

Having one or even several risk factors does not automatically mean that you will get cancer. In fact, most people "at risk" remain cancer-free. It does, however, mean that the probability is higher than for those who are not in a risk group.

Uterine Cancer

Cancer of the endometrium or body of the uterus is the most common pelvic malignancy in women. Fortunately, however, it can usually be diagnosed and cured while still confined to this area. Remember, the Pap smear was designed to detect cervical, not endometrial, cancers. Therefore, negative results are of little reassurance regarding endometrial cancer. If you are at risk, and/or have experienced some of the symptoms described in Chapter 4, even if your Pap test suggests no cancer, you should be sure to have further evaluation by either endometrial biopsy in your physician's office or ultrasonography.[8]

RISKS

The vast majority, about 90 percent, of uterine cancers are diagnosed in women who are age 50 or older. Abnormal or postmenopausal uterine bleeding are the most common warning signs. This means that bleeding a year or more after your last menstrual period should be immediately brought to the attention of your physician. While in 75 percent of women, the bleeding is of benign origin, in the other 25 percent a diagnosis of uterine cancer can be expected.

If you are taking oral contraceptives or are on an estrogen-progesterone replacement therapy, you normally should have bleeding just after the progesterone cycle is completed. If your bleeding is erratic or during the progesterone phase, this may signal problems and should be reported to your medical provider.

The **estrogen stimulation hypothesis** suggests that an excess of estrogen may lead to overgrowth, abnormalities, and possibly cancer of the endometrial tissue. This may occur because your body is producing too much estrogen or because you are receiving it from other sources in a way your body can't handle. The hypothesis was formulated because many of the known risk factors are associated with an overabundance of estrogen.

Women who are seriously overweight are more than three times as likely to develop uterine cancer than those who are of normal weight. Estrogen is stored in fat cells; thereby an overabundance of these cells may contribute to an overly generous amount of estrogen.

Those who had a late menopause, early menarche, have no children, are diabetic, have close family members with a history of uterine cancer, or have taken estrogen therapy without progesterone, or tamoxifen therapy for breast cancer, are also considered to be at high risk. Additional risk factors include having hormonally active ovarian tumors, polycystic ovary disease, prior pelvic radiation, and the absence of menstrual periods for long stretches during the years when menstruation should be a normal monthly event.[9]

Ovarian Cancer

The health of the ovaries may be assessed by palpation during a physical exam, through an ultrasound probe inserted into the vagina, pelvic ultrasound, or a blood test to determine the presence of the protein CA-125. However, the latter method is not recommended as a general screening test for cancer, since there is a high frequency of reported malignancies which are not present — thereby prompting unnecessary surgeries. The Pap smear, which is so effective in detecting cervical and vaginal cancers, is not useful with ovarian cancer. Since this cancer has no early warning signs, and no adequate screening test exists, cancer of the ovaries is a leading cause of death from malignancies in women.[10]

RISKS

Heredity appears to play a major role in the appearance of ovarian cancer. A registry to track family histories of cancer of the ovaries was established in 1981. It is now called the Gilda Radner Familial Ovarian Cancer Registry, after the late comedienne who died of the disease and had several close relatives similarly afflicted.

If you have two or more close relatives (sisters, mother) who had this cancer, the likelihood of your developing it in your lifetime is about 40 percent. In other words, almost half the women with several close relatives who had ovarian cancer also develop it. On the other hand, if you have only one relative with this disease, your chances are substantially reduced.[11]

Well-off women from highly industrialized countries more often have ovarian cancer than those who are less prosperous or come from other parts of the world. Sweden has the highest incidence, with Norway second, and white women in the United States third. Having no or just one child, eating a diet high in animal fat, and regularly drinking coffee for more than 40 years also are linked with a greater likelihood of developing ovarian cancer. Other associations include long-term habitual use of talcum powder in the vaginal area and chemical hair dyes.[12]

Factors That May Decrease Likelihood of Developing Ovarian Cancer · On the bright side, Dr. H. R. Barber of Cornell University Medical College reported that women who take the contraceptive pill for four or five years *decrease* their chances of getting ovarian cancer by 40 percent. He estimates that "the oral contraceptive pill can prevent approximately 1,500 ovarian cancers a year."[13] (You might recall, however, from our earlier discussion, that oral contraception is associated with an increased likelihood of cervical cancer. The reason for this may be that probably no physical barrier is used during intercourse. To resolve this apparent dilemma, you might want to use oral contraception *and* a condom or diaphragm with a new or nonexclusive sexual partner.)

Researchers at the Stanford University School of Medicine concluded from their work that "pregnancy, breast-feeding, and oral contraceptive use induce biological changes that protect against ovarian malignancy."[14] Other scientists found a lower incidence of ovarian cancer among women who had

had a tubal sterilization and those who had had a hysterectomy without removal of the ovaries.[15]

In essence, oral contraceptives, pregnancy, breast-feeding, hysterectomy, and tubal sterilization all contribute to a lower likelihood of developing ovarian cancer. While the Stanford University researchers attribute this benefit to biological factors, Dr. Ann-Louise Silver suggests that what these factors have in common is that they lessen the need for contraceptive gels and foams. She hypothesizes that these inserts may in some way *increase* the likelihood of ovarian cancer.[16]

Breast Cancer

Breast cancer is the most common cancer found in women. About 11 percent of all American women will develop this cancer in their lifetime. It is twice as likely to occur after the age of 65 than before.[17]

RISKS

Risk factors for breast cancer are similar to those for other cancers. Women who have a close relative with the disease are considered at risk. Those who had cancer in one breast have increased odds of getting it in the other breast. Additional risk factors include: never having children or having them after age 30, menstruating before age 12 or stopping after age 55, and being overweight — especially in the upper body. While caffeine does not appear to be related to the likelihood of developing breast cancer, the role of alcohol use, oral contraceptives, and hormone replacement therapy are still being studied.[18] Table 5 – 2 summarizes the risk factors for different gynecological cancers.

SIGNS AND SYMPTOMS

Gynecological cancers often make themselves known by particular symptoms. These should not be ignored, because the earlier diagnosis and treatment occur, the better the chances are of recovery. If any cancer signs, discussed in the following paragraphs, are present, you should see a physician as soon as possible.

While the symptoms listed must receive appropriate attention, they should not cause panic. Any of them may signify a benign condition. Only a properly trained medical person who obtains and examines suspicious tissue can make a reliable judgment.

Because signs and symptoms usually become apparent only in the more advanced stages, early detection, when you are symptom-free, is important. A regular Pap smear, although not 100% accurate, is an effective screening test for vaginal and cervical cancer.

TABLE 5 – 2
RISK FACTORS FOR CANCER

Vulva	Family history Previous other cancer Multiple sexual partners History of genital warts Cigarette smoking
Vagina	Family history Previous other cancer DES exposure prior to birth Multiple sexual partners History of genital warts Cigarette smoking Weakened immune system
Cervix	Family history Previous other cancer Sexual intercourse within a year of puberty Multiple sexual partners Cigarette smoking Sexually transmitted diseases History of genital warts
Uterine body (Endometrium)	Overweight Diabetes No children Prior pelvic radiation Taken estrogen without progesterone Treated with tamoxifen for breast cancer Postmenopausal bleeding Near or past menopause Late menopause
Ovary	Family history Previous other cancer No children High-fat diet Postmenopause Use of talcum powder in genital area Long-term coffee drinker Hair dyeing 4 to 5 times per year
Breast	Family history Previous other cancer No children Early puberty Late menopause Overweight

Sources: Patsner, 1993; Piver & Hempling, 1993; Tomatis, 1990, Rose, 1993; Veridiano, 1993.

VAGINAL BLEEDING

Irregular and increased vaginal bleeding are possible signs of uterine or vaginal cancer. Abnormal bleeding may occur between menstrual periods or as extra-heavy periods. It also may be apparent following sexual intercourse. If you are past menopause, have not had a period for a year or more, and then have vaginal bleeding, there is a 25 percent likelihood that this is symptomatic of uterine cancer.[19] While cervical cancer during pregnancy is not common, it does occur. If you notice vaginal bleeding during this time, you should notify your medical provider immediately.[20]

CHANGE IN BOWEL OR BLADDER FUNCTION

A large vaginal tumor may cause pressure on the bowel or bladder, resulting in constipation, diarrhea, or urinary problems. Bleeding associated with urination or defecation may also indicate that the bladder or colon is involved.[21]

BLEEDING OR PUS FROM THE VAGINAL LIPS

If a cancer exists in the vulvar area, it may signal itself by bleeding and/or a puslike discharge. Vulvar cancers also may cause discomfort or pain, because these external lesions may become infected. Regular self-examination of the external genitals with a mirror can alert you to suspicious irregularities.[22]

BLOATING OR PELVIC DISCOMFORT

The first sign of ovarian cancer may be a sense of bloating or a feeling that clothing is too tight around the abdomen. Even if it's likely that you've just been eating more and exercising less, you should be sure to report these observations to your physician.[23]

CHANGES IN THE BREAST

We have all been advised to engage in a monthly breast self-examination. Any discharge from the nipples or unusual lump should be brought to your health care provider's attention. Guidelines for breast examination are found in Chapter Three.

DEALING WITH THE NEWS

If tests confirm that you have cancer, you may enter a state of shock. Most people greet the news of a malignancy with confusion and denial. Once the diagnosis has sunk in, fear and anger are often felt. Questions such as "Will I die?" "Will I suffer?" and "Why me?" cause great anguish. Some individuals lapse into deep depression and give up on life. Most, however, learn to work with their physician to maximize their chances of recovery.[24]

COPING STRATEGIES

Andrew Slaby and Arvin Glicksman, practicing physicians and professors, describe ways in which people adapt to life-threatening illness. Their findings and those of others who have studied coping mechanisms should prove useful.[25]

1. Recognize that the outcome for most people diagnosed with cancer is positive. Cancer is usually *not* fatal. The odds are you will survive!
2. Learn what you can. Don't hesitate to ask your doctors for accurate information. Don't accept a brush-off. The reference list at the end of this chapter may offer a starting point for personal reading. Studies have shown that for most people, fear and anxiety are reduced when they know what is wrong and what can be done to help.
3. Know that you are not the first or only person with your diagnosis. Join a support group of others in your situation. Exchanging ideas, feelings, and experiences often is comforting and a source of strength.
4. Accept help and attention from family and friends. Those who want to give to you will get the satisfaction and pleasure of knowing that they are engaging in acts of kindness. You've been good to others; now may be the time to be on the receiving end. Do it graciously.
5. Be as independent as you can be. This may sound like a contradiction of the previous suggestion, but it's not. While it is good to accept, you should also try to do what you can for yourself.
6. Recognize that whatever has been important to you in the past may serve to bolster you now. Whether your pleasures have been cooking, carpentry, philosophy, or politics, continue to stay interested. This can keep you from dwelling on your own condition.
7. Recognize the emotions and needs of those around you. If you've been dependent on just one or two people for a considerable amount of care and attention, they may be experiencing fatigue or "burn-out." Encourage them to take time for their own activities. They will come back to help you refreshed and more effective.
8. Be open about your thoughts and wishes. Do not expect others to guess how you feel or what you want. Be forthright but considerate in asking for assistance and making plans. Don't sacrifice your own wishes in order to be a good patient. Never permit yourself to be hastily forced into a decision.
9. Don't be embarrassed to admit you are in pain. Pain is real and you are in no way less brave if you request medication to help alleviate your distress.
10. Recognize that your needs and coping mechanisms as a patient will be different at various stages of your illness. Some days you may feel helpless; on other occasions you may feel psychologically strong. Most people can muster the inner strength to confront serious illness peacefully and even cheerfully. It's worth the effort.

TREATMENT

Following a diagnosis of cancer, you may expect to undergo a series of treatments. Surgery, radiation, and chemotherapy are the primary therapies. Alternative approaches including diet and mental exercises are also options.

Primary Therapies

SURGERY

Women whose Pap tests show a **mild** dysplasia (CIN I or low-grade SIL) have a 30 – 50 percent chance of recovering without surgery or any other treatment! It is essential, however, that you stay in close contact with your physician for regular checkups.

Removal or treatment of the infected tissue is the most common approach to a clearly defined cancer (CIN II or III or high-grade SIL). The type and location of cell pathology determine the nature and extent of surgery.

Moderate to severe dysplasia, or vaginal or cervical lesions "in situ" — that is, limited to the surface cells — may be halted by excising only the cancerous tumors. The loop electrosurgical excision procedure (LEEP), an office procedure described in the previous chapter, as a diagnostic tool is often sufficient to eliminate these early cancer cells.[26]

When the disease is more advanced, and invasive cancer has been diagnosed in the cervix or body of the uterus, a hysterectomy and possible **oophorectomy** will be recommended. In these cases, the entire uterus, along with the fallopian tubes and often the ovaries, will be removed.

Whether to permit removal of healthy ovaries has been a subject of recent research. Dr. M. Parker and colleagues at Walter Reed Medical Center reported that 27 percent of the premenopausal women they studied who had their uterus removed, but retained their ovaries, lost hormonal function at an earlier age than normal or eventually required removal of the ovaries.[27] They conclude that women undergoing hysterectomy for cervical cancer should have both ovaries and fallopian tubes removed at the same time. They found no sexual diminishment or other ill effects. On the other hand, 73 percent of the premenopausal women who had hysterectomies in Parker's study and kept their ovaries retained normal ovarian function — so a case could just as easily have been made for retaining the ovaries!

A decade and more ago, it was standard procedure to remove the entire breast and lymph glands of a woman who had been diagnosed with breast cancer. Today, a lumpectomy or removal of just the tumor, if it has not spread, has been found to be just as effective in the large majority of cases.

The extent of surgery for cancer which is localized is a matter for individual judgment. If you hope to have children and are not in a risk group for other gynecological cancer, LEEP, or limited surgery combined with radiation therapy, might be the best decision. Regular follow-up is essential. On the other hand, more radical surgery may provide greater peace of mind in assuring that all the cancer has been removed and will not recur. You should be sure to discuss this issue fully with your doctor.[28]

RADIATION

Radiation therapy may precede or follow surgery. When it is used first, the goal is to limit the area that needs to be excised or to hopefully avoid surgery altogether. When radiation follows surgery, it is used to assure that all cancer cells have been destroyed. Sometimes **intraoperative radiation** treatment is used so that surgery is begun, radiation is applied, and surgery is completed all in a single session.

Radiation therapy has been available since the early 1900s; however, techniques have been markedly refined since that time. Radiation may be introduced either through beamed high energy rays or via the implantation of radioactive material in your body.[29]

External Radiation Therapy · If the decision has been made to use **external radiation**, you will participate in a procedure called **simulation** in which the radiation oncologist uses special X-ray equipment to determine precisely where radiation needs to be aimed — the **treatment port** or ports. These may then be marked on your skin with semi-permanent ink and will serve to guide treatment. They should not be washed off until the treatments are completed.

In external radiation therapy, **X-rays**, an **electron beam**, or **cobalt-60 gamma rays** are carefully directed at the tumors to be irradiated (the treatment ports) while other areas are shielded. You will be told to hold very still. The intention is to kill cancer cells while leaving surrounding healthy tissue intact. Although normal cells appear to recover from radiation more rapidly than cancer cells, well-focused treatment remains highly desirable.

Each treatment session may take between 15 and 30 minutes, while the actual time in which you are getting radiation probably will be only 1 to 5 minutes. You may expect to receive one treatment every day, except weekends, for one to two months. Weekends are usually excluded in order to allow normal cells a chance to recover.

Experiments are being conducted regarding reducing the dose of radiation by spreading the required amount out over more than one treatment per day. This is called **hyperfractionated radiation therapy.** The hope is that this procedure will produce fewer side effects.

Internal Radiation Therapy · **Internal radiation therapy,** or **implant radiation** is sometimes used instead of large external radiation machines. In implant radiation, a radioactive substance such as radium, cesium, iridium, iodine, or phosphorus is inserted in a small sealed container which is placed on or near the cancer site. For uterine cancer, the container may be located in the body of the uterus; this is called **intracavity radiation.**

Local or general anesthesia is normally required when the container is planted in your body. The actual radioactive material may be introduced later. The implant may be removed after one to seven days or left in place permanently.

Unlike external radiation treatment, in which the radiation is limited to the duration of each session, in internal therapy, radioactive material stays with you. The strength of the radiation diminishes with time, however, so that even if the capsule is not removed it will become inactive within a few weeks.

The radiation is most active for a few days following implantation. During that time you will probably be in a private hospital room and may be asked to restrict your movement. Visitors must remain at least six feet from you and limit their stay to 10 to 30 minutes a day. Children and pregnant women should not visit at all. Hospital staff will also be with you only briefly and may talk to you from a distance.

Side Effects · Radiation therapy may have some unpleasant effects. We have all experienced X-rays diagnostically for dental cavities, suspected bone fractures, and breast cancer (mammography). These are relatively low dose exposures, and leave us feeling as fine as we were before the procedure.

Radiation for therapeutic purposes, however, involves very high levels and may cause uncomfortable side effects. Within hours or days you may feel nauseous and need to vomit. The radiation treatment may also make you fatigued, and cause a skin irritation and/or loss of hair. Many of these problems are temporary and can be treated symptomatically. For example, avoiding spicy foods, and citrus fruits and juices prior to treatment may prevent nausea. Extra rest is appropriate to combat fatigue, and ointments may be used for skin irritation. Most women who have lost hair purchase wigs; others find colorful scarfs and hats more appealing.[30]

Research continues to improve radiation therapy. Small doses of external radiation have already been discussed. Another approach is "heavy-ion treatment" which has been developed by Japanese scientists. This may prove to be more effective than current methods in focusing destructive energy just on the cancer cells, thereby reducing side effects.[31]

CHEMOTHERAPY

A number of drugs are used in the treatment of cancer. In contrast to surgery and radiation therapy, drug or **chemotherapy** is systemic; that is, it acts on the entire human system. It may be introduced to attempt to shrink tumors before surgery and/or radiation, or after these treatments to eliminate cancers which might have spread. The goal in **antineoplastic** (anti-cancer) chemotherapy is to destroy cancer cells wherever they may be without doing damage to healthy tissue. While various agents successfully kill cancer cells, they unfortunately cut a wider swath and produce undesirable side effects.

Different chemicals, usually in combination, are used in the treatment of cancer at various sites. Several chemicals together usually have been found to be more effective than any single one. The nature of the tumor and its location influence its response to drug intervention. For example, fast-growing tumors are particularly responsive to **cell cycle specific** (CCS) agents such as vincristine, vinblastine, bleomycin and certain steroid hormones. "Solid tumors," or those not growing rapidly, are better treated by **cell cycle nonspecific** drugs.[32]

Cancer researchers continue to explore new drugs with limited success. **Taxol,** for example, reduced advanced ovarian tumors by more than half in 30 percent of women who participated in a recent trial. On the down side, the majority of women were not helped, and all suffered more severe side effects than with more standard chemotherapy. Taxol has also been helpful in some cases of breast and lung cancer.[33]

Chemotherapy may be administered orally, intravenously, or through infusion pumps which are generally also intravenous. Typically a patient will go to a hospital with a special cancer center. The chemicals are often introduced to the body slowly, so that you might expect to spend anywhere from an hour to overnight for each treatment. The chemotherapy schedule may be daily, weekly, or monthly. Sometimes periods of no treatment are interspersed to give your body a chance to rest and build healthy cells.[34]

Table 5 – 3 indicates the chemicals commonly used for various types of cancer.

Side Effects · As noted earlier, chemicals do not go directly just to cancer cells to wipe them out; they may do damage elsewhere as well. Whatever the drugs do to cancer cells, they may act in the same way to healthy tissue. This is the reason that CCS agents which are effective in combatting fast-growing tumor cells also attack normally fast-growing hair cells and cause hair loss.

Chemotherapy may interfere with the digestive process, causing nausea and vomiting. The body's immune system may also be weakened, so that people receiving chemotherapy are often more vulnerable to infections. While antibiotics are sometimes administered along with cancer-fighting agents, it is still wise to limit your interactions to healthy people as much as possible.[35]

TABLE 5 – 3
CHEMICALS USED IN THE TREATMENT OF CANCER

Site	Primary Drugs	Additional Drugs
Breast	Tamoxifen	Cyclophosphamide, doxorubicin, vincristine, methotrexate, fluorouracil, mitomycin, vinblastine, mitoxantrone, quinacrine, prednisone, megestrol androgens, aminoglutethimide, hydrocortisone, taxol
Cervix	Mitomycin, bleomycin, vincristine, cisplatin	Lomustine, cyclophosphamide, doxorubicin, methotrexate
Endometrium	Doxorubicin plus cyclophosphamide	Progestins, fluorouracil, vinblastine, cisplatin
Ovaries	Cyclophosphamide and cisplatin	Doxorubicin, melphalan, fluorouracil, vincristine, hexamethylmelamine, bleomycin, taxol

Note: Drugs are usually given in combination. Some, such as cisplatin, are considered "long-infusion" and require hydration therapy to protect the kidneys.
Sources: Kolata, 1993; Tierney, 1993.

Tamoxifen, used to treat breast cancer, has been suspected of contributing to endometrial cancer. Researchers suggest that the estrogenlike characteristics of this drug may account for malignant endometrial changes following long-term use. While tamoxifen is still being studied, nonhysterectomized women who are treated with it are advised to have annual transvaginal uterine ultrasonography and endometrial biopsy.[36]

While the thought of chemotherapy may be frightening, considerable scientific progress has been made in this area. Side effects can often be kept to a minimum, and the positive work of these chemicals, often in conjunction with other treatments, can often cure the cancer. Table 5 – 4 on page 92 provides some suggestions on minimizing the side effects of radiation treatment and chemotherapy.

EXPERIMENTAL TREATMENTS

Immunotherapy · The theory behind immunotherapy is that the human immune system normally counters foreign elements in the body. If a procedure could be found to make tumors seem "more foreign," the immune system's illness-fighting mechanism might be effectively activated.

Interferon is the best known of the drugs used to enhance the immune system's capabilities. It has been approved in the treatment of two rare types of cancer: hairy-cell leukemia and juvenile laryngeal papillomatosis. Regrettably, interferon has been shown to have serious, often fatal, side effects, and it can not be reliably used as a treatment for most cancers.

Interleukin-2, a protein produced by the cells of the immune system, showed some promise in the mid 1980s, but was later found to generally cause more harm than good. Research into enhancing the body's own defenses continues. Dr. Albert B. Deisseroth and colleagues at the University of Texas are exploring a method to genetically modify bone marrow cells, which are important in producing antibodies, so that they can tolerate increasingly higher doses of chemotherapy. He terms this "chemoprotection" and predicts the method will permit more powerful use of cancer-fighting drugs with reduced side effects.[37]

While we have listed immunotherapy as experimental, some researchers have suggested that it may become the fourth standard weapon against cancer, along with surgery, radiation, and chemotherapy.[38]

Alternative Approaches

Although the three mainstream treatment avenues for cancer are reasonably successful, dismay over side effects and their less-than-perfect track record especially in advanced cases, have led to a variety of alternative methods. Unfortunately, many of these have been found to be ineffective. Dependence on an unproven therapy may cause a cancer patient to not seek or delay more traditional treatment. This strategy may cost a life. We strongly recommend, therefore, that while alternatives may be considered, proven medical treatments should be given priority.

VITAMINS AND NUTRITIONAL SUPPLEMENTS

While a healthy diet alone, even with vitamin and mineral supplements, cannot cure cancer, it can help the treatment. If you are receiving chemotherapy, you may benefit by increasing your protein intake by 50 percent and your overall calories by 20 percent. Extra fluids are also advised to keep your kidneys functioning well. In addition, try to eat a well-balanced diet that includes whole grains and pasta, vegetables, fruits, legumes, dairy, and meat.[39]

Laetrile · Vitamin B-17, derived from apricot pits and more commonly known as **laetrile,** is probably the most familiar of the controversial cancer medicines. For many years following the early 1950s, when Dr. Ernest Krebs first endorsed laetrile as a cancer cure, thousands of people pinned their hopes on this drug.

Despite heavy promotional efforts and sincere testimonials from individuals who used laetrile, this product did not pass the careful scrutiny of medical research. Scientists at the National Cancer Institute, the Mayo Clinic, the Memorial Sloan-Kettering Center, the University of California at Los Angeles, and the University of Arizona all agreed that laetrile was not effective in stopping cancer cell growth and spread.[40]

Vitamin C · As we noted earlier, some cancers may be caused by microorganisms. Vitamin C has been advocated as an antiviral agent and has been used in limited experiments with cancer patients. The results of these trials were inconclusive, and Vitamin C has not been accepted as a cancer cure. Proponents of the Vitamin C treatment theory continue to recommend further investigation.[41]

Comfrey · **Comfrey** is an herb that is easily grown in most gardens. According to English folklore, it is helpful in the treatment of cancer. When submitted to the rigors of scientific study, however, comfrey was found to be of no use in the battle against cancer.[42]

VISUALIZATION THERAPY

Considerable attention in recent years has been given to the mind-body connection. Certainly our psychological state can affect our body's condition. When you are depressed, you may drag yourself around and feel achy all over. Conversely, physical pain can make you unhappy. But some proponents of the mind-body relationship take these interactions much further.

O. Carl Simonton, a medical doctor with a specialty in **oncology** (cancer), and his wife, Stephanie Simonton, have developed a program for cancer patients that involves relaxation, meditation, and visualization. They claim that relaxed concentration can serve as an *adjunct* to traditional therapy. For example, if a patient is experiencing radiation treatment or chemotherapy, they are counseled to focus on the therapy and visualize the X-rays or drugs attacking and killing the cancer cells.[43]

Bill Moyers has transcribed his lengthy interviews with many physicians and other health care providers on the connection between the mind and wellness. Mental focus appears to be a valuable supplement to traditional therapies.[44] For more information on psychological tactics to deal with cancer, see the Suggested Reading at the end of this chapter.

HYPERTHERMIA

Hyperthermia, or the application of heat to tumors, has been studied as a method of inhibiting cancer cell growth. Dr. Leon C. Parks experimentally removed blood from patients with advanced malignancies. The blood was heated to 106.7 degrees Fahrenheit and recirculated to the individual in a procedure taking approximately six hours. Dr. Parks reported some success with this treatment, but it should be noted that it was used as an adjunct to radiation and chemotherapy.[45]

TABLE 5 – 4
MINIMIZING RADIATION TREATMENT AND CHEMOTHERAPY SIDE EFFECTS

Side Effect	Management
Nausea and vomiting	Eat small, frequent meals Have liquids an hour before or after meals; not with meals Avoid sweet, fried, and fatty foods Eat slowly and chew carefully Have foods at room temperature Eat dry toast or crackers Try breathing through your mouth Take antimetic medications prescribed by your doctor
Diarrhea	Drink plenty of mild liquids, such as water, seltzer, or ginger ale, at room temperature Eat small, frequent meals Avoid coffee, beans, cabbage, broccoli, cauliflower, spicy foods, sweets, milk, and milk products
Constipation	Drink plenty of fluids Eat high-fiber foods Try to keep physically active
Dry, sore mouth	Drink plenty of fluids Suck on ice chips Eat soft, cold foods Avoid salty, spicy foods Keep your mouth and gums clean
Fatigue	Permit yourself adequate rest
Dry, itchy skin	Use hand creams or lanolin
Loss of balance or muscle strength	Move slowly and carefully, use handrails, grasp objects carefully

Source: U.S. Department of Health & Human Services, 1990.

PROGNOSIS

One in three Americans will eventually have some type of cancer. Nevertheless, if present trends continue, the vast majority of these people will achieve normal life spans.[46]

Almost 100% of women with cervical, endometrial, or breast cancer, when detected and treated early, live at least five more years. The "five-year survival rate" is the standard statistical index and suggests that the person is cured of cancer. Most of these women live a normal life span. A less optimistic outcome exists for women whose cancer has had time to spread. The key to a hopeful prognosis is early detection. Table 5 – 5 shows five-year survival rates for various types of cancers.

TABLE 5 – 5
PERCENTAGE OF WOMEN SURVIVING AT LEAST
FIVE YEARS AFTER CANCER DIAGNOSIS

Site	Survival Rate	
	Early Diagnosis	All Cases
Breast	almost 100%	92%
Uterine cervix	almost 100%	66%
Uterine corpus	almost 100%	83%
Ovary	87%*	40%

*Only about 23% of ovarian cancer is detected before it has spread.
Sources: American Cancer Society, 1993; National Cancer Institute, National Institutes of Health, Cancer Statistics Review, 1973-1989, NIH Pub. No. 92-2789.

For suggestions on making the most of the years following treatment, see Chapters Ten through Fourteen.

ENDNOTES

1. Benson, R. C., & Pernoll, M. L. *Benson & Pernoll's Handbook of Obstetrics and Gynecology,* 9th ed., New York: McGraw Hill, 1993.

2. Benson, R. C., & Pernoll, M. L. *Benson & Pernoll's Handbook of Obstetrics and Gynecology*, 9th ed., New York: McGraw Hill, 1993.

National Cancer Institute. *The National Strategic Plan for the Early Detection and Control of Breast and Cervical Cancers.* Atlanta, GA: U.S. Dept. of Health and Human Services, Public Health Service, Centers for Disease Control and Prevention, 1993.

3. Veridiano, N. P. Vaginal and vulvan cancer. *Emergency Medicine,* March 1993, 25 (4), 149 – 156.

4. Veridiano, N. P. Vaginal and vulvan cancer. *Emergency Medicine*, March 1993, 25 (4), 149 – 156.

5. Veridiano, N. P. Vaginal and vulvan cancer. *Emergency Medicine,* March 1993, 25 (4), 149 – 156.

6. Rose, P. G. Cervical cancer. *Emergency Medicine,* March 1993, 25 (4), 133 – 140.

7. Blakeslee, S. In research on cervical cancer, a wart virus is the prime suspect. *The New York Times,* Tuesday, January 21, 1992, C3.

Breit, E. B. You don't have to kiss a toad — HPV, genital warts, and cancer. *Our Sexuality Update,* Redwood City, CA: Benjamin/Cummings, April 1990.

8. Branch, Jr., W. T. *Office Practice of Medicine,* 3rd ed. Philadelphia: W.B. Saunders, 1994.

Feldman, S., Berkowitz, R. S., & Tosteson, A. N. Cost-effectiveness of strategies to evaluate postmenopausal bleeding. *Obstetrics and Gynecology*, June 1993, 81 (6), 968 – 975.

Patsner, B. Uterine cancer. *Emergency Medicine,* 25 (4), March 1993, 157– 161.

9. Patsner, B. Uterine cancer. *Emergency Medicine,* 25 (4), March 1993, 157– 161.

10. Bourne, T. H., Campbell, S., Reynolds, K. M., et al. Screening for early familial ovarian cancer with transvaginal ultrasonography and colour blood flow imaging. *British Medical Journal,* April 17, 1993, 306 (6884), 1025 – 1029.

Piver, M. S., & Hempling, R. E. Ovarian cancer. *Emergency Medicine*, March 1993, 25 (4), 141 – 148.

Rosenthal, E. Screening the tests that detect cancer. *The New York Times Magazine,* part 2, April 28, 1991, 8 – 12.

11. Piver, M. S., & Hempling, R. E. Ovarian cancer. *Emergency Medicine,* March 1993, 25 (4), 141 – 148.

12. Harlow, B. L., Cramer, D. W., Bell, D. A., et al. Perineal exposure to talc and ovarian cancer risk. *Obstetrics and Gynecology,* July 1992, 80 (1), 19 – 26.

Tzonou, A., Polychronopoulou, A., Hsieh, C.C., et al. Hair dyes, analgesics, tranquilizers and perineal talc application as risk factors for ovarian cancer. *International Journal of Cancer,* September 30, 1993, 55 (3), 408 – 410.

Whittemore, A. S., Wu, M. L., Paffenbarger, R.S. Jr., et al. Personal and environmental characteristics related to epithelial ovarian cancer. II. Exposures to talcum powder, tobacco, alcohol, and coffee. *American Journal of Epidemiology,* December 1988, 128 (6), 1228 – 1240.

13. Barber, H. R. Prophylaxis in ovarian cancer. *Cancer,* February 15, 1993, 71 (4 suppl), 1529 – 1533.

14. Whittemore, A. S., Harris, R., & Itnyre, J. Characteristics relating to ovarian cancer risk: collaborative analysis of 12 U.S. case-control studies. II. Invasive epithelial ovarian cancer in white women. Collaborative Ovarian Cancer Group. *American Journal of Epidemiology,* November 15, 1992, 136 (10), 1184 – 1203.

15. Hankinson, S. E., Hunter, D. J., Colditz, G. A., et al. Tubal ligation, hysterectomy, and risk of ovarian cancer: a prospective study. *Journal of the American Medical Association,* 1993, 270, 2813 – 2818.

Whittemore, A. S., Wu, M. L., Paffenbarger, R.S. Jr., et al. Personal and environmental characteristics related to epithelial ovarian cancer. II. Exposures to talcum powder, tobacco, alcohol, and coffee. *American Journal of Epidemiology,* December 1988, 128 (6), 1228 – 1240.

16. Silver, A. S. Tubal ligation, hysterectomy, and risk of ovarian cancer (letter to the editor). *Journal of the American Medical Association,* April 27, 1994, 271 (16), 1235.

17. National Cancer Institute. *Understanding Breast Changes: A Health Guide for All Women.* Bethesda, MD: National Institutes of Health Publication No. 93 – 3536, 1993.

18. National Cancer Institute. *National Institutes of Health, Cancer Statistics Review, 1973 – 1989.* NIH Pub. No. 92 – 2789, 1992.

Tomatis, L., ed. *Cancer: Causes, Occurrence and Control.* Lyon, France: International Agency for Research on Cancer, 1990. (Distributed in the U.S. by Oxford University Press, NY.)

19. Patsner, B. Uterine cancer. *Emergency Medicine,* March 1993, 25 (4), 157– 161.

20. Sivanesaratnum, V., Jayalakshmi, P., & Loo, C. Surgical management of early invasive cancer of the cervix associated with pregnancy. *Gynecologic Oncology,* January 1993, 48 (1), 68 – 75.

21. Veridiano, N. P. Vaginal and vulvan cancer. *Emergency Medicine,* March 1993, 25 (4), 149 –.156.

22. Veridiano, N. P. Vaginal and vulvan cancer. *Emergency Medicine,* March 1993, 25 (4), 149 – 156.

23. Piver, M. S., & Hempling, R. E. Ovarian cancer. *Emergency Medicine,* March 1993, 25 (4), 141 – 148.

24. Kubler-Ross, E. *On Death and Dying.* New York: Macmillan, 1969.

25. Slaby, A. E., & Glicksman, A. S. *Adapting to Life-Threatening Illness.* New York: Praeger, 1985.

Wardle, F. J., Collins, W., Pernet, A. L., et al. Psychological impact of screening for familial ovarian cancer. *Journal of the National Cancer Institute,* April 21, 1993, 85 (8), 653 – 657.

26. Blakeslee, S. Simplifying surgical removal of precancerous lesions. *The New York Times,* Wednesday, October 30, 1991, c13.

Patsner, B. Treatment of vaginal dysplasia with loop excision: report of five cases. *American Journal of Obstetrics and Gynecology,* July 1993, 169 (1), 179 – 180.

Rose, P. G. Cervical cancer. *Emergency Medicine*, March 1993, 25 (4), 133 – 140.

Rubin, S. C., & Curtin, J. P. Surgery for gynecological malignancies. *Current Opinion in Oncology,* October 1992, 4 (5), 923 – 929.

27. Parker, M., Bosscher, J., Barnhill, D., et al. Ovarian management during radical hysterectomy in the premenopausal patient. *Obstetrics and Gynecology,* August 1993, 82 (2), 187 – 190.

28. Averette, H. E., Nguyen, H. N., Donato, D. M., et al. Radical hysterectomy for invasive cervical cancer. A 25-year prospective experience with the Miami technique. *Cancer,* February 15, 1993, 71 (4 Suppl.), 1422 – 1437.

Averette, H. E., Hoskins, W., Nguyen, H. N., et al. National survey of ovarian carcinoma. I. A patient care evaluation study of the American College of Surgeons. *Cancer,* February 15, 1993, 71 (4 Suppl.), 1629 – 1638.

Barber, H. R. Prophylaxis in ovarian cancer. *Cancer*, February 15, 1993, 71 (4 suppl), 1529 – 1533.

John, E. M., Whittemore, A. S., Harris, R., et al. Characteristics relating to ovarian cancer risk: collaborative analysis of seven U.S. case-control studies. Epithelial ovarian cancer in black women. Collaborative Ovarian Cancer Group. *Journal of the National Cancer Institute,* January 20, 1993, 85 (2), 142 – 147.

Schwartz, P. E. The role of prophylactic oophorectomy in the avoidance of ovarian cancer. *International Journal of Gynaecology and Obstetrics,* November 1992, 39 (3), 175 – 184.

29. Berkow, R., ed. *The Merck Manual of Diagnosis and Therapy,* 16th ed. Rahway, N.J.: Merck Sharp & Dohme Research Laboratories, 1992.

U.S. Department of Health and Human Services. *Radiation Therapy and You: a Guide to Self-Help During Treatment,* (NIH Publication No. 91 – 2227). Washington, DC: Public Health Service, National Institutes of Health, October 1990.

30. Berkow, R., ed. *The Merck Manual of Diagnosis and Therapy,* 16th ed. Rahway, N.J.: Merck Sharp & Dohme Research Laboratories, 1992.

Editors of Time-Life Books. *Fighting Cancer.* Alexandria, VA: Library of Health, Time-Life Books, 1981.

U.S. Department of Health and Human Services. *Radiation Therapy and You: a Guide to Self-Help During Treatment,* (NIH Publication No. 91 – 2227). Washington, DC: Public Health Service, National Institutes of Health, October 1990.

31. Pollack, A. Japanese project aims to harness heavy ions to kill malignant cells. *The New York Times,* Tuesday, December 21, 1993, c3.

U.S. Department of Health and Human Services. *Radiation Therapy and You: a Guide to Self-Help During Treatment,* (NIH Publication No. 91 – 2227). Washington, DC: Public Health Service, National Institutes of Health, October 1990.

32. Tierney, Jr., L. M., McPhee, S. J., & Papadakis, M. A., eds. *Current Medical Diagnosis & Treatment 1994.* Los Altos, CA: Appleton & Lange, 1993.

33. Blakeslee, S. Race to synthesize cancer drug has photo finish. *The New York Times,* Tuesday, February 15, 1994, c3.

Kolata, G. The aura of a miracle fades from a cancer drug. *New York Times,* November 7, 1993, 1 & 28.

34. Benson, R. C., & Pernoll, M. L. *Benson & Pernoll's Handbook of Obstetrics and Gynecology,* 9th ed., New York: McGraw Hill, 1993.

Berkow, R., ed. *The Merck Manual of Diagnosis and Therapy,* 16th ed. Rahway, N.J.: Merck Sharp & Dohme Research Laboratories, 1992.

Branch, Jr., W. T. *Office Practice of Medicine,* 3rd ed. Philadelphia: W.B. Saunders, 1994.

U.S. Department of Health and Human Services. *Chemotherapy and You: A Guide to Self-Help During Treatment,* (NIH Publication No. 91 – 1136). Washington, DC: Public Health Service, National Institutes of Health, June 1990.

35. Brody, J. E. Tricks to ease the side effects of cancer drugs. *The New York Times,* January 22, 1992, c12.

U.S. Department of Health and Human Services. *Chemotherapy and You: A Guide to Self-Help During Treatment,* (NIH Publication No. 91 – 136). Washington, DC: Public Health Service, National Institutes of Health, June 1990.

36. Uziely, B., Lewin, A., Brufman, G., et al. The effect of tamoxifen on the endometrium. *Breast Cancer Research & Treatment,* 1993, 26 (1), 101 – 105.

37. Gibbs, W. W. Sentries and saboteurs: mutating patients' genomes to suit their medicine. *Scientific American,* October 1993, 269 (4), 21 – 24.

38. Moss, R.W. *The Cancer Industry: Unraveling the Politics.* New York: Paragon House, 1989.

39. U.S. Department of Health and Human Services. *Chemotherapy and You: A Guide to Self-Help During Treatment,* (NIH Publication No. 91– 1136). Washington, DC: Public Health Service, National Institutes of Health, June 1990.

40. Bricklin, M. *The Practical Encylopedia of Natural Healing.* Emmaus, PA: Rodale Press, 1976.

Moss, R.W. *The Cancer Industry: Unraveling the Politics.* New York: Paragon House, 1989.

41. Bricklin, M. *The Practical Encylopedia of Natural Healing.* Emmaus, PA: Rodale Press, 1976.

42. Bricklin, M. *The Practical Encylopedia of Natural Healing.* Emmaus, PA: Rodale Press, 1976.

Moss, R.W. *The Cancer Industry: Unraveling the Politics.* New York: Paragon House, 1989.

43. Bricklin, M. *The Practical Encylopedia of Natural Healing.* Emmaus, PA: Rodale Press, 1976.

Editors of Time-Life Books. *Fighting Cancer.* Alexandria, VA: Library of Health, Time-Life Books, 1981.

Moyers, Bill. *Healing and the Mind.* New York: Doubleday, 1993.

U.S. Department of Health and Human Services. *Radiation Therapy and You: A Guide to Self-Help During Treatment,* (NIH Publication No. 91 – 2227). Washington, DC: Public Health Service, National Institutes of Health, October 1990.

44. Moyers, Bill. *Healing and the Mind.* New York: Doubleday, 1993.

45. Editors of Time-Life Books. *Fighting Cancer.* Alexandria, VA: Library of Health, Time-Life Books, 1981.

46. American Cancer Society. *Cancer Facts & Figures — 1992.* American Cancer Society, 1599 Clifton Road, N.E., Atlanta, GA 90329 – 4251, 1993.

SUGGESTED READING

Brady, Judith, ed. *One in Three: Women with Cancer Confront an Epidemic.* San Francisco: Cleis Press, 1991.

Faschel, Marjorie. *Stop Dying with Cancer.* Van Treese, James B., ed. Salt Lake City, UT: Northwest Publishing, 1992.

Feldman, Gayle. *You Don't Have to Be Your Mother.* New York: W. W. Norton, 1994.

Fiore, Neil A. *The Road Back to Health: Coping with the Emotional Aspects of Cancer.* Berkeley, CA: Celestial Arts Publishing, 1991.

Frahm, David J., & Anne E. Frahm. *Cancer Battle Plan: Six Strategies for Beating Cancer from a Recovered "Hopeless Case."* Colorado Springs, CO: Pinon Press, 1992.

Greenwald, Howard P. *Who Survives Cancer?* Berkeley, CA: University of California Press, 1992.

Rosenblum, Daniel. *A Time to Hear, A Time to Help: Listening to People with Cancer.* New York: Free Press, 1993.

Temoshok, Lydia. *The Type C Syndrome.* New York: Random House, 1992.

Temoshok, Lydia, & Henry Dreher. *The Type C Connection: The Mind-Body Link to Cancer & Your Health.* New York: NAL/Dutton, 1992.

Chapter 6

TREATMENT OPTIONS

"When I was in my 30s I had trouble with my periods. Several local physicians recommended a hysterectomy. I sought a third opinion in New York City from an eminent gyn/MD. He said I had a fibroid tumor, but did not see any need for surgery as he felt there was much unknown about the hormones, etc., that would be missing. I had several D&Cs to relieve heavy bleeding and eventually the fibroids shrank." — Alice, age 42

"I am presently pregnant, following a successful myomectomy for fibroids."
— Tonda, age 35

DO YOU NEED A HYSTERECTOMY?

Check Your Options

SECOND AND THIRD OPINIONS

Based on your examination and test results, your gynecologist concludes that you need a hysterectomy. Now what?

Get a second opinion. It is most important that you see at least one other gynecologist, who is at least as fully qualified as your first doctor. Before you do this, contact your medical insurance provider. Some companies require a second opinion or they will not pay for your surgery. You may need to see a physician from their approved list, and insurance will likely cover this cost. Other companies conduct an independent investigation and may conclude that a second opinion is optional but will cover the expense.

Whether it is required or optional, it makes good sense to get a second opinion. Medical statistics reveal that when second opinions are obtained, elective hysterectomy rates decline.[1] Many women have had hysterectomies that were unnecessary because they never sought a second opinion.

If your insurance company does not provide a list of gynecologists for a second opinion, you might want to refer to the section in Chapter Three, "Selecting Your Health Care Provider," for help in choosing a second doctor.

Do *not* see a gynecologist in the same office or medical group as your doctor for this *impartial* second opinion.

Let the second doctor know that you have come for a second opinion. That is standard procedure. Prepare a list of questions to ask this new physician (see below for sample questions) so you can get the information you need to make an informed decision about your possible surgery. If your doctors disagree, or you are dissatisfied for any reason, do not hesitate to see a third doctor.

QUESTIONS TO ASK YOUR DOCTOR*

What exactly is wrong?
Can you draw a diagram for me?
What caused the problem?
Can I prevent it from happening again?
Are diagnostic tests needed?
Which tests?
Why? How will the results be helpful?
Can you explain the test results in plain language?
Is treatment or surgery needed?
How effective is such treatment or surgery?
What are the alternatives?
What are the risks associated with this treatment or surgery?
Is the treatment or surgery a painful procedure?
If I ignore this condition/problem, what might happen?
What effect will treatment or surgery have on my other medical problems?
What about the medication I am taking?

*New York/United University Professions Joint Committee on Health Benefits. *Report,* Fall, 1987, 4.

When second and third opinions concur with the original diagnosis, they provide you with reassurance. The big problem occurs when the opinions conflict.

There are a number of ways that we deal with such disparity. Some of us become self-educated as we search for "the answer" in articles and books; others turn to friends and family or go on "gut" instinct. A few of us seek out more and more medical opinions, while many follow the directions of a doctor we trust.

Sometimes the diagnosis makes the decision a little easier. For example, cancer of the uterus or very large fibroids that are pressing on other organs may make hysterectomy the clear choice. Other diagnoses may call for more consideration, and often less drastic therapy. Nonsurgical approaches are sometimes appropriate.

NONSURGICAL APPROACHES

The human body is remarkably resilient. When we are ill, time is often the best medicine. We can assist natural healing through diet, exercise, and home remedies.[2]

DIET AND DRUGS

If careful diagnostic assessment shows that your symptoms are not due to cancer or infectious disease, you may be able to treat your gynecological problems in benign ways. In Chapter Four we noted that excessive estrogen may contribute to menstrual problems. It follows that adjustment in our body's quantity of this hormone may help to alleviate some difficulties. Ingredients in products which we eat and drink can also have both general and specific effects on our well-being.

Eat Right and Watch Your Weight · The body stores estrogen in fat, so being overweight may contribute to gynecological problems. While not all abdominal or menstrually related difficulties will be resolved by shedding a few pounds, the side effects of feeling and looking better are added benefits.

Eating a balanced diet of grains, vegetables, fruits, and nonfat milk or yogurt and minimizing saturated fats, sugar, and salt will help you lose weight and will make you feel better. You might supplement this diet with multi-vitamins and minerals, particularly calcium, potassium, and magnesium. However, be cautious not to take toxic overdoses of vitamins and minerals. When you are appropriately nourished, your body tends to function more effectively.[3] Notice how restless you may feel if you've overindulged in sweets, or how irritable you might become when you've skipped a meal. Chapter Thirteen discusses diet in more detail.

Cut down on caffeine and alcohol. Coffee, tea, cola drinks, and chocolate are sources of caffeine. We enjoy these products in part for the "lift" they give us. But there is a down side. Caffeine may make us irritable and contribute to the cramping and breast tenderness associated with menstruation.

While a single alcoholic drink may ease cramps, larger amounts cause the body to retain fluid and may make you feel bloated. It is not a reliable treatment.[4]

Be aware of the food you eat. Herbs such as ginseng and cohosh are touted for their supposed ability to improve memory,[5] enhance libido, reduce fatigue, and ease depression.[6] They also contain estrogen-like chemicals, so some women take these herbs to help the body replace estrogen after menopause or a hysterectomy, thus avoiding other means of hormone replacement therapy. However, increasing the body's estrogen levels prior to menopause may contribute to menstrual problems.

Remember that endometriosis and uterine tumors, and the discomforts they cause, may be in part due to excess estrogen, especially prior to menopause. Therefore, during the premenopausal years you may want to try to lower your estrogen levels. After menopause, estrogen depletion is associated with osteoporosis and other health problems. At this time, you may wish to replace the estrogen that your body is no longer producing. (See Chapter Eleven for a discussion of hormone replacement therapy.)

Another — surprising — way we increase our levels of estrogen is through the composition of some of the foods we eat. For example, hormones are sometimes fed to cattle, chicken, and other animals in order to stimulate their growth and weight to make them more commercially marketable. As a result, traces of estrogen may remain in the meat we consume and in milk and other dairy products. Again, this may contribute to menstrual difficulties.[7]

Hormone Therapy · As previously noted, uterine fibroids and abnormal growth of endometrial tissue have been attributed to excessive estrogen within the system. Anti-estrogen medications have been used with limited success. One therapy under investigation is the use of **gonadotropin-releasing hormone (GnRH)**. GnRH is produced by the hypothalamus and works cyclically to stimulate the pituitary to either encourage or block the ovaries' hormone production. *Lupron,* a synthetic look-alike GnRH analog, acts to discourage estrogen production. It is taken through injections, but is still in the experimental stage. Another GnRH analog, *Synarel,* is administered as a nasal spray. Both may produce menopausal symptoms such as hot flashes and vaginal dryness. GnRH analogs are generally considered temporary measures either prior to gynecological surgery or pregnancy.[8]

Danazol, a synthetic steroid, is also an anti-estrogen drug. While it has been somewhat successful in the treatment of endometriosis, it may also cause facial hair growth, acne, weight gain and the retention of fluids. These negative side effects have limited its use.[9]

Rather than block estrogen as in the GnRH analogs described above, a combination of estrogen and progesterone is sometimes given to stimulate the uterine lining to shed and begin a new healthy cycle. Dr. Herbert Goldfarb terms this hormonal treatment "medical curettage," and notes that for women who do not have a cancerous or precancerous condition, this regimen may avoid the necessity for a D&C or hysterectomy.[10]

Caution! It is important to remember that estrogen is both useful (to help prevent osteoporosis, vaginal dryness, and heart disease), and potentially harmful, in that it encourages the growth of endometrial tissue and uterine fibroids.

Sometimes estrogen replacement therapy may be prescribed to alleviate menopausal symptoms, but ends up causing bigger problems such as fibroids. Dr. Mitchell Levine, a Boston area gynecologist, described the case of Mary P. At age 57, Ms. P. came to him seeking a second opinion regarding a recommendation of hysterectomy due to enlarged fibroids and abdominal discomfort. She reported that they started about a year ago — about the time she began ERT. Dr. Levine's recommendation was to stop the ERT and see if the fibroids would shrink by themselves. They did, and no surgery or other therapy was needed.[11]

Antibiotics · Pelvic inflammatory disease (PID) is sometimes considered an indication for hysterectomy. However, since it is usually caused by bacterial infection, it should first be treated by antibiotics. Incidentally, it is important for your sexual partner(s) also to be treated in order to prevent reinfection.

When PID is diagnosed early, antibiotics taken in pill form are generally sufficient to correct the problem. If PID is especially severe, hospitalization may be recommended. In these cases, antibiotics may be administered intravenously. In most cases, PID clears up. Unless it becomes chronic and there is damage to the uterus and fallopian tubes, surgery is unnecessary.[12]

Anti-Inflammatory Drugs and Antiprostaglandins · If your major complaint is extreme menstrual discomfort, remember that menstrual flow is the result of the shedding of the uterine lining. Prostaglandins, hormones secreted into our bloodstream, assist in shedding this unneeded tissue by encouraging uterine contractions. Sometimes, however, the prostaglandins are overzealous in their efforts, and the result is severe menstrual cramping. Over-the-counter medications such as ibuprofen (Motrin, Advil, Nuprin, or a generic form) and aspirin are useful, safe antiprostaglandins. These drugs also have anti-inflammatory and analgesic properties, which assist in relieving some of the other symptoms associated with menstruation such as muscle tension and pain.[13]

BODYWORK

The suggestions below may help alleviate some discomfort and can perhaps delay or avoid invasive treatment.

Stretch and Flex · Chapter Thirteen provides suggestions for exercises to make you strong and flexible. Even at the time of menstrual discomfort, gentle yoga stretches followed by a brisk walk may make you feel better.[14]

Do the Kegel · If a hysterectomy is recommended because of a prolapsed uterus and/or urinary problems, Kegel exercises, described in Chapter Ten, may be helpful.[15]

Warm Up · An old fashioned hot water bottle or heating pad on a crampy abdomen can do wonders. A long soak in the tub or even a hot shower often relieves menstrual cramps. (Incidentally, the old caution against bathing while you have your period is not valid.) While you're warming the outside, have some herbal tea for the inside.

Get Hot · Orgasm may provide some relief for menstrual discomfort. With or without a partner, this can be a useful therapy. See Chapter Ten: Let's Talk About Sex.[16]

Treat Yourself to Massage or Acupressure · Massage can be very relaxing and soothe aches and pains all over your body. Firm touch to a particular spot as in **acupressure** can also be beneficial.

Susan Anderson, president of the Los Angeles chapter of the Endometriosis Association, is an advocate of acupressure for endometrial pain. She advises to press as hard as you can in two places: (1) about two inches above the ankle on the inside of the leg, and (2) in your hand where the bones of the thumb and forefinger meet.[17]

Alexis Phillips, a medical massage instructor in New York City, recommends pressure in the depressions above both sides of the heel below the ankle for general relief of menstrual cramps.[18]

Author Susun Weed maintains that acupressure points to ease heavy menstrual flow are just under the nose and on top of the head. She also reports that acupuncture (the traditional Chinese treatment with needle pressure) is effective in shrinking fibroids.[19]

PESSARIES

Vaginal pessaries are sometimes recommended for women with a prolapsed uterus. Basically, this is a mechanical means for pushing the uterus up out of the vaginal area where it has intruded. Pessaries are inserted securely in the vagina by your medical caregiver; some are inflatable to assure a better fit. Pessaries may be left in place for four to six weeks and should be checked by your physician after that period of time — or sooner, if you experience problems. A slightly different shape or size pessary may be more effective. A diaphragm cannot be used for contraception while a pessary is in place.[20]

SURGERY: A COMPENDIUM OF APPROACHES

Following are descriptions of several surgical methods that have been developed to correct uterine problems. Some, such as LEEP, cryosurgery, cone biopsy, and D&C are performed as outpatient procedures either in the doctor's office or a hospital. Other more involved procedures, such as myomectomy, endometrial ablation, and hysterectomy, require hospitalization. As a prospective patient, you should be aware of how to make any of these experiences more palatable.

Transportation. Even the simplest procedures may make you achy and tired. Arrange to have a relative or friend drive you to and from the doctor's office or hospital. Same-day surgery does not mean same-day recovery. Both the anesthesia and the procedure itself will take a toll. Expect to need help.

Food. If you are having outpatient surgery, your hospital may not provide food following the procedure. Even if they do serve a meal, it may not suit your post-surgical palate. Consider bringing a little "picnic" lunch of food and beverage that appeal to you. A thermos of tea, some fruit, and crackers may go a long way to making you feel more comfortable.

Anticipate your needs when you get home. Whether your procedure is in the doctor's office or the hospital, you will not feel like cooking. Either prepare some dishes ahead or buy ready-to-eat food for your return. You will appreciate a refrigerator and freezer stocked with goodies that require minimal effort. Of course, your own living arrangements will influence this. Do you normally prepare food for others or is the situation reversed? A little planning can make your return home (after a few hours, a day, or a week) much more enjoyable.

Clothing and Incidentals. Wear comfortable but attractive clothing. Slacks with an adjustable waistband and an easy-to-put-on top are generally good choices. You may not feel like bending to tie shoes, so slip-ons (but obviously not high heels) and socks may be most serviceable. Doctors' offices and hospitals are often cool (but sometimes too hot). Dress fairly lightly, but take along a cotton sweater and a jacket.

Bring your toothbrush, toothpaste, comb, and usual cosmetics to fix yourself up as soon as you are able. You'll feel better when you look better. You may want to bring something to read to help the waiting time pass more pleasantly.

Depending on the procedure, you may need to wear menstrual pads for a few hours or days. The hospital, or doctor's office, will provide them while you are there, but you should have a small supply for your return home.

More hints for pre- and post-hospitalization are in Chapters Eight and Nine. The surgical procedures themselves are explained briefly below.

LEEP

The Loop Electrosurgical Excisional Procedure (LEEP) was described as a diagnostic technique in Chapter Four. LEEP may also successfully remove all precancerous cells, thus eliminating the need for further treatment. It is sometimes used when a Pap smear and subsequent biopsy show cervical dysplasia or CIN I or II (potentially precancerous cell irregularities). It is a relatively new but effective procedure, and is performed in a doctor's office.[21]

CRYOSURGERY

Cryosurgery, generally performed in a physician's office, freezes and thereby kills abnormal growths. Cryosurgery uses liquid nitrogen to destroy diseased tissue. A drawback to this technique is that the method is difficult to control, and **cervical stenosis** (narrowing of the cervical canal), or cervical scarring may occur. Healing following extensive cryosurgery generally takes three to six weeks.[22]

CONE BIOPSY OR CONIZATION

As the name implies, cone biopsy is primarily a diagnostic procedure to see whether cancerous cells are present. The technique involves surgically removing a cone-shaped mass of suspicious tissue from your cervix. Your physician may use a laser or the more traditional scalpel.

If your Pap test showed cervical intraepithelial neoplasia (CIN) I, II, or III — noninvasive cancer cells, cone biopsy can provide further information regarding their condition and extent. Sometimes, cone biopsy successfully removes all abnormal growths. If follow-up confirms the success of this procedure, no further surgery should be necessary.

Cone biopsy is an invasive procedure and is performed in a hospital operating room under general anesthesia.[23]

DILATION AND CURETTAGE (D&C)

We described dilation and curettage in Chapter Four as a diagnostic test, but it is also used as a method to control menstrual-related disorders.

When the endometrial lining is scraped, the tissue causing the problems may be removed and no further treatment may be necessary.

MYOMECTOMY

Myomectomy refers to the removal of uterine fibroids (the myomata) without damaging the endometrium or taking out the uterus. Since the uterus and all related organs are kept intact, future pregnancy is possible. Between a third and a half of women desiring a child successfully conceive and deliver following this procedure, regardless of the size of the fibroids and uterus.[24] However, attempts at conception should be delayed for two or three months following myomectomy, since this is a time of uterine healing.[25]

A disadvantage of myomectomy is that if multiple fibroids are present or if they are very large and deeply embedded in the endometrial wall, this technique may not remove them completely or they may grow back. A second drawback to myomectomy is that it is a new, fairly complicated procedure that requires "meticulous technique and experience."[26] It is advisable to

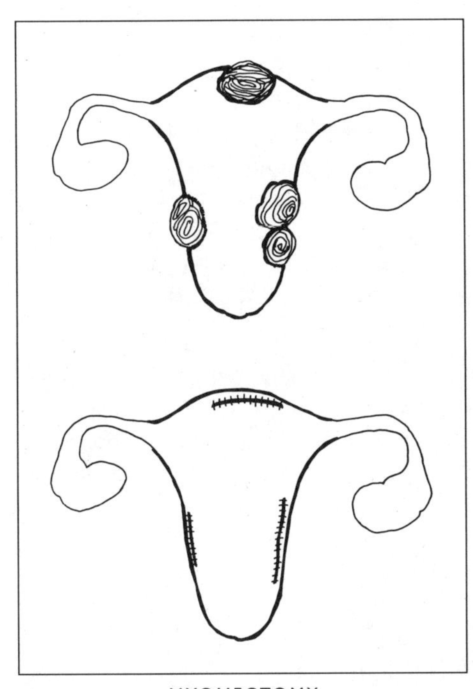

MYOMECTOMY

In a myomectomy, just the fibroids or myomata are removed. The uterus is preserved.

find a doctor who has a successful track record with it. Myomectomy can be accomplished in several ways.

Vaginal Myomectomy · After the area has been anesthetized, a **hysteroscope,** a viewing instrument, is placed in the vagina. Through fiber-optic technology, the surgeon is able to see **myomata** or **leiomyomatas,** the technical names for fibroid tumors. These then are removed by either surgical knife, laser rays, or the electrical current of a **resectoscope.** While the resectoscope is a fairly recent addition to gynecological technology, it has been employed safely for decades in the treatment of bladder problems.

All three methods of vaginal myomectomy have been used with good results. A team of physicians in Israel reported that just under 9 percent of the 46 women in their study needed a repeat vaginal myomectomy within five years; 6 percent required a hysterectomy.[27] Dr. M. H. Goldrath at Sinai Hospital in Detroit, Michigan, reported even greater success. Of 151 women who had vaginal removal of fibroids, less than 3 percent required later hysterectomy or abdominal myomectomy.[28] Similar findings were reported by surgeons at the University of Pennsylvania School of Medicine. Of 92 women who had resectoscopic myomectomy, only 3 percent required hysterectomy later.[29] Many physicians agree that this half-hour, outpatient surgical procedure is safe and effective under most circumstances. The risk is increased in those with large fibroids or serious bleeding problems.[30]

Laparoscopic Myomectomy · A **laparoscope** is an instrument used to view the inside of the abdomen.The laparoscope is equipped with a light and camera. The surgeon monitors his or her work on a video screen. Unlike the hysteroscope, which does not require an abdominal cut, the laparoscope is inserted through a small incision just below the navel. An additional tiny cut is made just above the pubic hairline. The uterus is entered through this second cut, and the fibroids are severed and removed by surgical scalpel or laser. Very large fibroids may be fragmented prior to excision.[31]

Although the laparoscope has been used successfully for several decades for tubal ligation, laparoscopic myomectomy has been criticized because some surgeons have used this technique without adequate training.[32] However, in the hands of a skilled and experienced physician, and especially if your fibroids are small, it is a useful alternative to myomectomy through a larger abdominal cut. The laparoscopic technique has the advantage of less visible scars and a shorter recovery time.[33] You would be wise to ask your surgeon how many laparoscopic myomectomies he or she has performed before you agree that this is the person to operate on you. Also, question your doctor about possible complications.

Abdominal Myomectomy · Either a vertical cut from the belly button down, or a horizontal incision just above your pubic hairline, is made in order to perform an abdominal myomectomy. The surgeon then inspects your uterus and removes only the fibroid growths. As with the laparoscopic technique, the fibroids may be destroyed by laser or more traditional surgical methods.[34]

Shrinking the fibroids before surgery. Some surgeons administer a gonadotropin-releasing hormone agonist, such as **leuprolide acetate,** either by injection or through an infusion pump. This blocks the production of estrogen, reducing the size of the fibroids prior to a myomectomy, thus allowing for simpler, more risk-free surgery.[35] We talked about the use of GnRH agonists in the section on hormone therapy earlier in this chapter.

A GnRH agonist, taken for three to six months, is more effective as preparation for myomectomy or hysterectomy than it is when used as a remedy by itself for fibroids, for the following reasons. First of all, GnRH agonists should not be used for long periods of time, since they may adversely affect the body's calcium balance and cholesterol levels, thereby increasing the likelihood of osteoporosis and coronary artery disease.[36] Second, when treatment with the GnRH agonist is stopped, tumors tend to grow back. This is far less likely if the fibroids are surgically removed following GnRH shrinkage.[37]

ENDOMETRIAL ABLATION

The procedures used in vaginal myomectomy may be used to **ablate**, or destroy, the endometrial lining in women who have heavy, painful periods due to fibroids, polyps, or hormonal imbalance. The techniques used to ablate the endometrium — laser surgery and electrosurgery — take about half an hour and usually are performed on an outpatient basis in a hospital. Since the entry is through the vagina, they do not require the cutting of skin, and therefore leave no visible scars. However, because the inner lining of the uterus is permanently destroyed, endometrial ablation is not an appropriate treatment for women wishing to become pregnant.

Laser Treatment · As in vaginal myomectomy, following a regional anesthetic, a hysteroscope is placed in the vagina. The physician, then, is able to see the inner surface of the uterus, which is normally collapsed, but has been inflated with a liquid or carbon dioxide gas. Laser rays, beamed through the scope, cut and seal the entire endometrial area.

Laser endometrial ablation reduces or eliminates both menstrual flow and premenstrual symptoms. It is safer than hysterectomy for several reasons. Endometrial ablation generally can be performed with regional anesthesia; it is performed in a shorter amount of time and with less bleeding than is associated with hysterectomy. Although side effects are uncommon, it carries a very slight risk of laser burn.[38] An additional, even more rare occurrence is gas embolism, which could result in cardiovascular problems. The likelihood of either complication, though remote, should be discussed with your physician.[39]

Electrosurgery · Endometrial ablation can also be performed through electrosurgery with a resectoscope. A hysteroscope is inserted into the vagina to permit viewing of the uterine lining. The resectoscope is then used to remove the entire endometrium.

It is less costly than laser endometrial ablation and may be more appropriate for women with symptoms which are not as extensive. Endometrial ablation with the resectoscope carries a very small risk of uterine perforation. This should be explored with your physician. In the vast majority of cases, however, the resectoscope is used safely and effectively.[40]

HYSTERECTOMY

Hysterectomy refers to the surgical removal of the uterus and usually the attached fallopian tubes. A **partial** or **subtotal** hysterectomy is when the cervix is left in place, but the body of the uterus is removed. In a **total** or **complete hysterectomy**, both the cervix and the body of the uterus are removed. It is possible to remove just the ovaries, and this is called an **oopherectomy.** Sometimes the term **"pan-hysterectomy"** is used to denote removal of the uterus, fallopian tubes, and ovaries; more precisely, this is a **hysterectomy with bilateral salpingo-oopherectomy.** A **radical hysterectomy**, performed in cases of cancer, is the removal of the uterus, fallopian tubes, ovaries, upper portions of the vagina, and the pelvic lymph nodes.

Excision of part or all of the uterus may be accomplished vaginally, using laparoscopic techniques, or through an abdominal incision.

Vaginal Hysterectomy · The medical term for vaginal hysterectomy is **colpohysterectomy; colpo** refers to the vagina. If the reason for your hysterectomy includes uterine prolapse or small fibroid tumors, it is likely to be performed through the vagina. Contrary to what you might think, vaginal hysterectomy is possible for women who have had previous Cesarean sections.[41]

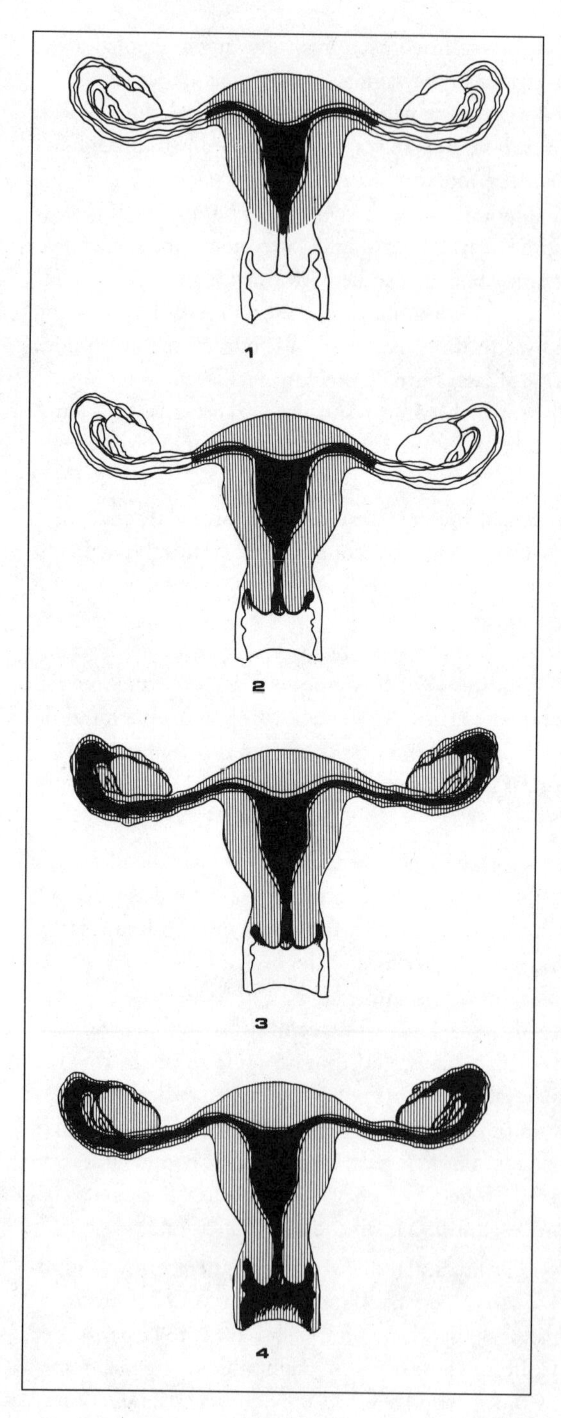

Partial Hysterectomy
In partial or subtotal hysterectomy, the uterus is cut and only the body is removed. The cervix is left in place.

Complete or Total Hysterectomy
A complete or total hysterectomy is the removal of the entire uterus.

Hysterectomy and Bilateral Salpingo-Oophorectomy
In this procedure, the uterus (usually including the cervix), the ovaries, and the fallopian tubes are removed.

Radical Hysterectomy
A radical hysterectomy includes removal of the uterus along with the cervix, ovaries, fallopian tubes, and probably upper portions of the vagina and affected lymph glands.

This procedure is used in about one-fourth of the cases in the United States in which hysterectomy is performed for reasons other than cancer.[42]

Vaginal hysterectomy is normally performed in the hospital and requires that you stay two or more days. It has also been performed with some success on an outpatient basis.[43]

Recovery tends to be more rapid in vaginal surgery, compared with the other techniques, and there is no visible scar. Kudo and his colleagues at Sapporo Medical College in Japan performed over 9,000 vaginal hysterectomies in a 32-year period for a variety of diagnoses. They reported only three cases of urethral injury (.03 percent) and concluded that this operation is safe, convenient, and less susceptible to complications than abdominal hysterectomy.[44]

On the negative side, however, this method may result in shortening the vagina and/or damaging the Grafenberg area, creating possible sexual problems both with intercourse and orgasm. These are problems which require further medical study, and you should discuss these concerns with your surgeon.

Just as the laparoscope with attached video monitor can be used for a myomectomy and other procedures, this technology is sometimes also appropriate for hysterectomy, and is called **laparoscopically assisted vaginal hysterectomy.** In this operation, the laparoscope is used to visually assist the surgeon while the uterus is removed through the vagina. The cost of the laparoscopic procedure is generally higher than that for either abdominal or non-laparoscopically assisted vaginal hysterectomy, due to a relatively longer operating time. It also requires special surgical skills. However, laparoscopically assisted vaginal hysterectomy tends to cause fewer complications than the abdominal approach and is gaining in popularity.[45]

Laparoscopic hysterectomy, requires three small external incisions: one in the navel and two in the lower abdomen. The laparoscope, really a miniature microscope, is placed into the abdominal cavity. The surgeon views the uterus and related organs on the video screen hooked up to the scope. Surgical instruments are introduced through the other tiny incisions, and the uterus is freed from connective tissue and removed through an internal incision in the vagina.

If your cervix is healthy, a single puncture in the navel may be used both for the laparoscope and for removal of the body of the uterus and the fallopian tubes, and ovaries if necessary. This is an alternative to the three-puncture method and is appropriate only if the cervix is to be retained.[46]

Laparoscopic hysterectomy takes places in the operating room of the hospital, and you are placed under anesthesia. Recovery time within the hospital is usually about two days. Most women are back to normal within a month.[47]

Laparoscopic hysterectomy is not risk-free. As with laparoscopic myomectomy, it is important that you find a surgeon who is skilled in this relatively new procedure.

Abdominal Approaches · Until fairly recently, almost all hysterectomies were performed through large incisions in the abdomen. This remains the most common method for removal of the uterus and related organs. However, new techniques are constantly being explored. For example, absorbable staples, in contrast to traditional sutures, speed surgery and reduce recovery time.[48] In general, you can expect to stay in the hospital for three to six days and to require four to six weeks before you can resume your normal life. Chapter Seven provides information on the risks and potential benefits of this surgical procedure, and Chapters Eight and Nine discuss the hospital experience.

If an abdominal approach seems appropriate, an important discussion must still occur between you and your doctor. You should know what type of abdominal incision your surgeon plans to make, and the reasons for this decision.

Vertical incision. The longitudinal abdominal incision cuts vertically from the belly button to the pubic hairline. It may be necessary to use this method to fully explore the internal organs and remove all diseased parts. Unfortunately, no matter how well it heals, a large scar will always be an obvious reminder of the surgery. (See Chapter Nine, pages 154 – 155, for hints on minimizing scar sensitivity.)

The bikini cut. The transverse or **Pfannenstiel incision,** otherwise known as the bikini cut, is done for reasons of vanity. Because the incision is made horizontally, directly above the pubic hairline, the resulting scar will be practically unnoticeable. The bikini cut generally requires more effort than the vertical procedure and may not always be appropriate. However, if scar placement is important to you, this should be an area in which you are assertive about your desires when you speak with your doctor.

WHAT'S COMING OUT: SAVING YOUR OVARIES

Remember, in medical terms, hysterectomy is the surgical removal of the uterus and usually the fallopian tubes. A separate operation, an oophorectomy, may be performed at the same time to remove the ovaries. You should be very clear about what surgery is planned for you.

Both surgical procedures may be necessary. However, when only the uterus is affected (such as fibroids with no ovarian involvement, or uterine prolapse), the ovaries may be able to be left in place.

The issue of removing the ovaries for those conditions which only involve the uterus is a sensitive one, with supporting research available to buttress arguments on both sides.

Cancer prevention. Physicians often recommend the removal of the ovaries to prevent the possibility of ovarian cancer later in life. A review of scientific literature suggests that 12 percent of ovarian cancers might be avoided if the ovaries were removed at the time of elective hysterectomy.[49]

If you are "at risk" for ovarian cancer (See Chapter Five), or if the reason for your hysterectomy is uterine malignancy, then removal of your ovaries along with your uterus is usually advisable. Similarly, the reverse: Removal of the uterus along with the ovaries is appropriate medical procedure in cases of ovarian cancer.[50]

On the other hand, in a study of 609 women who had their ovaries removed at the time of hysterectomy for benign reasons such as fibroids, uterine prolapse, and uterine bleeding, *none* were found to have malignant ovarian disease. There is no evidence that such women are more likely to develop ovarian cancer than non-hysterectomized women.[51]

Ovarian function. Chapters Two and Eleven detail the value of the ovaries' production of estrogen in preventing osteoporosis and coronary heart disease and in contributing to general health. We do not want to part with them frivolously.

How long can we hope to benefit from our ovaries? At menopause the ovaries decline naturally, so perhaps those of us who are near or past menopause at the time of hysterectomy might more easily agree to oopherectomy. In addition, about one in four women who have had their uterus removed but retained their ovaries quickly lose ovarian function anyway. This may be due to the decrease in blood supply and nutrients that the ovaries receive when there is no uterus.[52]

Contrary evidence, however, was reported by physicians at the Christchurch School of Medicine in New Zealand. They found no decline in ovarian function following hysterectomy, and concluded that the ovaries of women who have no uterus behave no differently from those of other women.[53]

Given the often negative impact of premature menopause, "preventive" oopherectomy may be as unjustifiable as removing any other healthy part of the body. When we recognize the importance of the ovaries and the hormones they produce for physical health and sexual well-being (See Chapters Two and Eleven), many experts agree that they should not be removed "to prevent the possibility of disease later on"— unless specific indications point to potential problems. You need to evaluate your own medical background before speaking out for retention or removal of your ovaries.

Table 6 – 3 summarizes surgical options.

TABLE 6 – 3
SURGICAL OPTIONS

Procedure	Indications
Loop excision (LEEP)	"Suspicious" cervical cells
Cryosurgery	"Suspicious" cervical cells
Cone biopsy or conization	"Suspicious" cervical cells
Dilation & curettage (D&C)	Menstrual problems
Myomectomy	Uterine fibroids
Vaginal	
Laparoscopic	
Abdominal	
Endometrial ablation	Uterine fibroids
Laser treatment	Benign uterine cysts
Electrosurgery	Heavy painful periods due to hormone imbalance
Hysterectomy	Uterine fibroids
Vaginal	Prolapsed uterus
	Endometriosis
	Vaginal cancer in situ
Laparoscopic	Fibroids
	Endometriosis
Abdominal	Fibroids
	Endometriosis
	Cancer in situ
Hysterectomy with bilateral salpingo-oopherectomy	Uterine or ovarian cancer or "at risk" for these

Note: In all cases, deciding whether to agree to a particular procedure is dependent on many factors. These must be discussed fully with your physician.

INFORMED CONSENT

All hospitals which are accredited by the **Joint Commission for Accreditation of Healthcare Organizations (JCAHO)** are legally required to obtain the informed consent of their patients. Therefore, when prospective patients enter a hospital, they are provided with an agreement to sign that summarizes the hospital's procedures and states inherent risks. The contents of the paper are usually explained and an opportunity for questions provided.

Since 1988, some states, such as California and New York, have laws requiring that women provide "informed consent" to a hysterectomy in addition to signing the general hospital release. The consent statement describes possible risks and complications of the surgery. At this time, you may be orally given information regarding usual length of stay in the hospital, full recovery time, costs, and alternatives to this procedure. You will be asked to sign a separate release for your anesthesia.

Does information increase anxiety? Several studies have confirmed that knowing what can go wrong does not significantly increase anxiety. Recognition of options provides each individual with a sense of self-determination and of control. Informed participation in medical decisions demonstrates a respect for the patient and contributes to better outcomes.[54]

If you have read this far in this book, you will clearly read all consent forms provided to you. In addition, you have the right — and responsibility — to ask pertinent questions right up to the moment when you are anesthetized. See Table 6 – 4 for suggestions. You are entitled to full information at every step of the way: before you enter the hospital, during your stay, and afterward.

Today's patients are "empowered participant(s) in decision-making processes";[55] we now have voices that must be heard.

TABLE 6 – 4
QUESTIONS TO ASK YOUR SURGEON

What are the risks involved with this particular surgery, and what is the success rate?
How long will I be in the hospital?
What type of approach will you use — vaginal, laparoscopic, or abdominal?
If you do an abdominal approach, what type of incision will you make — vertical or bikini cut? How big will it be?
Will the scar be noticeable?
How much does such an operation and follow-up care cost?
Will I need nursing care at home?
When can I go back to work?
How will this affect my sexual functioning?
Can this kind of surgery be done on an outpatient basis?
What might happen if I choose not to have surgery?
Can I wait and think about it?
How many of these surgeries have you performed? When was the most recent one?
How many of these surgeries have been done in this particular hospital?
What type of anesthesia will be needed?
Will the anesthesia be covered by my insurance? (In some but not all hospitals, Blue Cross/Blue Shield coverage includes anesthesia.)

THE DECISION IS MADE

As a result of a second (and if necessary a third and fourth) opinion, you have decided to have a hysterectomy. The next set of decisions concern which doctor and hospital to use.

SELECTING YOUR SURGEON

Several things should be considered in choosing a surgeon. Presumably, one of the prerequisites in your original choice of personal gynecologist was that he/she was board certified. In Chapter Three we described the importance of board certification for a specialist. Research has indicated better medical outcomes when surgery is performed by a board certified physician.[56]

Even if your doctor is board certified, you might want to check the subspecialty. For example, if you have endometriosis, you might seek a gynecologist who specializes in reproductive endocrinology; for cancer, you might look for a gynecological oncologist.

When you interview a prospective surgeon, you should ask how often he or she performs surgery. Like anything else, the more frequently you do something, the greater the likelihood of increased competence. Optimally you would like your surgeon to be performing approximately six to eight hysterectomies per month. Many more surgeries might indicate unnecessary operations; and fewer might mean insufficient experience with the procedure.

What are your surgeon's experiences with myomectomies and other options to hysterectomy? You want a physician who is open to the possibility of a variety of surgical procedures.

The normal stay for an uncomplicated abdominal hysterectomy is three to six days. Find out from your doctor how long his or her patients usually remain in the hospital.

Other factors which might influence your final choice of surgeon might include: whether the doctor is willing to talk and explain things without condescension; whether you are rushed in and out of the office; and finally, financial considerations. (See the section below on paying the bills.) One final note: The surgical team should consist of the surgeon, a first assistant, an anesthesiologist, a scrub nurse, and a circulating nurse.[57] You might want to confirm with your prospective doctor the proposed makeup of the team for your surgery.

SELECTING THE HOSPITAL

Hospitals are not all alike. There can be major differences between a proprietary (profit-making) and a not-for-profit hospital and between a hospital run by a religious order, a community hospital, and a university-affiliated hospital. In some cases, your chosen doctor will not have operating privileges in the hospital of your choice — which will leave you with a hard decision to make.

If you choose a community hospital, you might want to make sure that pelvic operations are performed there frequently. Dr. Robert Arnot suggests that several hundred pelvic procedures a year at a hospital is a desirable minimum. You should also confirm that the hospital has a surgical intensive care unit and a physician available 24 hours a day to respond to emergencies.[58]

If your hysterectomy is because of cancer, you might consider seeking a hospital with a reputation for excelling in the treatment of gynecological oncology. Another possibility would be a hospital that is designated a National Cancer Institute Center (see the list in the Appendix). You might also want to consult *The Best Medicine: How to Choose the Top Doctors, the Top Hospitals, and the Top Treatments,* by Dr. Robert Arnot, for his list of hospitals that have reputations as centers of excellence for gynecology.

In Chapter Seven we discuss mortality rates associated with hysterectomy. Your choice of hospital should have a comparable rate; for example,. approximately .2 percent for abdominal hysterectomy and .02 percent for vaginal hysterectomy.

Paying the Bills

INSURANCE: INS AND OUTS

It is important to know what the operation will cost and whether your medical insurance will cover the entire procedure or the main portion (that is, 80 percent) of the bill. Some HMOs will allow you to choose only a doctor who is enrolled within their plan, which might limit your options.

Be aware that major medical plans pay what they consider to be a "reasonable and customary amount for the procedure." That figure could be significantly lower than what the surgeon charges. If that is the case, you will be responsible both for a deductible and also for the difference between your insurance company's level of reimbursement and the doctor's price. When physician's fees are significantly higher than the "reasonable and customary amount," some women report success in negotiating a lower charge with their doctors. It certainly is worth a try.

A SOUVENIR

By the way, if you are interested in having your uterus as a memento — the time to ask for it is prior to surgery. Once informed, your doctor can take the steps necessary to preserve the structure.

ENDNOTES

1. Kramon, G. Medical second-guessing — in advance. *New York Times,* February 24, 1991.

2. Moyers, Bill. *Healing and the Mind.* New York: Doubleday, 1993.

3. Tkac, D., ed. *The Doctor's Book of Home Remedies.* Emmaus, PA: Rodale Press, 1990.

Weed, S. S. *Menopausal Years: The Wise Woman Way.* Woodstock, NY: Ash Tree Publishing, 1992.

4. Tkac, D. (Ed.). *The Doctor's Book of Home Remedies.* Emmaus, PA: Rodale Press, 1990.

5. Tkac, D. (Ed.). *The Doctor's Book of Home Remedies.* Emmaus, PA: Rodale Press, 1990.

6. Weed, S. S. *Menopausal Years: The Wise Woman Way.* Woodstock, NY: Ash Tree Publishing, 1992.

7. Hufnagel, V., with Golant, S. K. *No More Hysterectomies.* New York: New American Library, 1988.

8. Donnez, J., Schrurs, B., Gillerot, S., et al. Treatment of uterine fibroids with implants of gonadotropin-releasing hormone agonist: assessment by hysterography. *Fertility & Sterility,* June 1989, 51 (6), 947 – 950.

9. *Consumer Reports.* Hysterectomy and its alternatives. September 1990, 603 – 607.

Goldfarb, H. A. with Grief, J. *The No-Hysterectomy Option: Your Body — Your Choice.* New York: John Wiley, 1990.

Goldrath, M. H. Use of Danazol in hysteroscopic surgery for menorrhagia. *Journal of Reproductive Medicine,* January 1990, 35 (1 Suppl), 91 – 96.

10. Goldfarb, H. A. with Grief, J. *The No-Hysterectomy Option: Your Body — Your Choice.* New York: John Wiley, 1990.

11. Mitchell Levine, M.D., personal communication.

12. Tierney, Jr., L.M., McPhee, S. J., & Papadakis, M.A., eds. *Current Medical Diagnosis & Treatment 1994.* Los Altos, CA: Appleton & Lange, 1994.

13. Tierney, Jr., L.M., McPhee, S. J., & Papadakis, M.A., eds. *Current Medical Diagnosis & Treatment 1994.* Los Altos, CA: Appleton & Lange, 1994.

Tkac, D. (Ed.). *The Doctor's Book of Home Remedies.* Emmaus, PA: Rodale Press, 1990.

14. Hufnagel, V., with Golant, S. K. *No More Hysterectomies.* New York: New American Library, 1988.

15. Wigfall-Williams, W. *Hysterectomy: Learning the Facts, Coping with the Feelings, Facing the Future.* New York: Michael Kesend, 1986.

16. Haas, K., & Haas, A. *Understanding Sexuality,* 3rd ed. St. Louis, MO: Mosby-Yearbook, 1993.

17. Tkac, D. (Ed.). *The Doctor's Book of Home Remedies.* Emmaus, PA: Rodale Press, 1990.

18. Tkac, D. (Ed.). *The Doctor's Book of Home Remedies.* Emmaus, PA: Rodale Press, 1990.

19. Weed, S. S. *Menopausal Years: The Wise Woman Way.* Woodstock, NY: Ash Tree Publishing, 1992.

20. Benson, R. C., and Pernoll, M. L. *Benson and Pernoll's Handbook of Obstetrics and Gynecology,* 9th edition, McGraw-Hill, 1993.

21. Apgar, B. S., Wright, T. C. Jr., & Pfenninger, J. L. Loop electrosurgical excision procedure for CIN. *American Family Physician,* August 1992, 46 (2), 505 –520.

22. Goldfarb, H. A., with Grief, J. *The No-Hysterectomy Option: Your Body — Your Choice.* New York: John Wiley, 1990.

Hufnagel, V., with Golant, S. K. *No More Hysterectomies.* New York: New American Library, 1988.

Benson, R. C., and Pernoll, M. L. *Benson and Pernoll's Handbook of Obstetrics and Gynecology,* 9th edition, McGraw-Hill, 1993.

23. Carlson, K. J., Nichols, D. H., & Schiff, I. Indications for hysterectomy. *The New England Journal of Medicine,* March 25, 1993, 328 (12), 856 – 860.

Sobel, D. S., & Ferguson, T. *The People's Book of Medical Tests.* New York: Summit Books, 1985.

24. Brooks, P. G., Loffer, F. D., & Serden, S. P. Resectoscopic removal of symptomatic intrauterine lesions. *Journal of Reproductive Medicine,* July 1989, 34 (7) 435 – 437.

Gehlbach, D. L., Sousa, R. C., Carpenter, S. E., et al. Abdominal myomectomy in the treatment of infertility. *International Journal of Gynaecology and Obstetrics,* January 1993, 40 (1), 45 – 50.

Smith, D. C., & Uhlir, J. K. Myomectomy as a reproductive procedure. *American Journal of Obstetrics and Gynecology,* June 1990, 162 (6), 1476 –1479.

Verkauf, B. S. Changing trends in treatment of leiomyomata uteri. *Current Opinion in Obstetrics and Gynecology,* June 1993, 5 (3), 301– 310.

25. Beyth, Y., Jaffe, R., & Goldberger, S. Uterine remodeling following conservative myomectomy. *Acta Obstetrica Gynecologia Scandinavia,* December 1992, 71 (8), 632 – 635.

26. Garcia, C. R. Management of symptomatic fibroids in women older than 40 years of age: hysterectomy or myomectomy. *Obstetrics and Gynecology Clinics of North America,* June 1, 1993, 20 (2), 337.

27. Ben-Baruch, G., Schiff, E., Menashe, Y., et al. Immediate and late outcome of vaginal myomectomy for prolapsed pedunculated submucous myoma. *Obstetrics and Gynecology,* December 1988, 72 (6), 858 – 861.

28. Goldrath, M. H. Vaginal removal of the pedunculated submucous myoma. Historical observations and development of a new procedure. *Journal of Reproductive Medicine,* October 1990, 35 (10), 92 – 94.

29. Corson, S. L., & Brooks, P. G. Resectoscopic myomectomy. *Fertility and Sterility,* June 1991, 55 (6), 1041 – 1044.

30. Corson, S. L., & Brooks, P. G. Resectoscopic myomectomy. *Fertility and Sterility,* June 1991, 55 (6), 1041 – 1044.

Pace, S., Franceschini, P., & Figliolini, M. Myomectomy via hysteroscopy. Indications, techniques, results. *Minerva Ginecologica,* December 1992, 44 (12), 623 – 628.

Serden, S. P., & Brooks, P. G. Treatment of abnormal uterine bleeding with the gynecologic resectoscope. *Journal of Reproductive Medicine,* October 1991, 36 (10), 697 – 699.

31. Dubuisson, J. B., Lecuru, F., Foulot, H., et al. Myomectomy by laparoscopy: a preliminary report of 43 cases. *Fertility and Sterility,* November 1991, 56 (5), 827 – 830.

32. Altman, L. K. Standard training in laparoscopy found inadequate. *New York Times,* December 14, 1993, c3.

33. Andrei, B., Caltabiano, M., Crovini, G., et al. From laparotomy to pelviscopy. A new trend. *Minerva Ginecologica,* July-August 1992, 44 (7– 8), 345 – 348.

Foulot, H., & Lecuru, F. Other indications: tubal sterilization, medically assisted procreation, salpingitis, fibromas. *Revista Paulista de Medicini,* December 1, 1991, 41 (25) 2567 – 2569.

Nezhat, C., Nezhat, F., Silfen, S. L., et al. Laparoscopic myomectomy. *International Journal of Fertility,* September – October 1991, 36 (5), 275 –280.

Sutton, C. Operative laparoscopy. *Current Opinion in Obstetrics and Gynecology,* June 1992, 4 (3), 430 – 438.

34. Altchek, A. Management of fibroids. *Current Opinion in Obstetrics and Gynecology,* June 1992, 4 (3), 463 – 471.

Reyniak, J. V., & Corenthal, L. Microsurgical laser technique for abdominal myomectomy. *Microsurgery,* 1987, 8 (2), 92 – 98.

35. al-Taher, H., & Farquharson, R. G. Management of uterine fibroids. *British Journal of Hospital Medicine,* July 14 – August 17 1993, 50 (2 – 3), 133 – 136.

Christiansen, J. K. The facts about fibroids. Presentation and latest management options. *Postgraduate Medicine,* September 1, 1993, 94 (3), 129 –134, 137.

Letterie, G. S., Coddington, C. C., Winkel, C. A., et al. Efficacy of a gonadotropin-releasing hormone agonist in the treatment of uterine leimyomata: long-term follow-up. *Fertility and Sterility,* June 1989, 51 (6), 951– 956.

36. Christiansen, J. K. The facts about fibroids. Presentation and latest management options. *Postgraduate Medicine,* September 1, 1993, 94 (3), 129 – 134, 137.

Shaw, R. W. New approaches to the management of fibroids. *Current Opinion in Obstetrics and Gynecology,* December 1991, 3 (6), 859 – 864.

37. Friedman, A. J., Daly, M., Juneau-Norcross, M., et al. Recurrence of myomas after myomectomy in women pretreated with leuprolide acetate depot or placebo. *Fertility and Sterility,* July 1992, 58 (1) 205 – 208.

38. Hufnagel, V., with Golant, S. K. *No More Hysterectomies.* New York: New American Library, 1988.

39. Baggish, M. S., & Daniell, J. F. Catastrophic injury secondary to the use of coaxial gas-cooled fibers and artificial sapphire tips for intrauterine surgery: a report of five cases. *Lasers in Surgery and Medicine,* 1989, 9 (6), 581– 584.

Dallay, D., Tissot, H., & Portal, F. Endometrial ablation by fiberoptic hysteroscopy and YAG laser. *Journal of Gynecological and Obstetrical Reproduction* (Paris), 1992, 21 (4) 431– 435.

Lefler, H. T. Jr. Premenstrual syndrome improvement after laser ablation of the endometrium for menorrhagia. *Journal of Reproductive Medicine,* November 1989, 34 (11), 905 – 906.

Lomanno, J. Endometrial ablation for the treatment of menorrhagia: a comparison of patients with normal, enlarged, and fibroid uteri. *Lasers in Surgery and Medicine,* 1991, 11 (1), 8 –12.

40. Daniell, J. F., Kurtz, B. R., & Ke, R. W. Hysteroscopic endometrial ablation using the rollerball electrode. *Obstetrics and Gynecology,* September 1992, 80 (3 Part 1), 329 – 332.

Goldfarb, H. A. with Grief, J. *The No-Hysterectomy Option: Your Body — Your Choice.* New York: John Wiley, 1990.

McLucas, B. Intrauterine applications of the resectoscope. *Surgery, Gynecology and Obstetrics,* June 1, 1991, 172 (6), 425.

Petrucco, O. M., & Gillespie, A. The neodymium: YAG laser and the resectoscope for the treatment of menorrhagia. *Medical Journal of Australia,* April 15, 1991, 154 (8), 518 – 520.

41. Hoffman, M. S., & Jaeger, M. A new method for gaining entry into the scarred anterior cul-de-sac during transvaginal hysterectomy. *American Journal of Obstetrics and Gynecology,* May 1990, 162 (5), 1269 – 1270.

42. Tierney, Jr., L.M., McPhee, S. J., & Papadakis, M.A., eds. *Current Medical Diagnosis & Treatment 1994.* Los Altos, CA: Appleton & Lange, 1994.

43. Powers, T. W., Goodno, J. A. Jr., & Harris, V. D. The outpatient vaginal hysterectomy. *American Journal of Obstetrics and Gynecology,* June 1993, 168 (6 Part 1), 1875 –1878.

Stovall, T. G., Summitt, R. L. Jr., Bran, D. F., et al. Outpatient vaginal hysterectomy: a pilot study. *Obstetrics and Gynecology,* July 1992, 80 (1), 145 –149.

44. Kudo, R., Yamauchi, O., Okazaki, T., et al. Vaginal hysterectomy without ligation of the ligaments of the cervix uteri. *Surgery, Gynecology and Obstetrics,* January 30, 1991, 170 (4), 299 – 305.

45. Boike, G. M., Elfstrand, E. P., DelPriore, G., et al. Laparoscopically assisted vaginal hysterectomy in a university hospital: report of 82 cases and comparison with abdominal and vaginal hysterectomy. *American Journal of Obstetrics and Gynecology,* June 1993, 168 (6 Part 1), 1690 –1697.

46. Pelosi, M. A., & Pelosi, M. A., 3rd. Laparoscopic supracervical hysterectomy using a single umbilical puncture (mini-laparoscopy). *Journal of Reproductive Medicine,* September 1992, 37 (9), 777–784.

47. Ben-Rafael, Z., Dicker, D., Farhi, J., et al. Laparoscopic hysterectomy. *Harefuah,* December 1, 1992, 123 (11), 443 – 445, 508.

48. Beresford, J. M., & Moher, D. A prospective comparison of abdominal hysterectomy using absorbable staples. *Surgery, Gynecology and Obstetrics,* June 1993, 176 (6), 555 – 558.

49. Schwartz, P. E. The role of prophylactic oophorectomy in the avoidance of ovarian cancer. *International Journal of Gynaecological Obstetrics,* November 1992, 39 (3), 175 –184.

50. Barber, H. R. Prophylaxis in ovarian cancer. *Cancer,* February 15, 1993, 71 (4 Suppl), 1529 –1533.

Parker, M., Bosscher, J., Barnhill, D., et al. Ovarian management during radical hysterectomy in the premenopausal patient. *Obstetrics and Gynecology,* August 1993, 82 (2), 187– 190.

51. Loizzi, P., Carriero, C., Di Gesu, A., et al. Removal or preservation of ovaries

during hysterectomy: a six-year review. *International Journal of Gynecology and Obstetrics,* 1990, 31, 257 – 261.

52. Parker, M., Bosscher, J., Barnhill, D., et al. Ovarian management during radical hysterectomy in the premenopausal patient. *Obstetrics and Gynecology,* August 1993, 82 (2), 187– 190.

53. Metcalf, M. G., Braiden, V., & Livesey, J. H. Retention of normal ovarian function after hysterectomy. *Journal of Endocrinology,* December 1992, 135 (3), 597– 602.

54. Kerrigan, D. D., Thevasagayam, R. S., Woods, T. O., et al. Who's afraid of informed consent? *British Medical Journal,* January 30, 1993, 306 (6873), 298 – 300.

Reiser, S. J. Consumer competence and the reform of American health care. *Journal of the American Medical Association,* March 18, 1992, 267 (11), 1511 – 1515.

Searight, H. R. Assessing patient competence for medical decision making. *American Family Physician,* February 1992, 751–759.

Wu, W. C., & Pearlman, R. A. Consent in medical decision making: the role of communication. *Journal of General Internal Medicine.* January-February 1988, 3 (1), 9 – 14.

55. Zussman, R. Life in the hospital: a review. *Milbank Quarterly,* 1993, 71 (1), 167 – 185.

56. Brody, J. Surgery study aims criticism at nonsurgeons. *New York Times,* October 21, 1976.

57. Arnot, R. *The Best Medicine: How to Choose the Top Doctors, the Top Hospitals, and the Top Treatments.* Reading, Mass.: Addison-Wesley, 1992.

58. Arnot, R. *The Best Medicine: How to Choose the Top Doctors, the Top Hospitals, and the Top Treatments.* Reading, Mass.: Addison-Wesley, 1992.

SUGGESTED READING

Cox, Kathryn. *Well-Informed Patient's Guide to Hysterectomy.* New York: Dell, 1991.

Culter, Winnifred. *Hysterectomy: Before and After.* New York: HarperCollins, 1990.

Goldfarb, Herbert, with Judith Grief. *The No-Hysterectomy Option: Your Body — Your Choice.* New York: John Wiley, 1990.

Hufnagel, Vicki G., with Susan K. Golant. *No More Hysterectomies.* New York: NAL/Dutton, 1989.

Lee, Florence C. *Facts about Ginseng: The Elixir of Life.* Elizabeth, NJ: Hollym International Corporation, 1993.

Null, Gary. *Healing Your Body Naturally.* Avenal, NJ: Outlet Book Company (Division of Random House), 1993.

Payer, Lynn. *How to Avoid a Hysterectomy.* New York: Pantheon Books, 1987.

Prevention Magazine Staff. *Compete Book of Vitamins and Minerals.* Avenal, NJ: Outlet Book Company (Division of Random House), 1992.

Weed, S. S. *Menopausal Years: The Wise Woman Way.* Woodstock, NY: Ash Tree, 1992.

West, Stanley, with Paula Dranov. *The Hysterectomy Hoax.* New York: Doubleday, 1994.

Chapter 7

RISKS AND COMPLICATIONS

"I developed a skin rash in my body orifices and on my skin with itching and fever. This was totally unexpected." — Yvonne, age 51

"I could not urinate for a couple of days after the surgery. That made me nervous because I wouldn't be able to go home until I did." — Rhoda, age 53

"Eight months after the hysterectomy I had emergency surgery for adhesions, and this was not something I was prepared for or expected." — Pamela, age 47

RISK / BENEFIT DECISION

In Chapter Four we discussed the conditions which might indicate a need for surgical treatment. Only about 10 percent of hysterectomies are performed to save lives; the rest are intended to relieve symptoms and are considered to be elective surgery.[1]

When faced with making a decision as to whether to have an elective hysterectomy, you need to weigh the benefits against the risks. For example, be aware that research has *not* shown that it prolongs life or improves its quality — in terms of no further medical problems.[2] Also, it is not clear how many disorders now treated with a hysterectomy could be resolved with alternative therapies. Those alternative treatments represent a more conservative approach and may be less costly in terms of health dollars, morbidity (illness), and mortality (death). See Chapter Six for a description of the various treatment options.

The other factors to consider are discussed in detail in Chapter Twelve. They are the long-term after effects that might occur as a result of estrogen deficiency, such as early postmenopausal symptoms, increased risk of cardiovascular disease, osteoporosis, and cancer induced by hormone replacement therapy. Any woman who is premenopausal and whose surgery will involve oopherectomy must consider these specific risks as compared with the benefits.

It is said that some wise doctor warned "curing a pelvic disease with a hysterectomy is the equivalent of treating a mild headache with decapitation. Treat the disease, don't get rid of the organ."

Anti-Hysterectomy Hysteria

Because hysterectomy has been correctly cited as an abused procedure — one where needless numbers of women have had their uterus (and ovaries) removed unnecessarily; and because it involves the organ that is most involved with womanhood; and because there are risks, complications, and long-term problems; hysterectomy has become an easy target for criticism.

While negative publicity is important in making women aware of the risk/benefit choices they face, some of the negative media hype can be hurtful to those of us faced with hysterectomy decisions.

NOTE: Negative consequences do not *occur to all or even a majority of women who have hysterectomies. But when you read some of the publications and hear lectures by some anti-hysterectomy advocates, you may begin to wonder whether* any *condition warrants a hysterectomy.*

An example of hype and misinformation was evident in a lecture by Nora Coffey, president of *Hysterectomy Educational Referral Service* (HERS) and a leading anti-hysterectomy proponent. In the lecture Coffey stated, among other things, that hysterectomy widened her bones, changed her walk, destroyed her family life, and left her castrated. She further noted that she could identify other women who had hysterectomies by their unique walk.[3]

A woman in definite and appropriate need of a hysterectomy would be tempted to cancel the surgery after hearing this very convincing lecture. At the least she would come away seriously frightened.

While we recognize that hysterectomy is an overused operation, so is cardiac bypass surgery and carpal tunnel syndrome surgery, to name just a few procedures sometimes judged to be unnecessary. Yet a hysterical outcry is not heard against those surgeries as it is against hysterectomy.

We not only acknowledge that hysterectomy is performed many times unnecessarily, we also know the importance of publicizing this fact. What troubles us is the swing to the other extreme, which is the "no more hysterectomies" position. Hopefully, a middle ground will shortly be reached, where hysterectomies will be performed only for appropriate reasons.

SURGICALLY CAUSED PROBLEMS

Hysteria aside, we must recognize that hysterectomy is not a procedure to be entered into lightly. Even the simplest and most routine surgery can create problems and complications. In considering whether you should undergo a hysterectomy, keep in mind that unless the benefits are sufficient to warrant the risks, you might be better off keeping your uterus and seeking alternatives.

Real Dangers

Hysterectomy is major surgery. Under anesthesia, your abdomen will be penetrated and your interior organs will be probed and excised. Assuming all goes well on the operating table, you're still not out of the woods. During recovery you continue to face the possibility of suffering from complications that arise from the surgery or from being in the hospital. **Iatrogenic** problems "caused" by the medical care system include infections and surgical mishaps such as damage to surrounding organs. Infections, which appear to be hospital-generated, account for a substantial number of problems to patients. Once you're home, you face the possibility of complications developing over the course of the next several years. These are discussed in the following pages.

POSTOPERATIVE COMPLICATIONS

Complications causing illness and/or suffering are possible following hysterectomy. Postoperative complication rates are astounding! They are reported as 24 percent for vaginal hysterectomy and 43 percent for abdominal hysterectomies.[4] Although most studies point to the surgery as the cause of the problems, a recent study attributed the major cause to preexisting medical disorders rather than surgical complications.[5] This suggests that if you are reasonably healthy when you enter surgery, you are generally unlikely to experience problems.

What Can Go Wrong? · According to Dr. Robert Arnot, hysterectomy is major surgery with complications in up to half of all patients.[6] Postoperative fever and infections account for the majority of complications.[7] More serious problems include hemorrhage requiring transfusion, damage to surrounding organs such as the bowel and ureter, the sudden need for unintended surgery (to correct a problem caused by the hysterectomy), life-threatening cardiopulmonary problems, and complications of general anesthesia.

Blood transfusions, required by 8 to 15 percent of patients, carry the small risk of transmitting a bloodborne disease such as hepatitis or AIDS.[8] This can be prevented by making an **autologous blood donation.** You can prepare for surgery by donating blood for your own use should that be necessary. (See Chapter Eight for more information.)

Improving Your Odds · Lower complication rates can be found in large urban teaching hospitals (which you would expect after reading the discussion in Chapter Three). At these hospitals, major complications occur only in approximately 3 percent of hysterectomies for non-cancerous conditions.[9] This should be compared to the 24 to 43 percent incidence generally reported.

As noted earlier, vaginal hysterectomies have a lower complication rate than abdominal hysterectomies. Women who undergo abdominal hysterectomy have longer postoperative hospital stays and convalescent periods, experience more problems with fever, and receive more blood transfusions. Ask your surgeon whether a vaginal approach is appropriate for you. If it is, then you should request it.

While newer hysterectomy procedures such as laparoscopically assisted vaginal hysterectomy may lower postoperative complications, data to support this supposition is not yet available because these procedures are so new.[10]

LONG-TERM PROBLEMS

Many studies describe a variety of long-term effects from hysterectomy. Repeat surgery for complications related to the original hysterectomy is estimated to be necessary in as many as 15 percent of patients.[11]

Urinary Complaints · The major well-documented long-term effect experienced by women who have had hysterectomies arises from urinary problems. Problems include increased frequency of urination, urinary stress incontinence, urethral obstructions, and fistulas (abnormal passages between the urethra and either the outside body surface or the anus or vagina).[12] Two studies reported by Parys and colleagues support the view that damage to the pelvic parasympathetic nerves is responsible for chronic bladder dysfunction after hysterectomy.[13] Because the incidence of this is high (estimated to be from about 5 percent[14] to 20 to 30 percent of all hysterectomies[15]), Parys and colleagues stress that meticulous attention should be paid by the surgeon to operative techniques so as to avoid bladder problems.

Another common problem, urinary tract infection, was reported as occurring more frequently in women who had hysterectomies.[16] This was reflected in higher rates of physician visits by this group compared with two age-matched groups, one that had other surgery and one that had no surgery. The results of that research led the study's author to question whether hysterectomy had actually improved a woman's quality of life, given the more frequent doctor's office visits after the surgery.[17]

Hormone Deficiency · For many premenopausal women who have undergone a hysterectomy and oophorectomy, the long-term negative effects are related to the sudden drop in hormone levels. See Chapter Eleven for a discussion on hormone replacement therapy.

Early ovarian failure also occurs in some women who have not had their ovaries removed during hysterectomy. (About 60 to 65 percent of women retain their ovaries.) For a number of those women, a reduction in hormone production occurs within one to two years.[18] These women face early unexpected menopausal symptoms which frequently and repeatedly cause them to visit doctors.[19]

The uterus itself is also a source of hormones whose functions, although not yet fully understood, may play a more important role in female endocrinology and immunology than is currently realized. Further research will prove or disprove this conjecture.

Sexual Function · A small percentage of women report a lessening of sexual pleasure. This might be explained by the fact that the uterus normally contracts during orgasm, and its removal might affect sexual sensations. However, the findings of some studies comparing the same women before and after their hysterectomies suggest improvement or no change in sexual functioning after hysterectomy.[20] Further, even if one experiences some loss of sexual sensations, it does not have to lead to sexual dysfunction. For a more complete discussion of this topic, see Chapter Ten.

Depression and Psychological Stress · Studies comparing the same women before and after their hysterectomies for benign conditions have found no evidence that the operation leads to depression or greater psychological distress.[21] For further information on emotions following hysterectomy, see Chapter Fourteen.

Adhesions · Internal scar tissue, **adhesions,** can form following any type of surgery. For example, myomectomies may result in adhesions, especially if a considerable amount of blood has been lost.

Adhesions after hysterectomy sometimes cause obstructions affecting the intestines. These may result in chronic pain and eventually require corrective surgery.

When the ovaries have been left in place following hysterectomy, thick adhesions may form on them which prevent the development and release of eggs. Ovarian hormones may also be blocked. This condition is often painful and is called **post-operative residual ovary syndrome.**[22]

Some people seem more likely than others to develop adhesions, even when the operation was performed flawlessly. On the other hand, adhesions may often be blamed on less-than-meticulous surgical procedures. Again, this is a call to be diligent in selecting your physician and hospital. Unfortunately, adhesions may not become apparent until years after the initial surgery, so those responsible may be unaware of the damage they have caused.

DEATH

Reported mortality rates after hysterectomy range from 6 to 11 per 10,000 women when the surgery was for reasons not involving pregnancy or cancer, to 70 to 200 per 10,000 when performed because of a cancer diagnosis.[23] While the risk of death is relatively low compared to other surgical procedures, the fact that so many hysterectomies are performed brings the death rate to an estimated 600 to 2,000 deaths annually in the United States.[24]

Hysterectomy is second only to Cesarean section as the most frequently performed major operation in the United States. The tragedy here is that many women whose hysterectomies were elective and medically unnecessary die needlessly.

ON THE BRIGHT SIDE

Hysterectomy for most women is an elective procedure to treat a specific problem. For a long time, improvement of the "quality of life" was the major justification for the surgery. Once the specific gynecological problem was resolved, it was expected that these women's rate of contact with physicians and hospitals would return to that of the general population. The expectation was that the rate could be even lower than the general, nonhysterectomy population since gynecological problems account for such a high proportion of women's health needs. Data collected in Manitoba Province, Canada in 1974 confirmed this expectation for hospitalizations (though not necessarily doctors' office visits).[25] Women in this study, compared with matched controls, had sharply reduced rates of hospital admissions following their hysterectomies.

Furthermore, for many women menstrual disorders are the primary complaint prior to nonemergency, nonmandatory hysterectomy. Clearly, hysterectomy solves this problem. However, one researcher, Nora Roos observed that for this group, less than half (40 percent) had a D&C prior to admission for hysterectomy.[26] "This is of concern since good standards of practice would suggest attempting to control bleeding with a D&C before proceeding to hysterectomy."[27] In other words, the menstrual problems might have been resolved by a simpler procedure.

Although birth control alone is not a valid reason for hysterectomy, a recent study suggests that this surgery (as well as other sterilization procedures such as tubal ligation, and vasectomy for men) provides the greatest degree of contraceptive satisfaction. These procedures result in a justifiable feeling of confidence that sexual intercourse does not contain a risk of pregnancy.[29]

While we have outlined problems associated with hysterectomy, we reiterate that most women experience only minor if any complaints. In our study of 365 women, 77 percent of those who had hysterectomies reported that they were glad that they had the surgery. They enjoyed the freedom from menstrual discomfort and birth control concerns.

ENDNOTES

1. Arnot, R. *The Best Medicine: How to Choose the Top Doctors, the Top Hospitals, and the Top Treatments.* Reading, Ma: Addison-Wesley, 1992.

2. Roos, N. P. Hysterectomy in one Canadian province: a new look at risk and benefits. *American Journal of Public Health,* 1984, 74(1), 39 – 46.

3. Coffey, Nora. Lecture, SUNY at New Paltz, New Paltz, New York, November 5, 1992.

4. Dicker, R. C., Greenspank J. R., Strauss, L. T., et al. Complications of abdominal and vaginal hysterectomy among women of reproductive age in the United States: the collaborative review of sterilization. *American Journal of Obstetrics and Gynecology,* 1982, 144(7), 841– 848.

5. Boyd, M. E., & Groome, P. A. The morbidity of abdominal hysterectomy. *Canadian Journal of Surgery,* 1993, 36(2), 155 –159.

6. Arnot, R. *The Best Medicine: How to Choose the Top Doctors, the Top Hospitals, and the Top Treatments.* Reading, Ma: Addison-Wesley Publishing, 1992.

7. Carlson, K. J., Nichols, D. H., & Schiff, I. Indications for hysterectomy. *The New England Journal of Medicine,* 1993, 328(12), 856 – 860.

8. Tuomala, R. Hysterectomy. *The Harvard Medical School Health Letter,* May, 1988, 5 – 8.

9. Carlson, K. J., Nichols, D. H., & Schiff, I. Indications for hysterectomy. *The New England Journal of Medicine,* 1993, 328(12), 856 – 860.

10. Carlson, K. J., Nichols, D. H., & Schiff, I. Indications for hysterectomy. *The New England Journal of Medicine,* 1993, 328(12), 856 – 860.

11. Arnot, R. *The Best Medicine: How to Choose the Top Doctors, the Top Hospitals, and the Top Treatments.* Reading, Ma: Addison-Wesley, 1992.

12. Tancer, M. L. Observations on prevention and management of vesicovaginal fistula after total hysterectomy. *Surgical Gynecology and Obstetrics,* 1992, 175(6), 501– 506.

13. Parys, B. T., Haylen, B. T., Hutton, J. L., et al. The effects of simple hysterectomy on vesicourethral function. *British Journal of Urology,* 1989, 64(6), 594 – 599.

Parys, B. T., Woolfenden, K. A., & Parsons, K. F. Bladder dysfunction after simple hysterectomy: Urodynamic and neurological evaluation. *European Urology,* 1990, 17(2), 129 –133.

14. Parys, B. T., Haylen, B. T., Hutton, J. L., et al. The effects of simple hysterectomy on vesicourethral function. *British Journal of Urology,* 1989, 64(6), 594 –599.

15. Carlson, K. J., Nichols, D. H., & Schiff, I. Indications for hysterectomy. *The New England Journal of Medicine,* 328(12), 1993, 856 – 860.

16. Roos, N. P. Hysterectomy in one Canadian province: a new look at risk and benefits. *American Journal of Public Health,* 1984, 74(1), 39 – 46.

17. Roos, N. P. Hysterectomy in one Canadian province: a new look at risk and benefits. *American Journal of Public Health,* 1984, 74(1), 39 – 46.

18. Riedel, H., Lehmann-Willenbrock, E., & Semm, K. Ovarian failure after hysterectomy. *The Journal of Reproductive Medicine,* 1986, 31(7), 597– 600.

19. Roos, N. P. Hysterectomy in one Canadian province: a new look at risk and benefits. *American Journal of Public Health,* 1984, 74(1), 39 – 46.

20. Coöpen, A., Bishop, M., Beard, R.J. et al. Hysterectomy, hormones and behavior: a prospective study. *Lancet,* January 17, 1981, 126 –128.

Gath, D., Cooper, P., & Day, A. Hysterectomy and psychiatric disorder I. Levels of psychiatric morbidity before and after hysterectomy. *British Journal of Psychiatry,* 1982, 140, 335 – 342.

Puretz, S. L., & Haas, A. Sexual desire and responsiveness following hysterectomy and menopause. *Journal of Women and Aging,* 1993, 5(2), 3 – 15.

21. Ryan, M. M., Dennerstein, L., & Pepperell, R. Psychological aspects of hysterectomy: a one-year prospective study. *British Journal of Psychiatry,* 1989, 154, 516 – 522.

22. Hufnagel, V., with Golant, S. K. *No More Hysterectomies.* New York: New American Library, 1988.

23. Hysterectomies in New York State: a statistical profile. New York: New York State Department of Health, 1988.

Wingo, P. A., Huezo, C. M., Rubin, G. L., et al. The mortality risk associated with hysterectomy. *American Journal of Obstetrics and Gynecology,* 1982, 144, 841 – 848.

24. Arnot, R. *The Best Medicine: How to Choose the Top Doctors, the Top Hospitals, and the Top Treatments.* Reading, Ma: Addison-Wesley, 1992.

Easterday, C. L., Grimes, D. A. & Riggs, J. A. Hysterectomy in the United States. *Obstetrics and Gynecology,* 1983, 62, 203 – 212.

25. Roos, N. P. Hysterectomy in one Canadian province: a new look at risk and benefits. *American Journal of Public Health,* 1984, 74(1), 39 – 46.

26. Roos, N. P. Hysterectomy in one Canadian province: a new look at risk and benefits. *American Journal of Public Health,* 1984, 74(1), 39 – 46.

27. Roos, N. P. Hysterectomy in one Canadian province: a new look at risk and benefits. *American Journal of Public Health,* 1984, 74(1), p. 44.

28. Rosenfeld, J. A., Zahorik, R. M., & Saint, W. Women's satisfaction with birth control. *Journal of Family Practice,* 1993, 36(2), 169.

Chapter 8

GETTING READY

"I had never been in a hospital as a patient before the hysterectomy surgery. I didn't know to bring a sweater and socks — the hospital room was cold — and I had to ask my husband to bring me these things." — Judy, age 47

PREOPERATION PREPARATION

The decision has been made: you are going to have a hysterectomy. Now what?

MEDICAL INSURANCE

Probably the first thing you need to do is to contact your medical insurer. Even if you have already started the process under your medical plan of qualifying for reimbursement by having a second opinion consultation, you still must notify your insurance administrators that you are now planning to go ahead with the surgery. Your notification starts the process of preadmission certification. If you have not already done so, this may be the appropriate time to determine the extent of your medical coverage.

AUTOLOGOUS BLOOD AND IRON

The next thing to attend to is to prepare yourself for an **autologous blood donation.** Autologous means that you donate your own blood, which is then kept available for use for you in case it is needed during the surgical procedure. Although ordinarily the surgery will not cause any major loss of blood, it is wise to prepare by having your own blood available in case blood loss during surgery is extensive enough to require a transfusion. This occurs in about 8 to 15 percent of hysterectomies. In these times of anxiety about AIDS and hepatitis, having your own blood available eliminates a cause of needless worry.[1]

Autologous blood donations are made at blood banks, which are usually conveniently located in hospitals or laboratories. It is necessary to have your physician's okay — usually in the manner of a "physician statement of consent" form. You would be wise to donate two pints of blood — one pint on each of two visits.

The visits should be spaced approximately one week apart and no more than three weeks or less than one week before surgery. There usually is a fee involved (approximately $60.00 for the first donation and $40.00 for the second) which is nonrefundable and is not covered by many medical insurance policies. At the blood bank, one of the questions which you will be asked is "if you do not use your blood during surgery, can it be included as donated blood to be used for some other blood-needy individual?" Since this question raises the issue of civic responsibility to contribute to blood banks, this is an easy way to be involved.

To physically prepare for an autologous blood donation, you may be instructed to begin a regimen of iron supplements. This is to promote rapid blood regeneration following your donations. Recommendations of daily dosage vary, however, most blood banks recommend 325 mg., three times a day (usually in the form of ferrous sulfates). When taking the iron supplements, try to take the pills after eating to enhance their effectiveness. Also consider taking a Vitamin C supplement at the same time since ascorbic acid assists the effectiveness of iron absorption.

Two side effects of iron supplements to expect are: black stools — in this case, they are not indicative of a medical problem — and possible constipation or stomach problems (such as gastrointestinal upset). Constipation can usually be alleviated by varying your diet to include food which promotes bowel movement; for example, prunes, fiber, and more fluid. (For other recommendations, see Chapters Nine and Thirteen.) Avoid consuming large amounts of coffee, tea, eggs, milk, whole wheat breads or cereals before your blood donation and surgery, since they decrease iron absorption.

If you have not donated blood before, be assured that the process of donating blood is easy. Your blood pressure and iron count are checked by the nurse before blood is drawn. This is to confirm that your body is healthy enough to donate blood. The actual procedure usually takes less than ten minutes; however, because your body has lost one pint of blood, a short rest period followed by a liquid and cracker snack is routine before you are allowed to leave. If donating blood is a new experience for you, it might be advisable to have someone with you to drive you home. This is particularly important following your second donation, even if you are a regular donor.

The recommendations from the blood donor center usually will include reminders: to leave the dressing over the puncture for at least six hours and to keep the dressing dry; to drink at least one quart of fluid over the next 24 hours, to not smoke for at least one-half hour; to lie down or sit with your head between your knees if you feel faint, dizzy, flushed, too warm, or suddenly weak. If the latter symptoms persist, you are advised to return to the hospital or blood donor center. If you feel fine, you may resume your normal activities — within limits, that is. Do not go out and jog five miles, even if that is your normal activity!

DIETARY AND HEALTH CONSIDERATIONS

There is only one special precaution that you must take prior to your expected operation, and that is not to take any aspirin, which is a blood thinner, approximately five to ten days before surgery. However, you will want to be as healthy as you can be before going into surgery. Basically, that means analyzing your diet to make sure that you are getting your daily nutritional needs. According to the 1990 dietary guidelines issued by the U. S. Departments of Agriculture and Health and Human Services, a good daily diet consists of: 3 – 5 servings of vegetables; 2 – 4 servings of fruit; 6 –11 servings of bread, cereals, rice, pasta; 2 – 3 servings of milk, yogurt and cheese; and 2 – 3 servings of meats, poultry, fish, dry beans and peas, eggs or nuts. Servings vary, but some suggested equivalents include: for vegetables, 1 serving is roughly 1 cup of raw leafy greens or 1/2 cup of other vegetables; for fruit, one medium apple, orange, or banana; for grains, 1 slice of bread or 1 ounce of cereal; for milk, 1 cup of milk or 1.5 ounces of cheese; for meat and poultry, about 2 – 3 ounces of cooked lean beef or chicken without skin.

You also want to try, as much as possible, to avoid contact with people who have colds/flu or other contagious infections. Depending on your work and family life, this last recommendation may be hard to follow.

PRESURGICAL TESTING

Not so many years ago, all candidates for surgery were instructed to enter the hospital one or two days earlier for presurgical testing. In the current era of rising medical expenses and cost containment policies, presurgical testing generally is done on an outpatient basis for what is called **same day admission surgery.**

Once again, it is important to be aware of what your medical insurance plan covers. Many plans provide full coverage if the tests are done by a hospital (in outpatient service departments) but will not completely cover the same tests when done by an independent laboratory — even though the independent laboratory may be cheaper than the hospital laboratory. You may be left having to pay those private laboratories for tests which would have been at no cost to you if done in the hospital. If you have a family physician, you can request that all test results also be sent to him or her. This will ensure that your doctor has a complete medical record which can be used as a baseline in the future.

Minimum Tests Required · While hospitals have differing policies, many will require at least an **electrocardiogram** and a **hematocrit;** the hospital may also require a urinalysis.

Electrocardiogram. The purpose of this test (also known as **EKG** and **ECG**) is to evaluate heart function prior to surgery. You will be asked to recline on an examining table and electrodes (small pieces of metal on a rubber strip) will be placed on various parts of your body. A paste that conducts electricity is applied between the electrode and the skin to help pick up the heart's electrical activity. The electrodes are connected by wires to the EKG machine which records the impulses, detected by the electrodes, on a moving piece of graph paper. The various electrodes allow the heart to be evaluated from 12 different locations. The entire procedure will take approximately 15 minutes.

Hematocrit. This blood test measures the percentage of the blood volume that is made up of red blood cells. A low hematocrit percentage indicates that anemia is present. The blood for the hematocrit may be collected from a fingerstick (blood obtained from pricking the finger with a small sharp piece of metal — a lancet). This blood will be analyzed by a centrifuge designed for that purpose.

Urinalysis. A complete **urinalysis** may be requested by your physician and/or hospital. The complete urinalysis consists of a series of tests aimed at studying urine makeup. In addition to evaluating the general appearance of the urine (color, clarity, odor, appearance of foam), a dipstick analysis will pick up the presence of blood, glucose, ketones, bilirubin, protein, and urobilinogen — none of which are normally found in urine — and will measure the pH (acidity) of the urine. A urinometer is used to measure the specific gravity of the urine (the concentration of urine in comparison to plain water). Microscopic analysis is also part of the complete urinalysis.

Additional Tests · Do not be surprised if your physician requires additional tests, some of which are useful in establishing preoperation baselines and some of which may not be necessary. Those additional tests might include: a battery of blood tests, a pregnancy test, and a chest X-ray.

Blood tests. The battery of blood tests that will be run are from the blood obtained by both **venipuncture** (in which blood will be taken from a vein in the arm) and fingerstick. The blood tests could include the following:

Complete Blood Count (CBC). The CBC is one of the most commonly performed blood analyses and consists of several different tests that are automatically machine-analyzed. Of the tests, four are for the red blood cells, two are for the white blood cells, and one is a platelet test. The tests for the red blood cells are: Red Blood Cell Count, an actual measure of the red blood cells present; Hematocrit (HCT) — the one test required by the hospital — previously described; Hemoglobin (Hg), a measure of the amount of hemoglobin in the blood; and Red Blood Cell Indices, a measurement among other things of the actual size of the red blood cells.

The two CBC tests for the white blood cells include the WBC and the WBC Differential. The WBC (white blood cell count) will measure the number of white blood cells present in the blood, while the white blood cell differential will count the number of each of the five types of white cells present (neutrophils, lymphocytes, monocytes, eosinophils, and basophils) and report them as a percentage of the total number of white cells present.

The last test in the CBC is a test for the platelets (Platelet count) and is used to determine if adequate numbers of platelets are present to ensure proper clotting.

Since the mere presence of the platelets in adequate numbers does not ensure that they are working properly, the next two tests, *Prothrumbin Time* (PT) and *Activated Partial Thromboplastin Time* (APTT), are used as screening tests to measure blood clotting factors. The clotting of blood is a result of interactions between various proteins in the blood (clotting factors) and platelets. Normal ranges on these two tests are an indication that the blood will clot as expected. The PT value may reflect liver functioning since many of the clotting factors are produced by the liver. Vitamin K (which is absorbed from the intestines) is necessary for many of the clotting factors to be produced by the body.

As part of the routine blood work-up, your doctor might also direct the laboratory to do a *serology test.* Serologic testing analyzes your blood for antibodies, immune complexes and antigen-antibody reactions. In your case, the serology test will focus on the latter and will include a *Rapid Plasma Reagin* (RPR) or *Venereal Disease Research Laboratory* (VDRL). These two tests are the most common screens for syphilis — they detect an antibody-like substance in the blood which forms when an infection with syphilis is present.

A *Chem Screen,* also sometimes requested, is a multiple test panel which includes an analysis of approximately 20 items, many of which are indicators of electrolyte balance. Electrolyte testing provides important baseline information which can be referred to after surgery if problems develop. Usually included in the results are values for: albumin, bilirubin, calcium chloride, cholesterol, creatinine, glucose, magnesium, potassium, phosphorus, sodium, triglycerides, and uric acid. You might want to ask your physician to include an HDL/LDL Cholesterol analysis. This is not normally part of the Chem

Screen but can easily be included. The results will be important for later dietary recommendations, as discussed in Chapter Thirteen.

A pregnancy test and a chest X-ray may also be ordered; they may not be necessary. If you have no reason to suspect you are pregnant — for example, if you have used birth control carefully, consistently, and conscientiously, or if you have had a period within the previous two weeks, or if you have been medically sterilized, or if you have not had sexual intercourse in six months, then there is no reason for a pregnancy test, other than to increase the size of your medical bill. If a pregnancy test is demanded, then an inexpensive way to test for pregnancy is through an analysis of your urine — which is almost as sensitive as a blood test. While the Radioimmunoassay (RIA) — the blood pregnancy test — is more accurate and can be used to pick up tubal pregnancies, it is also double the price of a urine pregnancy test.

Similarly, if you have had a recent chest X-ray, or if you are in the low risk group for lung cancers, or if you have had a recent battery of X-rays (including the IVP — a high-radiation test described in Chapter Four) and are concerned about excess radiation exposure (and are also in the low-risk lung cancer group), then the chest X-ray is a procedure which is not necessarily in your best interests. However, please note that lung malignancies are detected as a result of this screening X-ray.

THE ANESTHESIOLOGIST

A presurgical interview with the anesthesiologist is part of the prehospital same-day admission policy. The interview will most likely be routine; however, this is the time to ask any questions you may have. Questions could include the type of anesthesia to be used and what you might expect during recovery as anesthesia-related side effects. The anesthesiologist will be most concerned about your medical history — for example, medications you are currently taking, allergies you may have, any family history of allergies, previous anesthesia experiences, or previous surgical experiences. You should explore local as compared to general anesthesia and their relative advantages and disadvantages. With general, you will be fully asleep and unaware of any pain or unpleasantness. With local, you will probably feel fairly relaxed following administration of Valium or a similar product. You will be numbed to the pain of surgery but may be awake and aware of your surrounding. General anesthesia carries a greater risk of complications. The choice of technique, however, is dependent on your feelings, your surgeon's and anesthesiologist's preferences, and the surgical procedure.

PACKING YOUR BAGS

Immediately after the surgery, you may feel as if you have been hit by a ten-ton truck. For that reason you can do yourself a favor by bringing to the hospital clothes which will make you feel psychologically better. A pretty nightgown and bathrobe may do wonders for the psyche. That is not to say that your old comfortable pajamas and knock-around bathrobe won't do — obviously they will. But a new outfit might help to make you feel better.

You should bring along a pair of slippers, preferably scuff slippers — the kind you can just slip your feet into. While other slippers may be warmer, your inability to bend after surgery precludes putting them on. You may want socks and a sweater, or bed jacket, since hospitals are sometimes kept fairly cool. An optional item to bring is underpants. If you do decide to bring them, bring a large pair with a loose waistband so that they will not bind or rub your incision.

Toiletries can consist of hand lotion, shampoo, lip balm, comb, brush, toothbrush and toothpaste. If you use makeup, bring it along. Consider also bringing some cologne — sometimes a change of odors (from hospital sanitize) is refreshing. Other belongings to bring could include pen and paper and something to read.

Most hospitals recommend bringing a minimum of money and leaving valuables (like jewelry) at home. If you plan to rent a television or telephone, payment by check is usually acceptable.

LEGAL ODDS AND ENDS

Although hysterectomy is a relatively safe and routine procedure, there is, as with any surgery, the danger of unforeseen complications. As a result, you should prepare for the worst scenario by making sure you have a Will and a Power of Health Attorney and/or Health Care Proxy form completed. They should be in an accessible place and the individuals you have designated should be informed of their role and know the location of the documents.

Wills · Do you need a Will? Absolutely yes! There is not one circumstance where it is advantageous to not have a Will. Even if your assets are jointly held or if you have no assets, a Will provides for the appointment of your personal representative (executor/executrix). A Will has to be signed and witnessed. Although most are prepared by a lawyer, you can make one yourself if you are prepared to do the necessary research to ensure that your document will withstand legal challenge. Keep in mind that you can avoid probate (a court-supervised process whereby an individual is appointed to distribute the assets of the estate in accordance with the Will) and its expenses if all of your assets are jointly held, held in trust for another (A in trust for B) or if you have a beneficiary named (A pay on death to B). Legal advice can provide guidance in making these decisions.

Living Wills and Health Care Proxies · While having a Will is very important, it is equally recommended to legally prepare for a health care emergency. The two documents which will cover your health and medical interests are the **Living Will** and the **Durable Power of Attorney** or a **Health Care Proxy.** States have varying legislation regarding these instruments, so it is best to find out the requirements for your state.

You must be at least 18 years old and of sound mind to make any of the documents. It's a good idea to keep your original documents in a safe place and to give a photocopy to both a friend or family member and your doctor. While in most states the documents are permanent from the time they are finalized, you can change your mind and revoke them. To do that you should destroy the old documents and inform your doctor or lawyer and anyone else with a copy of your change.

A Living Will (often called a Medical Directive or Directive to Physicians) is a document which lets you tell your physician in advance that you do not want your life artificially extended in certain situations.

The Durable Power of Attorney for Health Care or a Health Care Proxy should be prepared at the same time as the Living Will. Either document lets you choose a person to make medical or health care decisions for you if you become incapable of doing so. New York State was the first state in the union to pass a Proxy law, which became effective on January 18, 1991. Prototypical forms for these documents are available for a minimal charge (approximately $3.00) from The Hemlock Society, P.O. Box 11830, Eugene, OR 97402. You might check first with your hospital, since many states, such as New York State, require that they be made available to you, usually free of charge.

THE NIGHT BEFORE SURGERY

Emotions · Some people experience higher levels of anxiety than others. Make sure you speak to your physician about your concerns. Your doctor may prescribe some medication to be used in the days before surgery to help you feel more calm.

Physical Preparation · You will have been informed by both your doctor and the hospital of the procedure which you should follow the evening before surgery. Assuming that surgery is scheduled for early morning, you will be instructed to have a light meal no later than 6 PM. You also might be asked by your doctor to take a cleansing enema (purchased in a pharmacy for under $1.50). The enema acts to cleanse the lower colon, and directions for its use are contained within the package. You will be instructed not to drink any fluid (including water) or eat anything after midnight. Do not be surprised if you are thirsty when you awaken. The dry mouth is probably due as much to anticipation anxiety as to knowing that you are not allowed to drink. If you smoke, *do not* smoke the evening before. Also, refrain from having alcoholic beverages. If you are taking any medications for other conditions, you should have spoken with both the anesthesiologist and your surgeon about the advisability of taking these prior to the surgery.

THE HOSPITAL EXPERIENCE

Preoperation: (Surgery Day)

Who to Bring and What They Should Expect · It is helpful to have made arrangements with a support person (your husband, partner, relative, or friend) to bring you to the hospital on the day of surgery. First and most importantly, the emotional support and comfort will be helpful; second, many hospitals do not want you to leave your vehicle parked in their parking lots for several days. The person who brings you can leave at any time during the process that is about to be described, or can remain throughout. The support person who chooses to stay can expect to spend approximately four to five hours waiting. Usually an opportunity to speak with your physician about the surgery immediately after the operation will be available. Be sure to remind your companion to tell the receptionist/nurse to notify your doctor that there is someone waiting. Whoever accompanies you will be allowed to see you after surgery, once you are brought to your regular hospital room, but do not expect to be very social or conversational for several hours following the operation!

Signing In · You will be notified by the hospital, probably the day before, as to the exact time that you should arrive. At that time you will be formally admitted. While each hospital has its own method of registration, certain basic paperwork must be filled out (for example, insurance information, general consent for treatment, and a patient's bill of rights).

From the admitting office where you have signed in, you will walk to the ambulatory surgical area. Here you will be separated from the person who brought you to the hospital. Your companion must wait in the visitor's lounge while you are physically prepared for the operation.

Preparing for Surgery · In the surgical "prep" area, the nurses will prepare you for surgery. You will be provided with a hospital gown and a bag for your street clothes. The nursing staff, understanding your pre-op anxiety, will usually explain each of the steps in the process. First you will be given a hospital bracelet which will serve to identify you and to indicate by color code any medical problems, such as allergies, that the nursing staff should be alerted to. You will be instructed to lie on a stretcher and you may be fitted with elastic stockings — which you will probably wear for several days after the surgery. The stockings aid in circulation and help prevent thrombophlebitis. Your abdomen will be cleansed to remove sources of bacterial contamination and part of your pubic hair will be shaved. Then you will have an intravenous (IV) started which may contain fluids such as normal saline or Ringers Lactate, a fluid and electrolyte replenisher. The purpose of the IV is to provide access for anesthesia and medication during and after surgery. You will probably receive a sedative, either through the IV or injected intramuscularly. Versed, a short acting central nervous system depressant, is an example of a sedative that might be employed. You also may receive robinul, an anticholinergic drug which dries up excess secretions. Depending upon your doctor's orders, an antibiotic may also be given through the IV.

At this point and depending upon hospital policy and remaining time before the scheduled procedure, your companion can usually come into the surgical area to spend time with you until you are wheeled to surgery.

Before Going Under · It may be worth noting here that the more relaxed you are going under anesthesia, the more relaxed you will be coming out of it. The sedative that you are given will help but you can aid yourself with **positive imagery** or **visualization.** Positive imagery and visualization are new terms for old techniques of contacting the unconscious mind and harnessing its powers. These methods possibly had their roots in folk medicines, whereby an extremely vivid image was given to a patient in a deep trance as a means to cure a sick organ using the mind's power.

The image you choose should be one that you can see in your mind as clearly as something you can see with your open eyes. It should relate in a positive way to the procedure you are about to undergo and your hopes for a successful outcome. What you visualize should be a pleasant scene complete with color, texture, aroma, and sounds. Perhaps you are in a lovely garden surrounded by beautiful flowers and birds, or in an enormous balloon which will safely float you upwards through the clouds so you can observe leisurely the grandeur of the earth's panorama before descending back to earth; or you can be walking on a beautiful sunlit beach with the interplay of sand, water and sky.

THE OPERATION

The whole procedure, barring complications, will take approximately two hours. You will either be totally unaware of what is transpiring or only dimly aware, depending on the type of anesthesia used.

The surgery is now over, and your post-hysterectomy life begins. The remainder of this book deals with both immediate events and long-term concerns and issues.

ENDNOTES

1. O'Dwyer, G., Mylotte, M., Sweeney, M., et al. Experience of autologous blood transfusion in an obstetrics and gynaecology department. *British Journal of Obstetrics and Gynaecology,* 1993, 100(6), 571 – 574.

Chapter 9

RECOVERY

"I feel like a new person. I never knew what it was like to go three weeks in a row without pain." — Ellen, age 49

"My recovery went very well. I began an exercise program six weeks after surgery. By the eighth week I was back to running five miles." — Janet, age 52

POST-OPERATION (SURGERY DAY)

WHAT TO EXPECT

The surgery is over, and you are wheeled into the recovery room. Here your vital functions will be monitored as you recover from the anesthesia. You will most likely remain in the recovery room for several hours before being wheeled to your room. Although you will be quite groggy, you might be aware of things going on around you. For example, you must be shifted to your bed from the stretcher that has been used to wheel you to your appointed places, and you might be conscious enough to experience some discomfort during that process.

Nurses will be in and out of your room, checking on your condition and speaking to you — asking you questions or giving you instructions. How much you are conscious of these comings and goings is a very individual matter and depends on the anesthesia used. The same thing applies to your awareness of your companion who has completed a lonely vigil during your surgery and is now at your bedside — that is, unless you have decided you don't want to be seen in a groggy post-surgical condition and your companion respects your wish.

Recovery from anesthesia is gradual and there are many individual variations and reactions, ranging from mild to severe nausea and/or vomiting; slow to rapid recovery to consciousness; and little to extreme sensitivity to pain and/or discomfort.

When you do become conscious, you will notice at least two foreign bodies in you. The first is the IV (that had been inserted during the pre-op preparation), which now may contain plain saline, plain dextrose, antibiotics, or minerals and/or vitamins. While you might have been aware of the IV when it was being inserted, once it is in you it generally does not cause any discomfort. The second foreign body is a **catheter.** The catheter is a balloonlike device that was inserted into the bladder during surgery. It is connected to an external bag which collects your urine. The catheter might cause you to experience some discomfort in your urinary system. You may also have a nasogastric tube inserted in through your nose. This will make your nose and throat feel dry and uncomfortable, but it is used to prevent the nausea often brought on by general anesthesia. Because of these devices, and the fact that there is no need to get out of bed (your urinary needs are being taken care of and you will not have to defecate because you've used an enema), and because you will still be recovering from the anesthesia (and probably groggy), your mobility on the day of surgery could be nonexistent. However, some hospitals have a policy of getting you on your feet briefly the day of your surgery, so don't be surprised if you're asked to stand. It is to your advantage in achieving a quick recovery to get moving as soon as possible. The nurses are not being mean when they want you to get up. It really is for your own good.

Pain · As mentioned earlier, individual tolerances to pain and discomfort vary. However, when you are conscious, do not be surprised if all of your awareness is focused on your abdominal region. You will be offered medication to ease your suffering at this stage. It is generally recommended that you accept what is offered to "stay ahead of the pain."[1] On the other hand, these drugs may contribute to constipation, so you will need to weigh your options.

Food · You will most likely receive no solid food the day of surgery, but will be getting fluids and nourishment via the IV.

Odds and Ends · A respiratory therapist may see you late in the day of your surgery. He or she will bring you a "toy" which is an **incentive deep breathing exerciser.** The importance of this device is that it gets you to activate your lungs and keep them from filling with fluid. Depending upon your condition after surgery, playing with this toy might have to be deferred until the next day!

DAY 1 AFTER SURGERY

WHAT TO EXPECT

Full consciousness will gradually have returned overnight and you face Day 1 after surgery very aware of being connected to the IV, possibly nauseous because of anesthesia side effects, aware of the balloon in your bladder, and acutely aware of your abdomen.

The nurses will continue their monitoring (it never ceases!) of, among other things, your pulse, temperature, respiratory rate, blood pressure, and the dressing. If you were not conscious enough to use the air toy on the previous evening, you will be revisited and reminded of how to use the device and how important it is to activate your lungs and keep them from filling with fluid.

Your physician will probably see you early in the morning. What is done by your doctor is an individual practice issue. Most likely, bandages will be removed and the incision and stitches or staples will be checked (the incision will become another thing checked periodically by the nursing staff). Your doctor will probably ask to have your IV and catheter removed and will start you on oral pain medication. The recovery process has officially begun.

Do not be surprised if on that first morning following surgery, you are presented with breakfast. In all likelihood it will be a liquid breakfast — regular meals should gradually resume thereafter. You will appreciate your liquid breakfast because you may feel extremely dehydrated or dry-mouthed and crave lots of fluids.

During that first day, every time you move, you will be made aware of your abdominal region. If the discomfort is not from the incised fascia or skin, it might be from a general distention of the abdomen due to gas. You probably will have some vaginal staining. The hospital has maxi-pads (held in place by an elastic waist band) which the nurses will provide for you. Intermittent staining can occur for up to several weeks post-op.

Possibly for the first time, you will become aware of the role the abdominal muscles play in your life. The muscles we call abdominals consist of four groups (the rectus abdominus, the transverse abdominus, and the external and internal obliques). In textbooks on kinesiology, these muscles are listed as muscles of both the thorax and spine because of their functions as flexors of the trunk and depressors of the lower ribs — the latter used in vigorous exhalation. In addition, these four muscle groups together form a strong anterior support for the abdominal viscera, providing compression of the abdomen and also assisting in urination and defecation. During surgery there is no actual cut made in any of the muscles; however, the transversalis fascia, which lines the entire wall of the abdomen (and also covers the internal surface of the transverse abdominus muscle) is incised.

As a result of the surgery, the interconnectedness of muscles, ligaments, tendons and fascia become very evident when you cough, sneeze, or laugh. Exquisite abdominal pain will greet each of those events and it will feel as though every muscle has been cut in your abdomen, when in reality only skin, fascia, and peritoneum have been incised. Have a pillow handy so that you can place it over your abdomen. Press down on the pillow (and onto your belly) prior to coughing, sneezing, or laughing. Laughing and visitors will be discussed shortly.

Definitely at some point during the first day you will be encouraged by the nurses to walk. With your nurse's physical support, you will venture off your bed. Besides feeling like your legs are made of jelly, you will also feel that you are walking like a cavewoman. Standing erect will be painful, so you will have to be satisfied for a while with a stooped-over posture.

Your chief obligations on the first day after surgery are to get plenty of rest, sleep, and fluid; to exercise your lungs, and to do some walking. That is it! You owe it to yourself to do nothing more.

Doctor's Visits · Your doctor (or one of the members of the group if he/she is in a group practice) should visit you every day. This is the time to ask questions about what you are experiencing, anything that is troubling you, what you should expect, and so on. Write down your questions when they occur to you, or you are apt to forget them by the time the doctor arrives. You should expect, and insist upon, considerate answers from your doctor. Remember, all of your questions are intelligent and important.

You should ask your doctor to see the patho-histo (pathology-histology) report. This report should be ready by Day 2 or 3 after surgery and will serve to confirm the original diagnosis.

Visitors · Just as a reminder to you: The day of your surgery is "the pits," but you are pretty much "out of it." The first day after surgery may feel even worse, because your anesthesia has worn off and you may feel its after effects such as some nausea. By Day 2 after surgery, you are beginning to be aware of something other than your abdomen.

As a general rule: Friends and relatives should not come to visit until at least Day 2. If they "must" come to see you on Day 1, tell them ahead of time to keep their visits *very* short. It is definitely not in your interest to have to entertain visitors on Day 1. You will be amazed at how physically exhausting it is to interact with others.

It is tempting to even go so far as to say that visitors on Day 2 will also be a strain and should not be encouraged, although friends and family might view that as excessive. If visitors do come on Day 2, they should be advised to stay only a short time.

The same is true of telephone calls — believe it or not. Definitely no calls the day of surgery. Anyone who wants to make sure the operation was successful and that you are okay should call the hospital's information number for that confirmation. You probably will find that even calls on Day 1 after surgery will require a lot of effort on your part. Another problem created by the telephone is that its intrusive ringing may occur just as you are taking a nap — depriving you of some needed rest. You may also have trouble reaching the telephone. Ask a nurse or friend to place it in a handy spot, if possible.

Medication · At some point late on the day of surgery, you will probably be started on some oral pain medication which usually contains a narcotic combined with aspirin or acetaminophen. The medication's synthetic opiate will have analgesic and sedating properties, while the aspirin/acetaminophen it contains will have analgesic and antipyretic (fever-reducing) properties.

Do not be a martyr. Do not wait until you are in severe discomfort to ask for a pain pill — the pills do not take effect immediately and you will continue to be in severe discomfort for some time after taking the pills. Pain medication is most effective when it is used in anticipation of its need. At the same time, it is important that you do not become a pill popper. Remember, these drugs may contribute to constipation. On the other hand, they will help in healing. Be aware that side effects such as nausea, lightheadedness, or dizziness are not uncommon; however, you should notify the nurses immediately if you experience these symptoms.

Because your initial medication will be a potent narcotic with drug dependency a possibility, you will most likely be changed to a milder medication, for example Tylenol with codeine, as soon as your doctor thinks you can tolerate the shift.

Bowel Issues · One of the body functions that the nurses will be monitoring is **peristalsis.** Peristalsis is the muscular action which pushes food through the large intestine. That process produces sounds which indicate to the nurses that your gastrointestinal tract is functioning. It is not unusual for it to temporarily stop as a result of anesthesia.

The next event that is greatly anticipated by everyone (nurses and yourself) is your first bowel movement — which usually happens during Day 1. Drinking lots of water and juice as well as walking will help encourage that first bowel movement. If these don't do the trick, milk of magnesia or an enema or suppository may be required by Day 2 or 3.

To say that constipation and gas exacerbate your pain is an understatement. They aggravate the abdomen's already sensitive condition, so in addition to drinking fluids and walking, you should be aware of your diet. For some unfathomable reason, special menus for this type of surgical procedure are rarely created; you will probably have to select your meals after Day 1 breakfast from the regular hospital menu. Wise choices can help add bulk but not create gas (see "Nutrition During Recovery" later in this chapter for more advice).

As we noted earlier, and what the nurses might not tell you, is that the same medication which helps relieve pain may also cause constipation. Given this dilemma, the wise choice is probably to take less pain medication — but again, don't be a martyr.

DAYS 2 to 5 AFTER SURGERY

WHAT TO EXPECT

Your condition during the next few days will fluctuate from actual pain to mild discomfort — with your entire focus still on your abdomen. Having a bowel movements and minimizing bowel gas will be important considerations, and anything you can do toward these goals will be in your best interest. Thus proper nutrition, plenty of fluids, and exercise — walking — require your attention. It is also important to continue using your lung toy and to get as much rest as possible. You will gradually find how to use certain muscles that have not been affected by the surgery, to enable you to accomplish the movements you want with a minimum of pain and discomfort. For example, to get out of bed you will find it easiest to roll onto your side (in a semi-fetal position) and use your bottom arm to push yourself up — at the same time that you are assisting yourself by grabbing your knees with your top arm and pulling. Also, use your hospital bed to its maximum advantage in positioning you into a semi-upright position. Hopefully you will have received this type of instruction by the hospital nurses.

A note about hospital beds. You will find that the many positions that the hospital bed allows you to get into will help make you more comfortable. Do not be afraid to experiment with raising and lowering either your legs or torso by playing with the bed's controls.

On either Day 1 or Day 2 after surgery, you may be allowed to take your first shower. That event will serve as a real spirit-booster — enjoy! Incidentally, a decade and more ago, a first shower was not allowed until at least several days post-operation.

Hospital Routine · Hospitals have a life of their own, and you will find that you quickly become part of the routine. Meals are served usually around 8 AM, noon, and 5 PM (allow for individual variations between hospitals). Unlike the restricted visiting hours of yesteryear, most hospitals allow visitations from noon to 8 PM — but, as mentioned earlier, that may not be to your best advantage. Nurses usually work in eight-hour shifts that may run from 7 AM to 3 PM, 3 PM to 11 PM, and 11 PM to 7 AM. Expect to have a routine checkup when the nurses begin (and possibly end) their shifts. That means that you will probably be awakened around midnight and again early in the morning. Of course, those interruptions are felt most keenly by the early-to-bed people (who are in a comfortable sleep at midnight) and the late-morning sleepers (who suddenly are awakened to see dawn). In most cases, your body's need for sleep will allow you to quickly return to Morpheus after the nursing interruptions.

Money-Saving Tips · *Television.* If you want to rent a television, many hospitals have private contractors who will be around daily to oblige. Try the TV set in your room first, since you might be able to get one station without paying for it. The TV set is never disconnected — but your access to various channels is controlled. If you are not a TV addict, you might consider not renting one (the cost mounts up quickly, $4 to $8 per day).TV may help relax you, however, and its rental might make a thoughtful gift from a family member or close friend.

Telephone. Hospitals have different arrangements. Some have you pay for a bedside telephone and do not charge you for local calls. In other hospitals you are charged for daily local telephone service but are required to use your telephone credit card, call collect, or charge to a third party all other outgoing calls. If you are given a choice, it may be cheaper to reject the daily local telephone service and just charge those calls in the same way as described above. You know your phoning habits, but it's safe to say that you are probably not going to feel like making many calls for the first few days.

Hospital Discharge · Assuming no complications, somewhere between Day 3 and Day 5 you will be ready to leave the hospital. While each hospital has its own procedures, in general you can expect the following. Your doctor will be the official who will authorize your discharge (he or she is the only one who can legally do this). Once that has been done, a floor nurse should have a conference with you to review the post-op patient discharge instructions. Many hospitals have summarized those instructions, and you receive a copy of that printed information, which you and the nurse sign after your discussion. Once all the necessary paperwork is completed, you are free to leave. Expect to be asked to sit in a wheelchair, wheeled to the front door, and helped into the awaiting vehicle you arranged for — hospital regulations.

NOTE: You do not have to leave the hospital until you think you are medically ready. Presumably you will have discussed this issue with your doctor. However, if there is a disagreement, you can request a review of the discharge decision. Every hospital has a review agent who will speak individually with you and your doctor and check your medical record before rendering a decision. You will most likely be informed of these rights to review when you are being processed for discharge. Most hospitals have a discharge notice *form which you sign indicating that you agree or disagree with the decision by the doctor and the hospital that you no longer require care in the hospital and can be discharged.*

Doctor's Parting Orders · As part of your discharge, your doctor should discuss with you a set of recommendations as to what to do and not do during the ensuing weeks. It is in these instructions that we see medicine as an art rather than an exact science.

One doctor will prescribe bed rest, no stair climbing (or at the most only once a day), showers but no baths, no car rides, no driving by yourself until at least four weeks after surgery, and so on. Another doctor will suggest that you can bathe, climb stairs, ride in cars and drive when you feel comfortable. The reason for this discrepancy is that, unfortunately, research has not yet been conducted to substantiate or refute either approach. Each doctor, therefore, relies on personal experience, intuition, and feedback from patients.

Odds and Ends · Although most of your clothes will have remained with you in the hospital, request whoever is coming to get you to bring any additional items you may need. For example, you might consider wearing some loose-fitting garments (such as some type of sweatpants or at-home wear) for the trip home because of the sensitivity of your abdominal area.

Also ask the person who is taking you home to bring several pillows and possibly a blanket for the car. The pillows will be very handy in making yourself comfortable in what could be an otherwise uncomfortable ride home. If you must go home by yourself in a taxi, ask the driver to help you bring your things inside.

HOME AGAIN

WHAT TO EXPECT

The recovery process, both in the hospital and for the next two to four weeks at home, is a humbling experience — especially for those who are "superwomen," women who successfully juggle families and careers. For all women, recovery is a slow process. Remember, for those who had an abdominal hysterectomy, your entire abdomen has been incised and spread apart, and now the fascia and skin have to come back together and reunite. You will spend an inordinate amount of time sleeping — whether you call it napping, dozing, or shutting your eyes. Sleep is nature's way of providing the quiet time necessary for recuperation. Although household demands may make it difficult, do not fight it. Allow your body the rest it needs, and use your body judiciously between rest times.

Pain and Discomfort · Expect pain and discomfort to be with you for some time, but to lessen in intensity with each passing day. Because the pain pills that have been prescribed for you are both addicting and constipating, it is best to try to wean yourself off them as fast as possible once you are home.

Take as needed, trying to find the line between being overly brave and overly dependent.

You will continue to find that your entire focus will be on your abdomen, and it will feel like your bowels are your abdomen. Continue with a sensible diet which will promote defecation and minimize gas production (see this chapter's section on nutrition during recovery). Drink plenty of fluids and exercise sensibly.

Emotional Reactions · For the majority of women, the surgery is a relief. However, some experience a primal reaction to the removal of their uterus and the symbolic ending of their womanhood. See Chapter Fourteen for suggestions on improving your spirits.

Getting Around · It is hard to give a blanket prescription about exercising during recovery. The woman who runs marathons and climbs mountains has to be restrained, while the inactive woman has to be encouraged to push herself. General guidelines could include the following:

- Slowly increase your activity when you go home. Begin by walking five to ten minutes a day if you are able.
- Avoid heavy lifting (over ten pounds) until you are cleared by your doctor.
- Avoid bending at the waist; bend at the knees to pick things up.
- You may (depending upon your doctor's orders) go up and down stairs — but do not overdo this.
- You may (after clearing it with you doctor) want to start a series of basic exercises designed to gently ease your body "back into shape." A sample exercise protocol developed by William A. Smith, physical therapist, is described in Table 9 – 1.

TABLE 9 – 1

POST-HYSTERECTOMY EXERCISE PROTOCOL*

To strengthen the hip and lower extremity muscles:

1. Lie supine (on your back) with heels more or less together and toes pointed in opposite directions away from each other.

   Tighten and hold buttock muscles in a contraction for a slow count of from three to six. This is done three times in a group. Do one group every two hours. Add one group of three every other day until a total of six groups is reached.

   Pull feet and toes toward shins and then push feet down as if stepping on the gas, each for a slow count of three. Start with one and gradually add more until you can repeat three times (three ups and three downs).

2. Bend knees up with feet on the bed drawn up near the buttocks. You can do this exercise with or without a folded towel between your knees.

continued on next page

TABLE 9 – 1 *(continued)*

Squeeze knees and thighs together for a slow count of three, and rest for up to ten seconds. Do two groups of three, resting about one to two minutes between each group. Add one group every other day until you reach six groups of three.

3. Straighten knees out again and cross one leg and ankle over the other.

   With the blocking provided by the feet and ankles, try to push legs apart (rendered now impossible because of the leg-over-leg position). Push apart for a slow count of three, repeating three times. Add one group of three every other day until six groups of three are reached.

To recondition the abdominal muscles:

1. Lie down on your back and practice pursed-lip breathing: Take a slow breath in through the nose, swelling your belly, if possible, as you breathe in. Hold for a slow count of three and blow slowly out through pursed lips with your hand about eight inches in front of your face. Imagine your breath as making a candle flame flicker without blowing it out. At first you should try to make the flame flicker for four to five seconds as you blow, counting "a thousand and one, a thousand and two," so as to time the out breath. Rest about one minute and repeat one more time. Repeat every half hour to one hour, just two breaths each time. The length of the pursed lip exhalation or "breeze out" can be extended up to 10 to 15 seconds over the course of the next week, so as to help clear the lungs. If you place your fingertips on the abdomen, you'll feel the stomach muscles get harder and harder towards the end of the breath; this provides the strengthening. Remember, the candle never gets blown out, but only flickers.
2. When you think your abdominals are ready for more exercise, add a head and neck curl off the pillow by lifting your chin towards your chest. This should be done while lying on your back with your knees bent and feet flat on the bed.

   Add shoulders to the head and neck curl-up. Progress at your pace as it feels "okay."

---

*Developed by William A. Smith, physical therapist, New Paltz, NY.

It is normal to have soreness in and around the incision, which may increase as you become more active. Listen to your body — it will tell you when you have increased your activity too much.

Your abdominal muscles may occasionally go into spasm (knots) or cause a burning sensation. It most likely indicates that they are not ready for even the small amount of use that you are asking of them. You will experience muscular fatigue in other muscle groups, such as in the back, which are working overtime to compensate for the lack of abdominal cooperation. As you begin walking more, expect some fatigue in your legs.

Muscular exertion (even if it seems like very little compared to what you normally do) may lead to your feeling completely exhausted. Give in to that feeling and rest!

> Carol, age 48, reported to us that her diary entry for Day 12 after her hysterectomy reads: "Think I'm fine today so I'll shower and go downstairs to breakfast. One hour later — I hobbled back to my bed, humbled by my exhaustion."

Many women have indicated that one of the most difficult things is sitting up (not in bed but in a straight-backed chair with their feet on the floor) for up to two weeks after surgery. This is because the surgery and subsequent inactivity have weakened the abdominal muscles. Plan to have access to a bed or couch throughout your first few weeks of recovery. Keeping pillows handy to place under your legs (to elevate them and take pressure off your abdominals) will make you more comfortable.

After six weeks, when you start to escalate your physical activities to presurgery levels following your doctor's medical clearance, it is important to realize that your muscles are still weak and that you should not suddenly resume your prior physical workout routine. If you do, you will probably suffer from abdominal pain as a result of muscular fatigue from the sudden increase in exertion.

An important part of your recovery exercise/activity program should include abdominal exercises. This important muscle group has been affected by the surgery and your subsequent inactivity, and will need your careful attention to gradually bring them to a condition in which they are functioning optimally. Begin with the regimen described in Table 9 – 1 before you advance to the routine described in Chapter Thirteen.

Doctor's Appointments · At the time of hospital discharge, your doctor may instruct you to call the office and schedule an appointment for approximately one week later.

Keeping that appointment will likely be your first major outing since your departure from the hospital. During that session, the doctor will check your incision and maybe do a brief scan of the vaginal area. Depending upon the type of material and the suture that the doctor used to close your incision, your stitches or staples may be removed. For example, if a 4-0 dexon subcuticular suture was used, there will be no stitches to remove. If, however, other materials for the stitches or staples were used, they will be removed during this visit. Some doctors, however, remove them the day of hospital discharge. If you have questions, write them down as they occur to you prior to the visit so that you won't forget to ask them when you are with the doctor.

The next and final appointment will most likely be scheduled for four weeks later (approximately six weeks after surgery). At that time, the doctor will check the incision and examine your vagina. If everything seems to be healing as expected, your doctor will probably give you the okay to resume all your normal activities (including sexual intercourse).

Bathing · Some doctors recommend that you take showers and not bathe in a tub for about three weeks to avoid infection of the internal vaginal stitches. Whether you shower or bathe (with your doctor's okay), the external incision should be washed with soap and water each time.

Tending to Your Scar · Proper self-treatment of scar tissue is seldom discussed, but should be, according to Smith. It is possible that the area can remain hypersensitive or develop into **keloids**, or knotty scar, if it is left untended. Mr. Smith reports an example of a patient he was treating for low back strain problems. She happened to complain of the extreme sensitivity of her abdominal scar — from a hysterectomy fifteen years earlier. Instructed on how to properly self-treat the area, there was complete resolution of the ultrasensitive abdominal area scar and adjacent skin tissue in less than a month.[2]

To properly desensitize the scar, you should begin to massage the area, according to Smith, the same day as surgery and continue for the next six to eight weeks. See Table 9 – 2 for a description of the self-treatment.

TABLE 9 – 2

SELF-TREATMENT OF THE HYSTERECTOMY SCAR*

Self-treatment begins by placing both hands over the bandaged area several hours post-surgery, and simply allowing the weight of the hands to press down on the bandaged tissue overlying the incision. This should be done for appro::imately two minutes every two hours. Additionally, the outlying skin on the hips and upper abdominal area can be gently massaged in a kneading manner.

The day after surgery, the hands should be placed over the bandaged tissue, and instead of simply leaving the weight of the hands there, a very gentle, nonpainful up-and-down pressure can be applied, pressing down for a slow count of four (counting "a thousand and one, a thousand and two, a thousand and three, a thousand and four) and relieving the pressure to simply the weight of the hands for a slow count of four. This should be done for approximately two minutes every two hours. In addition to a kneading-style massage of the hip and upper abdominal area, a circular motion massage can be done. In this, the pads of the index, middle, and ring fingers are held in contact with the skin so as to not slide over it. Then you make silver-dollar-sized circles with your hands.

Day 3, the treatment is the same, with the undulating pressure gradually increasing, but never to the point of discomfort. The circular massages and kneading about the hips and abdominal area gradually get stronger as the tissue around the surgical area responds and is able to take more vigorous activity.

continued on next page

After clamps or sutures are removed, the surgical site can be massaged very gently in a circular pattern, using four, five, or six finger contact spots over the surgical scar in a very gentle motion. This should be done every two hours for one to two minutes. Continue circular massage in the other areas.

By three weeks post-surgery, a substantially deeper, more kneading-type massage of the entire abdominal area, including the scar, should be done for two to three minutes every two hours and continued for three to five more weeks.

---

*Developed by William A. Smith, physical therapist, New Paltz, NY.

Sex · Because of the nature of the surgery (see Chapter Six for a detailed discussion), the vagina has had stitches applied to it. As a result, most doctors do not recommend intercourse until after your second post-op appointment, anywhere from four to six weeks after surgery. It is very likely that you will not feel physically ready until that time anyway. However, your libido may return sooner than your body's physical recovery. It is not unusual for sex dreams and fantasies to occur — sometimes within the first two weeks — or for them to lead to nocturnal orgasm. The whole issue of females having nocturnal orgasms has been debated, but for those women who physically experience them — there is no debate. When your libido returns, creative sex which does not involve intercourse can and should be practiced. (See Chapter Ten.)

When the doctor gives you the okay to resume intercourse, there may be some pain and staining the first time. If either seems excessive or lasts for more than a few episodes — contact your doctor.

Nutrition During Recovery · After surgery, when your entire focus is on your abdomen, your digestive system plays an important part in your recovery and comfort. What goes in through your mouth will determine in part what occurs in the rest of the gastrointestinal tract and your whole body.

Two major foci during the days immediately following your surgery are: promotion of defecation and minimization of gas production. Although fiber has been recommended as a remedy for constipation, many nutritionists believe that the fiber content of foods may cause gas and distention. According to the *Manual of Clinical Dietetics*, this position has been poorly documented. The manual notes that the symptoms of gas and distention are more likely due to a change of diet, anesthesia, and the general effect of bed rest.[3]

Since the research on this controversy is inconclusive, it seems prudent, while you are healing, to adopt a diet which includes some fiber (to promote defecation) but in minimal quantities (in order to ease gas pains). The diet which follows (see Table 9 – 3) is comprised of soft foods which you should use as a transition between the liquid diet given to you immediately after surgery and a regular diet.

TABLE 9 – 3

POST-OP SOFT DIET

This diet is a transition between a full liquid diet and a regular diet. It consists of easily digested, non-irritating foods which are not difficult to assimilate by the digestive tract. It is appropriate for patients physically unable to tolerate a general diet after surgery.

This diet meets the recommended dietary allowances and provides a minimum of 2,000 Calories.

MEAT, FISH, AND POULTRY

FOODS ALLOWED: Baked or broiled tender beef, lamb, veal, liver, pork, lean ham, fish, chicken, or turkey

FOODS TO AVOID: Smoked, cured, pickled, or highly spiced meats, fish or poultry such as luncheon meats, frankfurters, sausage (except lean ham)

CHEESE

FOODS ALLOWED: Cottage cheese, mild American, Swiss, brick cream cheese, Muenster, ricotta, mild cheddar

FOODS TO AVOID: Cheese with seasonings; sharp or spicy cheeses

EGGS

FOODS ALLOWED: Scrambled, poached, or soft-cooked; plain omelets

FOODS TO AVOID: Spicy omelets

FATS

FOODS ALLOWED: Cream, butter, margarine, sour cream, and mayonnaise; gravy without pepper or onions

FOODS TO AVOID: Highly seasoned commercial salad dressings; highly seasoned gravy

VEGETABLES

FOODS ALLOWED: Cooked vegetables; asparagus, beets, carrots, celery, green or wax beans, peas, spinach, squash, tomato puree (no seeds); vegetable juices; lettuce (not iceberg) and tender salad greens

FOODS TO AVOID: All other raw vegetables; corn; cabbage family vegetables, such as broccoli, brussel sprouts, cauliflower, cabbage, and onions

POTATOES AND SUBSTITUTES

FOODS ALLOWED: mashed, boiled, or baked white or sweet potatoes; rice, spaghetti, noodles, macaroni

FOODS TO AVOID: Highly seasoned potato product snacks; spaghetti with highly seasoned sauce

FRUITS

FOODS ALLOWED: All fruit juices; ripe bananas, fresh orange and grapefruit sections; ripe peeled peaches, pears, or apples; canned or cooked fruit

FOODS TO AVOID: All fruits with edible seeds, fresh fruits with skins, melons

continued on next page

BREADS AND CEREALS

FOODS ALLOWED: Refined cooked cereals, cream of rice, cream of wheat, farina, oatmeal, corn flakes; white bread; soda and graham crackers, melba toast, zwieback

FOODS TO AVOID: Rolls or bread made with coarse grains, cracked wheat, seeds, nuts or dried fruits

MILK

FOODS ALLOWED: All milk combinations if you are not lactose intolerant

BEVERAGES

FOODS ALLOWED: Coffee, decaffeinated coffee, tea, juices

DESSERTS

FOODS ALLOWED: Custard, gelatin pudding, sherbet, plain cakes, cookies, and cream pies

FOODS TO AVOID: Desserts containing nuts, coconut, seeds, dried fruit; rich pastries

SEASONINGS

FOODS ALLOWED: Salt, sugar, cinnamon, mace, sage, nutmeg, vinegar, parsley, oregano, basil, vanilla, and other flavoring extracts

FOODS TO AVOID: Chili powder, mustard, garlic, seed spices; all commercial meat sauces such as A-1, Worcestershire

MISCELLANEOUS

FOODS ALLOWED: Cream or broth soups with allowed vegetable; jelly, honey

FOODS TO AVOID: Jam and preserves with seeds; chocolate

Source: Rosemary Mancuso, Dietitian, Kingston Hospital, Kingston, New York

The soft diet consists of easily digested, non-irritating foods which are not difficult to assimilate by the digestive tract.

If you decide to increase your fiber intake, make sure you drink additional quantities of liquids and try to substitute refined grains for coarse grains. Also try to eat those fibers primarily in the morning so you won't have to sleep with the possible gas they create.

If you have gas in the hospital, try to increase the frequency of your walks around the halls. Walking will promote defecation and ease the gas and distention. Once you are home, you might try to eat smaller and more frequent meals and continue walking to help prevent gas and distention during your recovery.

Nutritionists are in agreement that certain foods should be avoided during your recovery. These include, among other items: chocolate, spices/flavorings, raw vegetables including members of the cabbage family (for example, broccoli, cauliflower, cabbage), fruits with edible seeds or skins, fried foods, and sharp or spicy cheeses.

There are other approaches to nutrition which are at variance with standard medical orthodoxy. These counter-culture methods place great emphasis on holistic health, alternative medicine, and spirituality. Herbs are advocated by many who pursue self-sufficiency in female health care through the timely and preventive use of plant medicine. Texts are available, such as Susun Weed's *Wise Woman Herbal Healing Wise,* which describe philosophies and give specific information about these alternative approaches to nutrition.[4]

Reprise

The pain and discomfort gradually subside until one day you awaken unaware that for several weeks your abdomen has been the primary focus of your attention. Usually this occurs sometime after week three, but it varies with the individual. Until at least week four you should consider yourself a healing invalid who is gingerly attempting to regain her health.

ENDNOTES

1. Wilder-Smith, C. H., & Schüler, L. Postoperative analgesia: pain by choice? The influence of patient attitudes and patient education. *Pain*, 1992, 50(3), 257–262.

2. William Smith, physical therapist, personal communication, 1994.

3. American Dietetic Association. *Manual of Clinical Dietetics.* Chicago, IL: American Dietetic Association, 1988.

4. Weed, Susun S. *Wise Woman Herbal Healing Wise.* Woodstock, NY: Ash Tree Publishing, 1989.

Chapter 10

LET'S TALK ABOUT SEX

"I enjoy my sexuality so much more since my hysterectomy. My husband and I look forward to our lovemaking — kissing, caressing, as well as intercourse."

—Rachel, age 56

In Chapter Two, we pointed out that the organs needed for reproduction are also important in sexual gratification. Now that you no longer have a uterus and may also be lacking ovaries, how might this affect your sexual needs and feelings? In this chapter we explore and discuss these concerns, and also provide guidelines for sexual satisfaction.

"NO 'SEX' FOR SIX WEEKS?"

DANGER: SEXUAL ACTIVITY!

Following hysterectomy or similar surgery, you will likely be advised not to "have sex" for a period of four to six weeks. After this time you will probably be asked to return to your surgeon for a checkup. If all is well, you can then resume "normal relations."

How important is it to follow this medical recommendation? If we define "sex" as intercourse, the answer is *very*. Dr. John W. Huffman, a Professor Emeritus of Obstetrics and Gynecology at Northwestern University Medical School in Chicago, describes a situation in which a 28-year-old married woman clearly did not follow his prescription for temporary sexual abstinence.

> Ms. X and her husband engaged in coitus ten days after an abdominal total hysterectomy. Ms. X immediately suffered from profuse vaginal bleeding, rupture of the vaginal vault (which had been closed during surgery), and shock. She developed a severe pelvic infection, the tear had to be repaired, she required 16 units of blood in transfusion, and had to be hospitalized for three weeks.[1]

While not all sexual intercourse within six weeks of surgery has such drastic results, coitus is definitely *not* advised. The sutures need time to mend, and the entire vaginal area is more vulnerable to infection.

You probably won't feel much like having sexual intercourse for the first two weeks following surgery. Your abdomen will be sore, you will doubtless have a vaginal discharge, and you may feel generally weak. We do not know in the example of Ms. X, above, whether she actually desired intercourse or was simply obliging her husband.

Individuals, however, vary. Suzanne Morgan, author of the book *Coping With a Hysterectomy*, describes another 28-year-old woman who masturbated *in the hospital* several days after hysterectomy and oopherectomy. While she was clearly sexually motivated, she reported only a "superficial" orgasm. Morgan does not mention medical problems as a result of masturbation or orgasm days after surgery.[2]

To adequately address the question of "sex" during the first month or so following surgery, we need to define our terms much more precisely than the average surgeon is likely to do. What exactly are we advised *against*? Is it no intercourse, no orgasm, no masturbation, no arousal? What harm can befall us in each of these cases? Unfortunately, most physicians equate "sex" with intercourse and therefore provide their patients with limited information. Most of us as patients are much too embarrassed or not quick enough to ask "What do you mean by 'no sex'?" In short, perhaps due to social inhibitions, the risks of various sexual activities are not well documented.

Intercourse? No · It is plain that sexual intercourse is dangerous for about one month following hysterectomy. The internal incisions and sutures have not had time to heal. Insertion of anything (including a penis, fingers, a dildo, bath or douche water) into the vagina may introduce bacteria resulting in infection. The pressure of intercourse may also cause rupture of the surgical repair.

Genital Stimulation and Orgasm? Maybe · Although not adequately studied, there is some evidence that women may be satisfactorily stimulated to orgasm as early as two weeks following surgery with no ill effects. This may be accomplished through masturbation of the outer genitals by finger or vibrator or similar manipulation by the woman's partner. It does not include actual intercourse. In our study, nine women (almost 10 percent) of the 92 women responding to the question on this issue reported that they engaged in genital stimulation within two weeks of surgery. The same number and proportion reported achieving orgasm. It is probable that most women do not attempt genital stimulation at least in part because they are warned against "sex."

Can orgasm within the first two weeks cause internal stitches to rupture? We have seen no reports indicating ill effects.

Sexiness? Perhaps · If you are inclined to act sexy, why not? When you come home from the hospital you may want to engage in some sexy, noncoital activities. Remember necking and petting? If you feel like it, go to it.

You can dress and groom yourself appealingly. Just because you are home recuperating doesn't mean that you must look sick. Attention to your appearance can help you feel better, too.

If your partner desires sexual stimulation to orgasm and you are in the mood, you can accommodate in many ways. You may use your mouth, your hands, your breasts, your thighs, your underarms (and baby or massage oil) to glide your partner to satisfaction. You may find that this gives you pleasure as well.

Tenderness and Closeness? Yes · If you are fortunate enough to have a partner with whom to snuggle and exchange endearments, by all means, don't hold back. Your recovery will be so much more pleasant if you show love and accept loving. An offer of a body or foot massage is a wonderful gift to anyone, especially someone who is recuperating from serious surgery. (Leave this book open to this page if you want to drop someone a hint!)

Hugs and kisses, special attention, and little acts of thoughtfulness are all more than welcome as you convalesce. Be open to these offerings and consider yourself lucky if there is someone who can be there for you.

SEX AFTER SIX WEEKS — THE LONG-TERM OUTLOOK

We will consider how hysterectomy and oopherectomy affect sexuality from two perspectives. First, we note what might be expected as a result of the absence of key anatomical parts. Second, we examine the research that has investigated how these surgeries do affect sexuality. In this second section, we also discuss women's reports of their sexual feelings and experiences.

STAGES OF SEXUAL RESPONSE

The uterus and ovaries normally play a part in sexual arousal and orgasm. An understanding of the four stages of sexual response described by Masters and Johnson may help you predict what to expect after hysterectomy and oopherectomy.[3] You may also wish to review Chapter Two.

Excitement · During the first stage, excitement, two biological processes occur: **vasocongestion** (increased blood flow to the sexual organs) and **myotonia** (bodily muscle tension). For women, this increased blood flow results in some enlargement of the clitoris and the vaginal lips. The vaginal walls moisten and breasts and nipples become more sensitive and erect. Myotonia causes the uterus to be internally pulled up with the likely result of positioning it to receive sperm. Heart rate, blood pressure, respiration, and perspiration increase. You feel physically and psychologically aroused.

Excitement may be the result of direct touch to the genitals, and it is most often preceded by the brain signaling sexual interest. The signals come from what you see, smell, touch, and think. In fact, your mind is significantly responsible for how receptive you are to sexual arousal. (Visualize how *unaroused* you would be in response to uninvited direct touch!)

Androgens produced in the adrenal glands and the ovaries play a part in the physiology of arousal. As a result of oopherectomy or aging and atrophy of the ovaries, a now-limited amount of these hormones may slow down arousal time. Similarly, estrogen, produced by the ovaries, is indirectly responsible for the moistening of the vagina during arousal. This moisture serves as a lubricant for intercourse, and its absence or sparseness is sure to be noted.

After hysterectomy there is no uterus to be pulled into a receptive position, so the uterine aspect of the excitement phase will be lacking. This is not noticed by many women.

Plateau · During the second stage of the sexual response cycle, the increase in blood flow and bodily tension continue, resulting in a heightened sense of erotic readiness. The specific signs we mentioned in the preceding section become more pronounced. More than half of all women also experience a "sex flush," during which skin color deepens in patches in various parts of the body.

The inner two-thirds of the vagina expands during the plateau phase, and the uterus continues to elevate in a process called "tenting." Again, post-hysterectomy, the uterine activity will be lacking but not necessarily missed.

Orgasm · According to the studies by Masters and Johnson, the uterus and outer third of the vagina contract several times during the third stage of sexual response. This process is seen as integral to the pleasurable feelings of climax. How, then, can a hysterectomized woman feel the release and joy of orgasm?

Physiologically, hysterectomy and/or oopherectomy should not impair your orgasmic potential. Women who were previously aware of uterine contractions may indeed miss these climactic surges. However, most women (60 percent) do not notice a difference with their uterus missing.[4] Instead, they continue to experience the satisfactions obtained from stimulating any number of responsive areas in the vagina, including the G-spot (see Chapter Three), and clitoris.

Ultimately, it is the clitoris that acts as the central neurological focus of the good feelings that are built up by exciting that organ itself and/or various areas within the vagina, or almost anywhere on the entire body (breasts, thighs, abdomen, lips, hair). Thus, the removal of the uterus may make orgasm feel a little less complete for some women, but most do not notice a difference.

Resolution · During the final stage of sexual response, which lasts between five and fifteen minutes, the body returns to its prearousal state. The ovaries, hormones, and uterus are least likely to be missed in this phase. Some researchers suggest that this "afterglow" period may be shorter than before because the sexual changes themselves were less intense.[5]

WOMEN'S OBSERVATIONS FOLLOWING HYSTERECTOMY / OOPHORECTOMY

Does the physiology of sex match women's own perceptions? How do women describe their sexual desire, vaginal lubrication, and overall sexual satisfaction?

SEXUAL DESIRE

Dr. Wulf H. Utian studied 85 healthy, married women in Cape Town, South Africa to determine the effect of hysterectomy, oopherectomy, and estrogen therapy on sexual desire.[6] The women gave detailed histories regarding their sexual interest, activity, and satisfaction for up to two years post-surgery. Dr. Utian concluded, "The operation of hysterectomy *per se*, irrespective of whether the ovaries are removed or not, is shown to be associated with a significant reduction in libido. Moreover, estrogen replacement therapy is shown to be of no benefit in the treatment of decreased or absent libido." The latter is not surprising since it is *androgen,* not estrogen which contributes to libido. However, it is important to note that estrogen provides vaginal lubrication, and therefore may be important in maintaining sexual satisfaction, as well as the perception of sexual arousal.

In our study, we asked women to "estimate how frequently, on average, you desire sexual activity." Responses to this question were given by 181 premenopausal, 56 post-hysterectomy, and 61 naturally post-menopause women. We found the premenopausal group to desire activity most often, followed by the hysterectomized group, and the naturally menopausal women (see Table 10 – 1). About half (53 percent) of the premenopausal women said they wanted sexual relations more than once a week, compared to 41 percent of the hysterectomized women and 31 percent of the postmenopausal women. Similarly, 25 percent of the postmenopausal wanted relations once a month or less, compared to 14 percent of the hysterectomized women and 12 percent of the premenopausal women.

TABLE 10 – 1

DESIRED FREQUENCY OF SEXUAL RELATIONS IN PREMENOPAUSAL, HYSTERECTOMIZED, AND POSTMENOPAUSAL WOMEN

	N = 298 Desired frequency of sexual relations		
	more than once a week	once a week	once a month
GROUP			
Premenopausal 181 (61%)	95 (53%)	64 (35%)	22 (12%)
Post-Hysterectomy 56 (19%)	23 (41%)	25 (45%)	8 (14%)
Post-Menopausal 61 (20%)	19 (31%)	27 (44%)	15 (25%)
Totals	137 (46%)	116 (39%)	45 (15%)

X = 11.08971 with 4 degrees of freedom. $p < .05$

When we looked closely at our findings, we found that it was *age* more than surgery or menopause which accounted for the differences in sexual desire (see Table 10 – 2). In fact, what we found was a clear age-related pattern regarding desired frequency of sexual relations. More than two-thirds (71 percent) of women in their 20s, regardless of whether or not they have had hysterectomies, desire relations more than once a week. The proportion of women seeking this degree of frequency decreases with each advancing decade. In their 30s, 58 percent of women desire sex more than once a week; only 44 percent of women in their 40s, 39 percent of women in their 50s, and 24 percent of women over age 60 express this frequency of desire.

The question remains, "What causes sexual desire to decrease as we get older?" Is it the surgical absence of the uterus and ovaries? Is it the naturally decreasing activity of both organs and their diminishing hormonal contribution? While physiological factors are important, we feel that they are not the whole story. Although in general the desire for sex declines as a woman grows older, at all ages there is considerable variability. Some women desire sexual activity frequently; others desire it rarely. Let us look at some individual cases to see if this may help explain these differences.

> Betty M., a 40-year-old hysterectomized grade school teacher, reported, "I desire sexual intercourse much more now; I never need lubrication." She attributes her *increase* in sexual desire to her hysterectomy *and* to having a husband who is desirable to her (as opposed to her previous spouse).

TABLE 10 – 2
DESIRED FREQUENCY OF SEXUAL RELATIONS
IN WOMEN AT DIFFERENT AGES

	N = 296 Desired frequency of sexual relations		
	more than once a week	once a week	once a month
AGE RANGE			
20-29 17 (6%)	12 (71%)	4 (24%)	1 (6%)
30-39 81 (27%)	47 (58%)	27 (33%)	7 (9%)
40-49 108 (36%)	48 (44%)	45 (42%)	15 (14%)
50-59 49 (17%)	19 (39%)	21 (43%)	9 (18%)
60-85 41 (14%)	10 (24%)	19 (46%)	12 (29%)
Totals	136 (46%)	116 (39%)	44 (15%)

$X^2 = 21.44013$ with 8 degrees of freedom. $p. < .01$

Jean, who is 68 years old, postmenopause, and a retired teacher noted, "I would like sex more often, but I'm a widow."

Sara, age 59, had a vaginal hysterectomy at age 43 and has taken estrogen replacement since that time. She reported "lessening of desire, more difficulty reaching orgasm." Sara has been divorced for 15 years, but has had two lovers. She attributed this change to the "aging process in both my partners and myself."

Forty-six years old, married, and in her own home business, Diane had her uterus and both ovaries removed three years before. She is taking estrogen replacement and noted "a decrease in libido since my hysterectomy."

Martha, now 50, has been married to her husband for 29 years. She rates herself in excellent health and reported "no current interest in sex *due* to the cessation of periods (as a result of natural menopause)."

In essence, then, women who are older and postmenopausal and women who have had hysterectomies are likely to desire sex less frequently than other women. But this is not true in all cases! Many older and post-surgical women have the same frequency of desire as younger, non-hysterectomized women. While physiology does contribute to our sexual desire, life situations, behaviors, and attitudes are also important. We will describe methods for overcoming limited sexual desire later in this chapter.

VAGINAL LUBRICATION

As would be expected based on physiology, our research confirmed that following hysterectomy with or without oopherectomy about half of all women experience a lessening of vaginal lubrication. Similarly, older and postmenopausal women are more likely to have less adequate vaginal lubrication than other women.

Researchers Lin S. Myers and Patricia J. Morokoff also found that postmenopausal women are likely to have less vaginal lubrication than other women. They did an interesting experiment. The investigators showed three ten-minute videotapes to women falling into three groups. Twenty women were premenopausal; 14 were postmenopausal, and another 14 postmenopausal were receiving estrogen replacement therapy. The first and last videos were non-erotic; the second was of a woman and man engaged in passionate kissing, breast and genital stimulation, and intercourse. This video had been rated as sexually arousing by women during the scientists' preliminary investigations.

Following each video, the women were asked to report on a four-point scale their degree of vaginal lubrication. Women who were premenopausal and those taking estrogen replacement reported significantly more vaginal lubrication in response to the erotic film than those women falling into the remaining group. The researchers conclude that estrogen appears to be "important in maintaining vaginal lubrication and the perception of sexual arousal."[7]

We will follow up on the idea of estrogen and other hormone replacement therapy in Chapter Eleven.

SEXUAL SATISFACTION

The concept of sexual satisfaction is more difficult to define than either frequency of sexual desire or vaginal lubrication. Some women may view it as ease of orgasm, others as climactic intensity, and still others as overall pleasure and affection associated with sexual activity.

Perhaps partly because of these differences in interpretation, when we asked, "in general, rate your current level of sexual satisfaction," we found relatively slight differences between premenopausal, hysterectomized, and postmenopausal women. Two-thirds (65 percent) of the premenopausal women, 58 percent of the hysterectomized women, and 46 percent of the postmenopausal women gave ratings of "good" or "excellent."

Our findings agree with those of the late science writer and sex researcher Edward Brecher, who found only "negligible" differences in satisfaction in the proportion of women with uterus and ovaries, compared to those without. He concluded, "the impact of hysterectomy (and oopherectomy) on sexual activity and enjoyment is quite modest." [8] It is important to point out that Brecher noted that for women without ovaries, estrogen replacement is often necessary for maintaining sexual satisfaction.

Further encouraging findings were reported by Dr. Helstrom and colleagues at University Hospital in Uppsala, Sweden. This team interviewed over 100 women one month before and one year after hysterectomy. Over half the women reported improvement in their sexuality, while only about one-fifth noted a decline.[9]

Orgasm · Before discussing this further, it is important to note that many women report that they typically do *not* experience orgasm as a result of intercourse.

The research on the proportion of women having orgasms after hysterectomy and menopause is quite limited. Phillip M. Sarrel and his colleagues studied 178 postmenopausal women, all of whom were married.[10] Of the women between the ages 35 and 62, 73 percent reported that they were often able to reach orgasm. It is unclear whether this was by coitus or masturbation. It may be worthwhile to note here that studies show that while from 30 to 50 percent of women reach orgasm during intercourse, from 75 to 95 do during masturbation.

Susanne Morgan in her book *Coping with a Hysterectomy* quotes a 51-year-old woman, Gayle, who recently had a hysterectomy due to fibroid tumors.

> Gayle reported, "There is less urgency. Before my hysterectomy I had two types of orgasms — clitoral and cervical — but afterward my orgasms were mainly clitoral. I'm not saying a clitoral orgasm isn't nice, because it is . . . but I just miss the combination of the two." [11]

Similarly, Mary Lou, a 52-year-old woman responding to our survey reported, "Following hysterectomy, orgasm just doesn't feel the same. I feel hollow inside. When I do 'come,' it is just a small clitoral climax."

Drs. Leon and Shirley Zussman and their associates reviewed a number of studies related to women's sexual response following hysterectomy with and without removal of the ovaries. They summarize their findings as follows:

> "For some women, the quality of the orgasm is related to the movement of cervix and uterus, and for these women the intensity of orgasm is thus diminished when these structures are removed. For other

women, orgasm is achieved mainly by clitoral stimulation, so that the loss of the internal structures does not have a comparable effect. Evidence that women experience one or both types of orgasm, sometimes blended, has been reported over many years and conforms with our clinical observations. The percentage of women for whom the cervix and uterus are sexually important is unknown."[12]

As noted earlier, sexual satisfaction is not restricted to orgasm; it may also include feelings of warmth and tenderness. Barbara L., age 45, noted, "I've never had a satisfactory sex life — it doesn't seem important to me — I only like the feeling of closeness." Similarly, Robin, age 52, wrote, "I have less desire for sexual intercourse but more need for intellectual stimulation and physical shows of affection."

The differing reports about orgasm and sexual satisfaction following hysterectomy and menopause may be partially due to individual variations in past behavior and current expectations. We suspect that virtually all women can have orgasms and experience sexual satisfaction, and we will offer some helpful suggestions later in this chapter.

WHAT CAN YOU EXPECT SEXUALLY AS A RESULT OF HYSTERECTOMY, MENOPAUSE, AND GETTING OLDER?

We have learned from the women who responded to our questionnaire and from the studies of other researchers that some patterns exist. These might help you predict how you may feel sexually following hysterectomy or natural menopause as you age. Surely some uncertainty remains. Every rule and description will not fit you perfectly, but they should help you understand your own experiences and feelings.

GOOD SEX EARLY LEADS TO GOOD SEX LATER

With some degree of confidence, we can tell you that if you desired sex more than once a week prior to surgery or menopause, you have about a 40% chance of continuing to have that frequency of desire. If you desired sex less than once a month, it is possible but unlikely that your desire will increase (see Table 10 – 3).

Similarly, if your vaginal lubrication prior to hysterectomy or menopause was adequate or good, it is far more likely to continue so compared to women who complained of scant lubrication at an earlier time.

It is worth noting that the Swedish researchers mentioned earlier similarly reported that preoperative sexual activity appears to be the best predictor of postoperative sexuality.[13]

TABLE 10 – 3

DESIRED FREQUENCY OF SEXUAL RELATIONS IN WOMEN BEFORE AND AFTER HYSTERECTOMY AND MENOPAUSE

	Current desired frequency of sexual relations		
	more than once a week	once a week	once a month
Prior Desired Frequency			
more than once a week 68 (63%)	30 (44%)	28 (41%)	10 (15%)
once a week 32 (30%)	6 (19%)	19 (59%)	7 (22%)
once a month 8 (7%)	2 (25%)	2 (25%)	4 (50%)
Totals	38 (35%)	49 (45%)	21 (19%)

$X^2 = 11.33684$ with 4 degrees of freedom. $p < .05$

OVERALL HEALTH AND FITNESS RELATE TO SEX

We found that women who consider themselves in good health and are physically fit desire sex more often and are more satisfied than those whose health and fitness are only adequate or poor.

PARTNER SUPPORT MAY INFLUENCE SEXUAL FEELINGS

Following hysterectomy or menopause, some women have reduced sexual pleasure because they fear their partner has a negative attitude toward their sexuality. Linda Anne Bernhard, in her report, "Black women's concerns about sexuality and hysterectomy," noted that almost half of the women in her study did not tell their regular sexual partner that they were having a hysterectomy prior to surgery. These women generally did not inform their partners because they believed that "men think women who have hysterectomies are 'different,' 'not complete,' and 'can't function sexually.'"[14]

> Beth, age 49, recently had a hysterectomy and reported that her husband told her he "missed the feeling of (his) penis against her cervix during intercourse... (he) tried to get the same stimulation against the head of the penis by moving in different positions, but it was not the same."

Some women report that their partners are unhappy with the poor vaginal lubrication which is a result of the lack of estrogen following surgical removal of the ovaries or menopause. The man may believe that this suggests

TABLE 10 – 8

DESIRED FREQUENCY OF SEXUAL RELATIONS IN WOMEN REPORTING DIFFERENT LEVELS OF HEALTH

	Desired frequency of sexual relations		
	more than once a week	once a week	once a month
Reported Health			
Poor 8 (3%)	2 (25%)	3 (38%)	3 (38%)
Adequate 30 (10%)	14 (47%)	8 (27%)	8 (27%)
Good 133 (45%)	63 (47%)	46 (35%)	24 (18%)
Excellent 126 (42%)	58 (46%)	59 (47%)	9 (7%)
Totals	137 (46%)	116 (39%)	44 (15%)

X = 16.19837 with 6 degrees of freedom. $p < .05$

the woman is not aroused. While this is not necessarily true, undiscussed, it may lead to the man's lessening of sexual interest, thereby reducing the woman's desire and resulting in a vicious cycle of withdrawal from sexual activity.

In our survey, we asked our respondents how their husband or partner reacted to menopause and gynecological surgery. We found that slightly more than 65 percent of the women reported that their husbands were supportive. Less than 3 percent reported negative responses from their husbands, and the remainder said their partner did not react either positively or negatively.

We found that women who report partner support are often likely to have a better sexual relationship as well. The impact of support is dramatically expressed by Delores.

> "In retrospect, I needed a lot more attention and understanding from my husband. All he wanted to know from me was — where he was going to get his sex while I recovered from surgery.... He claims the operation caused me to be frigid. I believed this until I left the marriage and found that I'm a very sexual person. I now live with a man and our sex life is excellent. At age 59, I find the only sexual problem I have is making up for lost time with my new companion for life."

WHAT TO DO TO IMPROVE SEXUALITY

SEXUAL DESIRE

Premenopausally, hormones released during the ovulation phase of the menstrual cycle may relate to sexual interest.[15] However, as you probably remember, this time of the month — midway between your period — was not the only time you were interested in sex. The desire for sex is influenced by many things. We may be stimulated by hormones, or a person, fantasy, movie, book, or exercise.

Hormone Replacement Therapy · Assuming that you have had your ovaries removed or are past menopause so that your ovaries are no longer producing hormones, you may opt for hormone replacement therapy (HRT). Strongly recommended by many health care providers, estrogen combined with progestin (if your uterus is still intact) may enhance all aspects of sexual function.

> Theresa, a 61-year old high school English teacher, noted, "I went through menopause when I was about 50. At that time I had been in a relationship for about ten years that had its ups and downs. The best part of the 'up' was the sex. Around the time of menopause, sex stopped being good. I first thought it was due to the craziness that Leonard and I were going through. I mentioned this to my regular gynecologist, who knew me fairly well. He didn't seem to want to talk about sex, so I went to see another gynecologist who had been recommended because he was also a sex therapist. This second physician put me on hormone replacement therapy and sex between Leonard and me became as good as ever. Unfortunately, the 'crazies' continued, so we are no longer together. I'm in a new relationship right now and the sex is great."

We will talk more about specific hormones and benefits and risks of HRT in Chapter Eleven.

The Power of the Mind · The mind is probably the most powerful sexual organ. We are stimulated by our thoughts, by seeing someone we feel is sexually desirable, by reading erotic stories, by surrounding ourselves with sensuous material and clothing, and by listening to certain music. Dr. John W. Huffman of Northwestern University Medical School points out in speaking of post-hysterectomized women that "it matters very much that the patient and her sexual partner understand that sexual pleasure is a child of the psyche."[16]

We can put ourselves "in the mood" for love. If you feel that your desire for sex has diminished, and you are unhappy about this, try to do things that will make you feel sexier. Go to see a romantic or even pornographic movie, read a love story, set your imagination free. Some women find buying new satiny underwear or negligees is arousing. Indulge yourself in a bubble bath or sprinkle on a new cologne. All of these may help.

Think about your partner, if you have one. Remind yourself of all the loving and tender things about this person. What brought you together in the first place? What do you admire about your lover? How can you show you care? Try to do nonsexual extras to please this person. A special meal, a little love note, or an unexpected gift may all help bring back romance. Spend intimate time together; take a walk in the evening or a drive on the weekend. Listen to your partner; rekindle your understanding and appreciation of this human being. As your thoughts turn toward affection, you may be surprised that your body may become aroused. What begins as hugs and touching to show closeness may lead to sexual foreplay.

Have you ever noticed how much of popular music is about love or sex? Play music that appeals to you. Sing along. Dance around the house. See if your partner will dance with you. Our world is full of potential sexual stimulation. Be aware of the resources available to you and take time to use them to your advantage.

Finding a Partner — or Not · The projected life expectancy for women is almost 80 years, and for men not quite 73.[17] Since women tend to live longer than men, many of us become widowed. Others of us lose husbands through divorce. In any gathering of older people, there are always far more women than men. Often the women seem to be competing for the few unattached men around.

Your first decision is whether you really want a partner. This is a very personal matter. If you've had a good relationship in the past, you may want to try again. On the other hand, a good past relationship may be something that you prefer to treasure in memory.

If you have decided that you want to enter the competition for a partner, you must admit that this is your objective. Then, let everyone know; you might have a chance of being introduced to someone great.

Go to activities that interest you and you may find a kindred spirit. While sexual relations between a man and a woman are most common, it is worthwhile to recognize that people, in fact, are sexual beings. This means that we are capable of being stimulated in a variety of ways. Sex researchers have reported that about one in four women has leanings toward, has participated in sexual activity with, or is currently in a sexual relationship with another woman.[18/19] Some women who have been with a man for most of their adulthood find a sexual partnership with another woman later in life quite wonderful.

Can you keep sexual interest alive if you do not have a partner? Should you? The second answer is really up to you. If you want to remain sexually vital as you age, you probably can be reasonably successful. Read on for some helpful advice. (Also see "Going It Alone," later in this chapter.) If, on the other hand, you feel that sexual desire without a partner is handicapping, then perhaps it is best to permit your sexual feelings to become dormant. You might wish to skip ahead to the next chapter.

Kegel Exercises · Sexual interest may be maintained by "working" the sexual organs as soon after surgery as is comfortable. (Generally, waiting a week is advisable.) Arnold Kegel, a gynecologist, devised a set of exercises to help women who suffered from urinary incontinence. These exercises turned out to be helpful not only in preventing the release of urine with coughs, laughs, and sneezes, but they also had a sexual benefit. The Kegel exercises, as they are now called, improve vaginal tone and can enhance all aspects of sexual functioning. Kegel exercises are often prescribed for women of various ages to alleviate an assortment of sexual problems involving arousal, responsiveness, and orgasm.

The focus of the Kegel exercises is to strengthen the **pubococcygeal** (PC) muscles (the muscles which encircle and support the vagina). Here is how they work.

1. For several days, practice stopping your urine flow and starting it again. This will help to make you aware of the PC muscle. As you stop your urine you will be contracting the muscle, as you permit the flow you will be letting the muscle relax.
2. When you have mastered step 1, tense your PC muscle for about three seconds, then relax it for another three seconds. You should do this about a dozen times three or four times a day for two or three weeks.
3. When you are comfortable with step 2, you are ready for step 3. This is similar to step 2, except rather than holding the tension or relaxation for three seconds, you alternate rapidly between the two. This is called the "flutter."
4. After about two months of moving through steps 1 through 3, you are ready for step 4. Concentrate on moving an *imaginary* object such as a finger, penis, or dildo up from the outside of your vagina to a place deep inside. You should have a drawing-in sensation.
5. The last exercise is the opposite of the previous one. In step 5, you bear down, focusing on pushing an imaginary object out of your vagina. Visualizing a large tampon may be helpful.

When you have gone through all 5 steps, continue to do all of the exercises several times a day. An advantage to Kegel exercises is that you can do them anywhere, anytime. While waiting in line at the grocery, watching television, driving a car, or reading, no one need know that you are working on your sexuality![20]

VAGINAL LUBRICATION

You can expect to have less vaginal lubrication as the result of removal of your ovaries or normal menopause. Fortunately, some good solutions to this problem exist.

Estrogen · Estrogen replacement therapy has been found to be highly beneficial in reducing vaginal dryness. Estrogen may be introduced into your system in a number of ways. You may take estrogen (possibly with other hormones) in the form of a pill or capsule. Some physicians prescribe estrogen "**transdermally**." This means that you wear a patch which slowly releases **estradiol** (a form of estrogen) into your bloodstream. A third way to obtain estrogen is through the use of a vaginal cream which contains **conjugated estrogen** in a nonliquefying base. This cream is inserted directly into your vagina through the use of a plastic applicator and/or spread on the inner and outer vaginal lips with your fingers. Estrogen creams should *not* be used in the vagina immediately prior to intercourse. While the long-term effect is to improve vaginal moistness, these creams are neither intended or effective as lubricants. In addition, if used just before intercourse, some may be absorbed through the man's urethra. While probably not harmful, the effect has not been adequately studied.[21]

The method that you choose is for you and your physician to decide. We talk more about hormone replacement therapy in the next chapter. If you decide to use estrogen in any form, you will probably find that it is helpful in relieving vaginal dryness.

Vaginal Lubricants · Whether or not you use estrogen, you may feel the need for extra lubrication for satisfactory sexual intercourse. *K-Y Jelly*™ is a commercial water-soluble lubricant that many women find very useful. A squish of about an inch or so from the tube may be smoothed on your partner's penis. You might also like to put a small amount directly into your vagina. This jelly is not harmful, will not degrade a condom, and is usually effective. One drawback, however, is that some couples find this product somewhat messy. Simple saliva is also a harmless and generally worthwhile lubricant.

If your partner uses a condom, petroleum-based products such as *Vaseline*™ or baby oil are not a good idea since they can damage the condom. (Condoms may be used to prevent sexually transmitted diseases and conception. Remember, occasionally women who have a uterus conceive during their menopausal years, and neither menopause nor hysterectomy protect you from STDs.) If no condom is used, as with an exclusive partner, oils may be used and can be very pleasant.

Moisturizing products, such as *Replens*™ and *Lubrin*™, are available without a prescription at local pharmacies. *Lubrin*™ is a capsulelike gel which is inserted into the vagina. It should be applied at least five minutes before intercourse so that it is dissolved prior to intromission. Moisturizers do not have to be used exclusively in relation to sexual activity. *Replens*™ is recommended to replenish vaginal moistness when inserted about twice a week. These products consist primarily of water, glycerin, mineral oil (and no hormones). No ill effects have been reported.

You should keep in mind that antihistamines and decongestants which you might take to combat colds or allergies serve to dry out *all* mucous membranes, not just the ones in your nose. If vaginal dryness is a problem, you might want to avoid these medications, since the vagina is composed largely of mucous membranes.

ORGASM

As you well know, if you have ever suffered from menstrual cramps, the uterus is a powerful organ. You have felt its contraction as part of your monthly cycle and possibly also as part of your sexual climax. Can you have a complete orgasm without a uterus?

The Masters and Johnson research team found that for *all* women, orgasm consists of contractions of the uterus, the outer third of the vagina, and the anal sphincter.[22] In addition, muscles in various other parts of the body also contract, and brain waves show a departure from their normal patterns.

Following hysterectomy, there is no uterus to contract. Women who were keenly aware of uterine contractions during orgasm prior to hysterectomy are most likely to miss this feeling. However, the pelvic muscles, vagina, and brain waves continue to mark sexual climax just as before.

If you feel that you are not adequately orgasmic, you may be able to help yourself in several ways.

Increase Clitoral Stimulation · If you find that following hysterectomy or menopause, orgasm is harder to reach than before, additional clitoral stimulation may be helpful. This may be achieved be encouraging your partner to use hand or tongue on the clitoris. Or you may rub your clitoris yourself while your partner enters your vagina from the rear. An additional option is to apply an electric massager or vibrator to the clitoris. Many women who do not climax readily in other ways respond surprisingly well to this device. The choice is yours, and you should feel free to experiment. Whatever technique or combination brings you satisfaction is okay to use. There are no rules as to what is "right," "mature," or "loving."

According to the research of Masters and Johnson, "all female orgasms follow the same reflex response patterns, no matter what the source of sexual stimulation."[23] This means that the physiological response will be the same whether a hand, mouth, or vibrator provides direct clitoral stimulation leading to orgasm, or a penis in the vagina during intercourse results in climax.

Explore the "G-Spot" · The Grafenberg area, more commonly known as the "G-spot," is an area in the front portion of the vagina that is supposed to be especially sensitive to stimulation. You may find that during intercourse, certain positions are especially exciting. This is likely because these permit the penis to contact the Grafenberg area.

Sexologists J. D. Perry and Beverly Whipple claim that the G-spot is the trigger point for orgasm.[24] Other sex researchers disagree and maintain that less than 10 percent of women have a sensitive area in the front part of the vagina.[25]

You can form your own conclusions for yourself. Explore your G-spot by placing a finger in your vagina and pressing toward the front. Your partner can help.

Sensate Focus · Masters and Johnson use a procedure known as "sensate focus" to help couples who are having sexual problems.[26] You can use it too. Begin by setting a time when you and your partner will be uninterrupted. Prepare a comfortable spot such as your bed or couch. You will have several sessions of touching one another *without* sexual intercourse.

In session one of sensate focus, you should simply touch your partner's body in a nonsexual way. Do *not* touch the genitals or breasts! Do *not* guess what will please or arouse your partner. Simply touch to explore the contours, temperatures, and textures of your partner's body. The goal is *not* arousal; it is simply exploratory.

In session two, your partner touches you in the same way that you did in the first session. You should try not to talk, but do make each other aware of what touch may be pleasant or uncomfortable.

Sessions three and four include the breasts and genitals. Begin with general touch and then move to exploration of the more sexual parts of the body. Do not try to arouse your partner; the focus continues to be simply to get to know the other person's body better. You may use the hand-over-hand, or "**hand-riding,**" technique in which the person being touched places his or her hand on top of the partner's. This way the person receiving the touch may *gently* guide the firmness, speed, and locations of touch.

In the next sessions, you and your partner touch one another simultaneously. You no longer take turns being the toucher and the receiver of touch. You do not engage in sexual intercourse, but concentrate on the sensations of touching your partner's body.

If the preceding session went well, you may move to the final stage, where you lie on top of your partner. You may permit your partner's penis to enter you after you have engaged in rubbing your genitals against his.

You may think of this as a kind of foreplay. In fact, it has been successful in increasing the feelings of arousal for both women and men and leading eventually to orgasm and general sexual satisfaction.

On a recent television talk show, host Phil Donahue asked women in the audience when they would like foreplay to begin. One woman responded "in the morning." "For sex that night?" asked Donahue. "You bet," was the response, which was met with enthusiastic audience applause. The point is that women are often slower to arouse and reach orgasm than men. This is especially true as we age. Engaging in sensate focus, as described above, permits the foreplay to begin days before sexual intercourse is even attempted.

Goal-Free Pleasuring · It is commonly believed that the "goal" of sex is orgasm. Even the term "foreplay" suggests that hugging, kissing, sweet words, or whatever, come before the "main" sexual activity — which is intercourse culminating in orgasm. Men may report the number of times "sex" took place on a particular occasion by the frequency of *their* orgasms. Women, too, often view "sex" as a step-by-step procedure with orgasm at the top rung. Partners move from hugging, to kissing, to caresses, to genital touch, to oral- genital activity, and finally to intercourse resulting in orgasm.

Sex need not be goal-directed, however. Sex therapist Helen Kaplan suggests that a goal-free approach encourages partners to enjoy every aspect of their intimacy without focusing on a magical end point. Instead of going up the ladder to climax, lovers may hug and kiss, then engage in oral-genital activity, go back and talk and caress, engage in intercourse, then hug and kiss, and simply orient themselves to provide and receive pleasure.

The idea behind goal-free pleasuring is that you do not have to experience orgasm to enjoy sex. Knowing and accepting that, many couples who remove the single-minded pursuit of orgasm from their intimate times, find that they may climax almost in spite of themselves. Whether or not this happens for you, simply enjoying sensuous interaction can be a delight in itself. You do not need to orgasm to enjoy sex.[27]

SEXUAL SATISFACTION

A decade or so ago, the late Edward Brecher set out to write a book about sex and aging. He designed a survey which was advertised in the magazine *Consumer Reports*.[28] Responses were received from 4,246 women and men between the ages of 50 and 93. As he began to read through the completed questionnaires, he realized that he would have to broaden his book.

For almost all respondents, sex and aging could not be discussed without also talking about love.[29] Sexual satisfaction is based on a number of factors.

Good Relations · Good sex does not begin in bed. It may begin at the breakfast table discussing the day's plans. Cooking a meal together, or cleaning up afterward, may kindle the embers that lead to sexual closeness.

One couple we interviewed always took a walk after dinner. In fact, they were known in their community as evening strollers. They could be seen regularly, arm-in-arm or holding hands; sometimes talking, often just enjoying the weather, scenery, and their special ritual.

Good relations means having positive thoughts about your partner. Accentuate in your mind those things that you like and admire. Don't harp on what irks you. Try to shrug off petty annoyances. Sometimes as we live with the same partner for many years we develop routines that may be helpful or harmful. A helpful routine may be the sincere compliment that comes without fail following the completion of some task. A harmful routine is an argument that you have repeatedly.

Do not expect to be mirror images of one another. If one of you is always early and the other tends to run late, this may be a source of routine fighting. Recognizing and accepting your differences can go a long way toward improving your relationship.

Love and Tenderness · Think of ways to express your love. Little notes, special meals, or small gifts can all say, "I love you. I value you."

> LuAnn, a postmenopausal woman who responded to our survey, wrote that her marriage of 42 years remained sexually "vibrant" because "we never take each other for granted." LuAnn wrote that she and her husband had been through some hard financial times and had experienced both sadness and joy in raising a disabled child. Their sex remained good "even after menopause" because they "never stopped appreciating one another."

> Rosemarie, a 68-year-old retired teacher, told us "we wish each other a happy birthday every morning. This means that we want the other to have a happy day every day. Then we shake our fingers at each other and say 'don't go away.' This doesn't mean don't leave, it means stay healthy, don't die...be with me always.... While the fireworks have dimmed somewhat, sex is still very sweet.... My husband doesn't orgasm every time anymore, although I do but more gently.... Somehow that part of sex matters less than it used to."

> Sharon, a 44-year old who had a hysterectomy in her early 40s, reported that her partner was always making her laugh. "He constantly does things that crack me up. I think it's his way of telling me that he

loves me.... Our sex is tender and loving, but I always need to use a vibrator to reach orgasm. I often think it would be better if I didn't, but we've both sort of accepted it as the way things are."

Is love essential for good sex? Edward Brecher received answers from 1,789 women and 2,377 men, all aged 50 or over, to the question "Is sex without love better than no sex at all?" About 28 percent of the women and 67 percent of the men agreed. Brecher quotes one 51-year-old woman: "If sex without love is the only thing available to an individual, then I see no problem — but it should never be understood as more than half a loaf."[30]

Massage and Other Goodies · Laura, a 49-year-old woman who reported that she "thinks (she is) going through menopause now," told us that "intercourse isn't as important as it used to be.... We do a lot of nonsexual but very sensuous stuff together.... We have an oversized bathtub and often soak together and still soap each other up. It's fun. It used to always lead to sex, but it doesn't anymore. Sometimes I care and feel we're getting old, but other times it's okay. Anyway, when we do have sex, it still feels great...it's just that it's not as often. I've been with my present husband for almost 15 years now.... I can't imagine soaking in a bathtub with my first husband."

> Bea, a 54-year-old hysterectomized woman who lives in Southern California, told us "our hot tub saved our marriage.... When the kids were little, our special time alone was when they were in bed and we could soak, look at the stars, and have time to talk.... It often got us worked up sexually, too. The hot tub is still our thing. We often use it consciously to help us get in the mood for sex.... I think as you get older you have to work more to get interested. This is true for both my husband and me."

Other women wrote us about the use of massage to just make one another feel good. You can massage any part of the body or the whole body. Some people really enjoy giving or receiving a foot massage. You apply pressure and rub or knead your partner. You might consider receiving a professional massage and then applying what you've experienced at home. There are also courses, workshops, and books which teach the art of massage. Remember, the objective is not sexual but sensual. Sexual feelings may be aroused, but they are not the purpose of most massage.

Going It Alone · According to Brecher, 47 percent of women in their 50s reported that they currently masturbate, compared to 37 percent aged 60 to 69, and 33 percent over age 70. Unmarried women are more likely to masturbate than married women. And more men than women of all ages report that they masturbate.[31]

Whether or not you have a partner, stimulating yourself sexually can be a highly effective way of maintaining sexual energy.

Betty Dodson is the author of an excellent little book (now also available as a home video), *Selflove and Orgasm*, which can serve as a guide for female masturbation.[32] Ms. Dodson, an artist, writes about her experiences with masturbation as a child, an adult, and a leader of selflove workshops. She describes how most of us feel reluctant to masturbate, especially if we are married or in a sexual relationship.

Going it alone requires, first of all, accepting your sexuality. This means recognizing that, contrary to many traditional beliefs, masturbation is fine. Although it is not usually talked about, masturbation is not something shameful. It can't hurt (or blind) you. It will make you more sexually responsive and aware, and may be considered a celebration of the female body.

You might want to begin by examining your genitals. Dodson has sketches of different women's external sexual organs. We all look a little different, but each is beautiful. This self-appreciation may be work after all the years of thinking about this part of our body as "dirty." Even the ancient Greek artists glorified the male penis in sculpture but ignored the female counterpart. Georgia O'Keeffe and Betty Dodson are two twentieth-century artists who encouraged women to see their genitals as lovely flowers rather than the "pussies" or "beavers" of male slang. Use a hand-held cosmetic mirror and take your time exploring your own body.

If masturbation has not been part of your sexual life for many years, give yourself permission to start again. Experiment with touch that feels good. Use your fingers to rub, pull, and pinch. Enter your vagina with one, two, or three fingers while rubbing your clitoris with your thumb. Try a two-handed approach. You may have both hands on your genitals or one there, the other on your breasts. Some women like to place an object, such as a large pillow, between their thighs and build up sexual pressure in this way.

Electric or battery-operated massagers may be placed on the genitals and moved or held as you desire. Betty Dodson reports the comments of a woman who was in one of Dodson's "Bodysex" groups. "...I've been using the vibrator since last summer...but I never masturbated before then. And would you believe it? I actually came in about three minutes after 25 years of not coming!"[33] Many women who do not climax easily any other way find that stimulation with a vibrator or massager provides an almost guaranteed orgasm.

Do not forget that sexual excitement is stimulated outside of the genitals, too. Even if you are alone, you may dress for sex. Silks and laces may help to arouse you. Look in the mirror to see how good you look. Romantic or pornographic movies, books, or magazines may put you in the mood.

Music may also help. Alone time may be prime fantasy time. Nancy Friday has written about women's fantasies, and reading about these may inspire some of yours.[34] Remember that age, menopause, and hysterectomy need not be barriers to sexuality. Betty Dodson writes about her telephone call to her 69-year-old widowed mother. The younger Dodson brashly started the conversation with, "'Mother, are you masturbating to orgasm?' and received the response, "Why Betty Ann, of course not! I'm too old for that sort of thing.'" Betty Dodson then lectured her mother on the relationship between good health and orgasm, telling her that masturbation would help to keep the lining of the vagina lubricated and stimulate hormone secretion. It was also a way to relax.

Dodson reported that in their next conversation, a couple of weeks later, "(her mother) had successfully and very easily masturbated to orgasm. Mother said it had been pleasant, and she felt that afterward she had slept more soundly. Then she chuckled and said it could never compare with the 'real thing.'"[35]

ENDNOTES

1. Huffman, J. W. Sex after hysterectomy. *Medical Aspects of Human Sexuality*, July 1985, 19, 174.

2. Morgan, S. Sex after hysterectomy — what your doctor never told you. *Ms.*, March 1982, 82.

3. Masters, W. H., Johnson, V. E., & Kolodny, R.C. *Human Sexuality, 4th edition*. NY: HarperCollins, 1992.

4. Goldfarb, H. A., with Grief, J. *The No-Hysterectomy Option: Your Body — Your Choice*. New York: John Wiley, 1990, p.175.

5. Morgan, S. *Coping with a Hysterectomy*. New York: Plume, 1986.

6. Utian, W. H. Effect of hysterectomy, oophorectomy, and estrogen therapy on libido. *Obstetrical and Gynecological Survey*, 1976, 31, 319 – 321.

7. Myers, L. S., & Morokoff, P. L. Physiological and subjective sexual arousal in pre- and postmenopausal women and postmenopausal women taking replacement therapy. *Psychophysiology*, 1986, 23 (3), 283 – 292.

8. Brecher, Edward M. *Love, Sex, and Aging*. Boston: Little, Brown, 1984, p. 278.

9. Helstrom, L., Lundberg, P. O. Sorbom, D., et al. Sexuality after hysterectomy: a factor analysis of women's sexual lives before and after subtotal hysterectomy. *Obstetrics and Gynecology*, March 1993, 81 (3), 357– 362.

10. Brody, J. E. On menopause and the toll that loss of estrogens can take on a woman's sexuality. *New York Times*, May 10, 1990, B15.

11. Morgan, S. *Coping with a Hysterectomy*. New York: Plume, 1986, p. 138.

12. Zussman, L., Zussman, S., Sunley, R., & Bjornson, E. Sexual response after

hysterectomy-oophorectomy: recent studies and reconsideration of psychogenesis. *American Journal of Obstetrics and Gynecology*, August 1, 1981, 140 (7), p. 729.

13. Helstrom, L., Lundberg, P. O. Sorbom, D., et al. Sexuality after hysterectomy: a factor analysis of women's sexual lives before and after subtotal hysterectomy. *Obstetrics and Gynecology*, March 1993, 81 (3), 357– 362.

14. Bernhard, L. A. Black women's concerns about sexuality and hysterectomy. *Sage*, Fall 1985, II (2), 25 – 27.

15. Masters, W. H., Johnson, V. E., & Kolodny, R.C. *Human Sexuality, 3rd edition*. Glenview, IL: Scott, Foresman, 1988, p. 105.

16. Huffman, J. W. Sex after hysterectomy. *Medical Aspects of Human Sexuality*, July 1985, 19, 166.

17. U.S. Bureau of the Census. *Statistical Abstract of the United States: 1994* (114th edition). Washington, D.C., 1994.

18. Hunt, M. *Sexual Behavior in the 1970s*. Chicago: Playboy Press, 1974.

19. Kinsey, A.C., Pomeroy, W. B., & Martin, C. E. *Sexual Behavior in the Human Female*. Philadelphia: W. B. Saunders, 1953.

20. Haas, K., & Haas, A. *Understanding sexuality, 3rd edition*. St. Louis, MO: Mosby-Yearbook, 1993.

21. *Physicians' Desk Reference*, 48th edition. Montvale, NJ: Medical Economics Data, 1994.

22. Masters, W. H., Johnson, V. E., & Kolodny, R.C. *Human Sexuality, 4th edition*. NY: HarperCollins, 1992.

23. Masters, W. H., Johnson, V. E., & Kolodny, R.C. *Human Sexuality, 3rd Edition*. Glenview, IL: Scott, Foresman, 1988.

24. Perry, J. D., & Whipple, B. Pelvic muscle strength of female ejaculators: Evidence in support of a new theory of orgasm. *Journal of Sex Research*, 1981, 17 (1), 22 – 39.

25. Alzate, H., & Londono, M. L. Vaginal erotic sensitivity. *Journal of Sex and Marital Therapy*, 1984, 10, 49 – 56.

26. Masters, W. H., Johnson, V. E., & Kolodny, R.C. *Human Sexuality, 4th edition*. NY: HarperCollins, 1992.

27. Haas, K., & Haas, A. *Understanding Sexuality, 3rd Edition*. St. Louis, MO: Mosby-Yearbook, 1993.

28. Brecher, Edward M. *Love, Sex, and Aging*. Boston: Little, Brown, 1984.

29. Edward M. Brecher, personal communication.

30. Brecher, Edward M. *Love, Sex, and Aging*. Boston: Little, Brown, 1984, pp. 244 – 245.

31. Brecher, Edward M. *Love, Sex, and Aging*. Boston: Little, Brown, 1984.

32. Dodson, Betty. *Selflove and Orgasm*. P.O.Box 1933 Murray Hill Station, NY, 10156: Betty Dodson, 1983.

33. Dodson, Betty. *Selflove and Orgasm*. P.O.Box 1933 Murray Hill Station, NY, 10156: Betty Dodson, 1983, p. 54.

34. Friday, N. *Women On Top: How Real Life Has Changed Women's Fantasies*. New York: Simon & Schuster, 1991.

35. Dodson, Betty. *Selflove and Orgasm*. P.O.Box 1933 Murray Hill Station, NY, 10156: Betty Dodson, 1983, p. 23.

SUGGESTED READING

Banner, Lois W. *In Full Flower: Aging Women, Power, and Sexuality. A History*. New York: Alfred A. Knopf, 1992.

Barbach, Lonnie, & David L. Geisinger. *Going the Distance: Finding and Keeping Lifelong Love*. New York: Plume, 1993.

Brecher, Edward M. *Love, Sex, and Aging*. Boston: Little, Brown, 1984.

Butler, Robert N., & Myrna I Lewis. *Love and Sex After Forty: A Guide for Men and Women for Their Mid and Later Years*. New York: Bantam Doubleday Dell, 1987.

Dodson, Betty. *Selflove and Orgasm*. P.O.Box 1933 Murray Hill Station, NY, 10156: Betty Dodson, 1983.

Friday, N. *Women On Top: How Real Life Has Changed Women's Fantasies*. New York: Simon & Schuster, 1991.

Greenwood, Sadja. *Menopause Naturally: Preparing for the Second Half of Life*. San Francisco: Spinsters-Aunt Lute Book Co., 1988.

Lloyd, Joan E. *If It Feels Good: Using the Five Senses to Enhance Your Lovemaking*. New York: Warner Books, 1993.

Ransohoff, Rita. *Venus After Forty: Sexual Myths, Men's Fantasies and Truths about Middle-Aged Women*. Far Hills, NJ: New Horizon Press, 1990.

Semmens, James. *Mid-Life Sexuality: Enrichment and Problem-Solving*. Durant, OK: Essential Medical Information systems, Inc., 1991.

Shapiro, Constance H. *When Part of the Self is Lost: Helping Clients Heal After Sexual and Reproductive Losses*. San Francisco: Jossey-Bass, Inc., 1992.

Sheehy, Gail. *The Silent Passage*. New York: Random House, 1992.

Sipan, Sipan N. *Sex Drive at Any Age*. New York: Vantage Press, 1991.

Westheimer, Ruth. *Dr. Ruth's Encylopedia of Sex*. New York: Continuum Publishing Co., 1994.

TAPES

Barbach, Lonnie. *Sex After 50*, videotape. Institute for Health and Aging (800-866-1000), 1991.

Zilbergeld, Bernie, & Lonnie Barbach. *An Ounce of Prevention: How to Talk with a Partner About Smart Sex*. Audiotape. Fay Institute (800-669-0156), 1988.

Chapter 11

HORMONE REPLACEMENT THERAPY

Live in each season as it passes; breathe the air, drink the drink, taste the fruit, and resign yourself to the influences of each. — Henry David Thoreau

HORMONE REPLACEMENT THERAPY

Sixty years ago, postmenopausal women didn't have to make a choice — there was no such thing as hormone replacement. Now that we have the option, we are torn between two points of view, each with excellent documentation and each claiming to be looking out for our best interests.

The conflicting points of view can be expressed as a simple question: should we (or should we not) take hormones as a replacement for those our body once produced? The information we're presenting in this book is not intended to be an answer. We are not taking sides; instead, in this chapter you will find a careful consideration of the latest information in support of and against **hormone replacement therapy** (HRT).

Although numerous studies have been published, many are recognized to have flaws which invalidate their conclusions. As a result, researchers are eagerly awaiting the findings from two projects which are currently underway. The National Institutes of Health's Postmenopausal Estrogen/Progestin Interventions Trial is nearing completion. The project has been examining the effects of different hormone replacement regimens on risk factors for heart disease, osteoporosis, some cancers, and diabetes. The other study on which much hope is placed is the federally funded project called The Women's Health Initiative.

The dilemma of whether or not to take hormones is a real one and faces all of us. We hope this chapter clarifies the issues and provides you with the information you need. Discussion with your physician is also an important part of the decision-making process. With all the various input, the informed decision will be yours to make.

HISTORY AND DEFINITIONS

Premarin, an equine estrogen, has been available and prescribed for postmenopausal women since 1941. However, it was not until the 1960s that the use of estrogen received wide publicity, mostly through the writings of R. A. Wilson. He coined the phrase "feminine forever" and strongly advocated that women take **estrogen replacement therapy** (ERT) for the remainder of their lives. Millions of women heeded his call.

In the 1970s, however, estrogen received bad publicity. Studies were revealing that the estrogen in the contraceptive pill used by women may have contributed to blood clots.[1] That information, combined with new revelations of estrogen increasing the risk of endometrial cancer,[2] caused many women to stop using estrogen — as birth control or replacement therapy.

In the mid 1980s, estrogen replacement therapy came back into favor. The increased usage was due to a convergence of three factors. First, new research indicated that estrogen has a beneficial effect in preventing bone loss. Second, studies showed a strong positive effect against cardiovascular disease. Finally, it was demonstrated that if progestin was used in combination with estrogen, it could protect the uterus from estrogen-induced hyperplasia and carcinoma.[3]

The new combined estrogen and progestin regimen prompted the change of nomenclature from estrogen replacement therapy to the broader term — hormone replacement therapy (HRT). In the discussion that follows, we will use the inclusive term *HRT* as a general term for *any* hormonal therapeutic intervention (that is, estrogen replacement with or without progesterone). When we want to refer to the therapeutic use of *only* estrogen, we will use the term *ERT*.

CHOICES OF THERAPY

Today, hormone replacement therapy may consist of estrogen alone or estrogen combined with progestin. Remember (from Chapter Two) that estrogen is a general term for a group of naturally occurring estrogens in the body: estradiol, estrone, and estriol. It also describes two other types of estrogens that are administered clinically: the **conjugated estrogens**, derived from the urine of pregnant mares; and the **synthetic estrogens**, like **diethylstilbestrol (DES)** and **chlorotrianisene (Tace)**, which don't have the same chemical steroid structure, but have an estrogenic effect. Progestins is the term used to refer to both the natural (progesterone) and synthetic chemical (progestogen) agents which act on the uterine endometrium. All three terms (progestin, progesterone, and progestogen) are often used interchangeably.

Estrogen · Estrogen, either conjugated or natural, may be taken orally in pill form, through vaginal cream, or via a transdermal patch.

Oral estrogen pills are usually taken daily for 25 days. They are available under both brand and generic names. A woman without a uterus usually takes the estrogen **unopposed** — the term used to denote the fact that progestin is not included. In the **combined opposed** regimen, progestogen is usually taken for 10 days. When progestogen is taken at a lower dose for the entire time that estrogen is taken, it is known as a **combined opposed continuous dosage** regimen. Taking estrogen in pill form has the possible disadvantage that it might induce gallstones or changes in liver metabolism. The advantage of oral estrogens is their ease and convenience of use.

Vaginal estrogen cream is inserted into the vagina with an applicator, or it may be applied to the vulva and vagina with the fingers. Estrogen is well-absorbed through the vaginal mucosa. While it has its greatest influence at that location, it also finds its way throughout the body. Vaginal cream provides the quickest relief of symptoms of what doctors call **atrophic vaginitis** such as vaginal irritation, **pruritis** (intense itching), vaginal dryness, and **dyspareunia** (painful intercourse). It makes sense to use this method if these are your primary symptoms. Some women taking oral estrogen may still need to supplement their pills with vaginal cream to maintain their vaginal mucosa.

Unlike estrogen in pill form, estrogen in the cream initially bypasses the liver as it enters the circulation. This method has its advantages and disadvantages. On the plus side, estrogen in vaginal cream form is unlikely to aggravate medical conditions such as gallstones and liver dysfunction. On the negative side, however, use of the vaginal cream won't increase HDL cholesterol (the good kind) — which seems to require action by the liver. Another disadvantage, though minor, is that if you still have your uterus, you should also take your progestogen pills.

Transdermal estrogen (the patch) was developed to provide a route for estrogen replacement that would avoid the liver but at the same time enter the blood more quickly than through vaginal cream. A small patch that looks like a round Band-Aid is applied to the skin of the abdomen or other area at 8 AM Monday and changed at 8 PM Thursday (or any other time regimen which divides the week in half). This time-controlled patch allows specified doses of estrogen to be absorbed gradually by the skin. The advantage of this method is that bypassing the liver avoids such negative side effects as exacerbating some preexisting medical conditions; for example, gallstones. Drawbacks of the patch include possible skin irritation and rashes, and problems with adhesion in hot wet climates. For some women this method may not allow for enough absorption, so that dosages have to be increased. A final weakness — transdermal estrogen may not have any effect on cholesterol levels because it bypasses the liver. Similar to the other non-oral estrogen delivery methods, if you are on a combined treatment regimen, you will have to remember to take your progestogen pills for the prescribed number of days each month.

Other estrogen delivery routes exist, but they are used less frequently. These include estrogen-saturated vaginal rings and estradiol subcutaneous pellets. The rings are saturated with sex steroids and inserted into the vagina. The pellets are implanted just under the skin and provide long-term slow release of estradiol. While an advantage of pellets or rings over the patch is you do not have to be bothered changing patches frequently, you will still have to take progesterone by pill if you are on combined hormonal therapy.

Progesterone · In hormonal therapy, progesterone is used in two ways. It is used cyclically to oppose estrogen's effect, and it is used clinically in a procedure known as the **progestogen challenge test**. This test is recommended by some on an annual basis for postmenopausal women with intact uteri (who are on *ERT*). It assesses potential natural or medicinal estrogenic stimulation of the endometrium which could result in a higher risk for developing abnormal or cancerous cells.[4]

Progesterone was introduced into cyclical estrogen therapy in the 1970s to counteract the effects of unopposed estrogen treatment; that is, the increased risk of endometrial cancer. One major drawback of taking progesterone is that most women with intact uteri will experience the recurrence of a menstrual period or spotting. If that occurs, it lasts only two or three days, produces only a very light to moderate flow, and generally ceases after several years.

NOTE: Experts are still divided about the benefits of progesterone therapy for women who have had hysterectomies and have no worry about endometrial cancer. While the consensus is that the addition of progesterone is not necessary, some feel that its use is a good idea because of its possible protection against breast cancer.[5] However, the experts who are opposed to its use say that the addition of the progesterone might actually contribute to the risk of breast cancer.[6]

Dosage Levels and Costs · A wide spectrum of dosages is available and includes the following:

Estrogen. The lowest available dosage of oral estrogen is 0.1 mg. However, studies have indicated that the minimum amount necessary for osteoporosis prevention in 90 percent of women is 0.625 mg. The cost of a month's supply of a 0.625 mg dosage is approximately $16.00. That dosage is also usually sufficient to control hot flashes and other symptoms; if not, the dosage can be increased to 0.9 mg or to 1.25 mg. Women who have had their ovaries removed during their reproductive years and those with osteoporosis usually require doses of 1.25 mg or higher.

For women with hysterectomies whose ovaries are preserved, menopausal symptoms are usually delayed until the expected time of natural menopause, at which time a dosage of 0.625 mg can begin.

The patch is currently available at 0.05 mg and 0.1 mg. The lower dose is equivalent to oral conjugated estrogen pills of 0.3 to 0.625 mg while the higher dose is approximately equivalent to 0.9 to 1.25 mg. The cost for a month's supply of patches is approximately $22.00.

The usual dosage for vaginal cream is one gram two to three times per week. However, because of individual differences in absorption of estrogen from vaginal cream, a variety of other doses is available. The price for a 42.5 g tube (which will probably last two months) is approximately $37.00. If you want this method and the original prescribed dose is not working (your symptoms of dryness and painful intercourse have not diminished), schedules and dose levels can be modified in consultation with your doctor.

Progesterone. The recommended dosage is quite variable, depending upon individual preference, physician preference, and reaction to the progesterone. Dr. R. D. Gambrell, Jr., Clinical Professor in the Medical College of Georgia's Department of Obstetrics and Gynecology and Physiology and Endocrinology, suggests that women taking oral estrogens for 25 days should take the progestogen from days 13 to 25.[7] For women on continuous estrogen, injectables, or estradiol implants, he recommends progestogen the first 13 days of each month. Dosage recommendations include 5 mg a day for 10 days, or for continuous low dosage 2.5 mg for 25 days. If you are postmenopausal and have not had a hysterectomy, you may expect irregular spotting during the first months of therapy. If withdrawal bleeding continues, dosage levels of estrogen may be decreased or another progesterone may be substituted. You will be advised to carefully monitor your bleeding. If you bleed, it should occur the day after having taken your last progesterone dose, and this pattern should be the same month to month. You are also advised that while not bleeding in any month is not a danger sign, any other variation in timing or flow should be considered abnormal and indicative of the need for a medical consultation.

For women who cannot tolerate any oral progestogen, progesterone suppositories (25 – 50 mg daily) are available.

TABLE 11 – 1

SUMMARY OF CHOICES OF HORMONE THERAPY

DRUGS AVAILABLE

Unopposed Regimen = only estrogen
Combined Opposed Regimen = estrogen and progestin

METHOD OF DELIVERY

Oral Pills
- Estrogen alone
- Estrogen and progestin
- Progestin alone

Vaginal Estrogen Cream
Transdermal (Patch) Estrogen
Vaginal Estrogen Rings
Subcutaneous Estrogen Pellets

DOSAGE LEVELS *and* TYPICAL MONTHLY COST*

	Approximate Monthly Cost**
Oral Estrogen	
Mg 0.1; 0.3; 0.625; 0.9; 1.25; 2.5	$16.00
Vaginal Cream	
Mg 0.01; 0.5; 0.625; 0.1; 1.0; 1.5	$19.00
Patch	
Mg 0.05; 0.1	$22.00
Progestogens	
Mg 0.075; 0.35; 2.5; 5; 10; 20; 40	$25.00

* Not a complete list.
**Price varies depending upon dosage and amount. Generics are available for some and are approximately half the cost. Some insurers will cover most of this expense.

SIDE EFFECTS

Some women experience side effects from either estrogen or estrogen-progesterone replacement therapy. Nausea is common, as is breast tenderness, edema, bloating, premenstrual irritability, lower abdominal cramps, and the return of menses in women with intact uteri. These problems sometimes can be managed by changing drugs, dosage levels, or delivery methods, and are handled in consultation with your doctor. Taking a mild diuretic or vitamin B_6, or cutting down on salt may alleviate bloating. A prostaglandin-inhibiting analgesic such as aspirin or ibuprofen should help with general aches and pains.

Many women find the side effects unacceptable and discontinue HRT. **CAUTION!** Never quit "cold-turkey" (abruptly), because of a possible rebound response from the pituitary and hypothalamus. This could result in severe problems with your temperature-regulating mechanisms. In consultation with your doctor, you should follow a regimen of gradual withdrawal.

STARTING HRT

Before you start HRT, you should expect that your doctor will establish a baseline health profile. As part of that procedure, you should have:

1. A thorough physical examination, including blood pressure, height and weight, a pelvic and breast examination, and a Pap smear.
2. A complete blood analysis. This will provide information on blood sugar, liver function, cholesterol (including HDL and LDL breakdowns), triglyceride levels, thyroid function, and calcium and phosphorus levels.
3. A vaginal smear to determine your current estrogen status.
4. A mammogram.
5. A test for existing osteoporosis, if deemed necessary.
6. A complete family history with emphasis on osteoporosis and cancer should already be part of your file. If not, expect your doctor to take one.

NOTE: If you have not had a hysterectomy, you might expect your doctor to do either a biopsy of the endometrium or a progesterone challenge test to rule out hyperplasia or cancer.

Depending on your physician, expect a follow-up appointment anywhere from one to three months after starting hormone therapy. At that checkup you may have another physical examination as well as an additional vaginal smear. If you have any questions or problems, be sure to discuss them at this time. With your input, the doctor can make adjustments in the drug, dosage, or delivery method. Do not be afraid to ask every question, no matter how trivial or embarrassing you may think it is, and make sure you get satisfying answers. (Don't forget the things we talked about in Chapter Three.)

After this initial visit, you should return for a checkup every six months. If we can remember to do preventive maintenance on our car, we owe it to ourselves to extend it to our bodies as well!

HRT: YES OR NO

The arguments pro and con which follow are technical and detailed. Do not be daunted by the in-depth analysis. It is included to provide you with some of the documentation supporting each point of view. As a help you might want to first look at the summary sheet (Table 11 – 2) which we present before the discussion. This will provide an overview of the differing opinions.

TABLE 11 – 2

SUMMARY OF THE PROS AND CONS OF HRT

Benefits / Advantages
Reduced risk of osteoporosis
Possible decreased risk of heart disease
Reduction or elimination of hot flashes
Reduction or elimination of vaginal dryness or soreness
Reduced risk of insomnia or irritability (if they are caused by interruptions in sleep due to night sweats)
Possibly helpful in preventing or reducing the severity of Alzheimer's disease
Consistent medical supervision (every six months)
Protection from urinary tract infection

Risks / Disadvantages
Periods or spotting
Possible increased risk of breast cancer (although this conclusion is controversial)
Possible increased risk of gallbladder problems
No regularly scheduled medical visits
Expense of prescription

NOTE: A good way to calculate for yourself the advantages or disadvantages is to take this list and rate each item as:

0 = not important to me
1 = somewhat important to me
2 = very important to me

Compare the scores for the two sections. Is it in your best interest to take or avoid estrogen? (Be aware that there are more items under the Benefits section and that might affect your score.)

THE YEA SAYERS

Experts who recommend that postmenopausal women use HRT mainly base their judgments on the protection afforded by estrogen against cardiovascular disease and osteoporosis.

Cardiovascular Disease · Estrogen's preventive effect on coronary heart disease was suggested as far back as 1952 by animal studies showing that baby chickens fed a high-fat diet and estrogen had a reduced risk of coronary artery lesions.[8] During that same year, a study was published which illustrated the ability of estrogen to influence lipid and lipoprotein levels.[9]

In the 1980s, studies began appearing which confirmed estrogen's strong cardiovascular protective effect.[10] Some researchers categorically stated that the most important long-term health effect of ERT is to lower cardiovascular disease morbidity and mortality.[11] In 1991, the *Journal of the American Medical Association* published "Estrogen and Coronary Heart

Disease in Women," by Barrett-Conner and Bush, which reviewed the accumulated relevant studies.[12] Their findings were that "the evidence suggesting that unopposed oral estrogen reduces the risk of coronary heart disease is strong, reasonably consistent, and biologically plausible. The degree of putative protection is clinically significant and exceeds any known risks."[13]

Osteoporosis · Osteoporosis is covered in detail in Chapter Twelve. Let it suffice here to state that rapid bone loss occurs at sites of **trabecular bone** (the honeycombed network of bone plates that give elasticity and strength to the bones) in the early postmenopausal period.[14] It is now accepted that the use of estrogens immediately after menopause prevents the loss of bone due to estrogen deficiency.[15] The effect is maintained for at least 10 to 15 years, and benefits will accrue even if hormone therapy is started several years after menopause.

NOTE: For women who had an oophorectomy as well as a hysterectomy, the younger you are when you had your surgery, the more years you will be estrogen-deficient. You might want to give special consideration to your risks of developing osteoporosis when you decide whether or not to use HRT.

Cancer: Not a Problem · The focus of the debate revolves around estrogen's potential carcinogenic effect for endometrial and breast cancer compared to its other benefits. While studies have reported high cancer risk levels, their findings have been challenged because of flawed methodology. First, the studies were carried out when larger doses of estrogen than currently prescribed were typical. Second, they examined estrogen replacement and not the combination of estrogen and progesterone now being used. While studies have found that unopposed estrogen has a risk of promoting endometrial cancer, progestogen added to the regimen seems to reduce the risk of endometrial adenocarcinoma to lower than it is for untreated women.[16]

Regarding breast cancer and HRT, statistical analysis of the results of several breast cancer studies has found the average relative risk to be very low.[17]

NOTE: While women who have had hysterectomies are not concerned with developing endometrial (uterine) cancer, fears about breast cancer do remain. A recent comprehensive review found no support for an overall increased risk of breast cancer in women who have ever used postmenopausal estrogens.[18] This study and others have led many experts in the field to recommend HRT for women who have no history of and are not in the high-risk group for breast cancer, as the increased risk (probably less than twofold), if any, is low and is not enough to eclipse the benefits of ERT in protecting women from cardiovascular disease and osteoporosis.[19] However, as mentioned previously, experts are divided on the relative risk or benefit provided by using progestins in women who have had hysterectomies. Thus, it is especially important for women on HRT to receive annual mammograms.

William H. Hindle, MD, professor of clinical obstetrics and gynecology and director of the Breast Diagnostic Center at Women's Hospital, University of Southern California School of Medicine, Los Angeles, summarizes the pro-HRT position as follows: "If all the reported risks associated with estrogen replacement therapy are taken at their maximum, and all the documented benefits are taken at their minimum, the benefits are overwhelming."[20]

THE FENCE STRADDLERS

Cardiovascular Disease: Maybe · Barrett-Connor and Bush, in their excellent review (cited earlier under cardiovascular disease), took pains to point out the necessity for a clinical trial which would analyze the effectiveness of oral estrogen as a method of heart disease prevention for postmenopausal women.[21] Because of the inability to answer the question of whether estrogen actually *prevents* heart disease, Barrett-Conner and Bush are concerned that a large number of women "may be prescribed extended estrogen replacement to prevent cardiovascular disease, but without the supporting data usually required for the widespread use of any other drug recommended for disease prevention."[22] They recommend that the prescription of estrogen solely or primarily to prevent heart disease be on an individual basis, for example to treat only women at high risk associated with low HDL or high LDL cholesterol levels.

Cancer: Maybe · Hysterectomized women face one conundrum in resolving the question of whether or not to use HRT. Since they do not have uteri, they do not need to take progestin to protect them from endometrial cancer. Yet, as previously mentioned, some experts think that using progestin conveys probable protection against breast cancer — while others think the opposite.[23]

THE NAY SAYERS

Cardiovascular Disease · Women with a personal history of a stroke or thromboembolism problems would be advised not to take oral estrogen.

Cancer: A Major Risk · Unlike the researchers cited in the section "Cancer: Not a Problem," some scientists believe cancer is a major risk. According to them, hormone-related cancers account for more than 40 percent of all newly diagnosed female cancers in the United States.[24] For women who have had hysterectomies, the question of benefits from HRT must be balanced against the risks, specifically an increased risk of breast cancer. Nearly all the breast cancer studies to date have evaluated risk attributable to ERT alone, not to combination HRT. However, data from a study in Sweden have suggested that risk associated with combination HRT is higher than for ERT alone.[25]

The "estrogen-augmented-by-progestogen" hypothesis posits that breast cancer is increased by estrogen alone but is increased further by simultaneous exposure of breast tissue to estrogen and progestogen.[26]

"Despite more than 50 epidemiologic and clinical studies and several meta-analyses. . . , there is still no consensus on which women should not take supplementary estrogen because of a suspected increased risk of breast cancer."[27]

For women with breast tumors that are not estrogen-dependent, HRT is often used as a treatment. However, HRT is definitely not recommended for women who have had uterine cancer or estrogen-dependent breast cancer. The rationale behind that proscription is that although estrogen is not a carcinogen, it is a growth accelerator and as such could act on cancer cells that may be present. The recommendation against the use of HRT is also usually extended to women who have a strong family history of estrogen-dependent breast cancers (although there are some doctors who do not use this as a criterion and prescribe HRT for women with family breast cancer histories).

NOTE: We repeat, it is important to receive annual mammograms and do regular breast self-examination if you are on a hormone replacement regimen.

ANOTHER WAY TO LOOK AT RISKS

Sometimes quantifying the multiple risks and benefits of HRT provides clarification and might point you in a particular direction. Jane Brody in her "Personal Health" column did just that for readers of the *New York Times*.[28] Citing an analysis by Dr. Lee Goldman and Dr. Anna N. A. Tosteson, Brody put it this way. The chance that a white woman from 50 to 94 years old will die: of heart disease is 31.0 percent;
of breast cancer is 2.8 percent;
of a hip fracture is 2.8 percent;
of endometrial cancer is 0.7 percent.

Looking at those percentages, one quickly realizes that without other known risk factors, even a small benefit of HRT on heart disease risk would outweigh the threat of a relatively large increase in cancer risk.

OTHER CONSIDERATIONS

OTHER BENEFITS OF HRT

Additional possible beneficial effects may accrue from HRT. Women going through menopause, including hysterectomized women whose ovaries were not removed, have been shown to experience fewer and decreased symptoms when on HRT. The alleviation of problems such as incontinence, hot flashes, or painful intercourse can result in a better quality of life for all women, whether they are surgically or naturally menopausal.

Hot Flashes and Night Sweats · One of the main benefits of HRT is the reduction of the occurrence of hot flashes. Hot flashes (or flushes) are described by women as a sensation of heat in the face and/or the upper half of the body, sometimes accompanied by profuse sweating. Variability exists in occurrence, duration, and manifestation. For example, some women report flushes only once or twice in a 24-hour period, while others have up to five to seven per hour. The flashes can last from less than a minute to as long as an hour, although the average is about three minutes. They range from mild — a warm feeling that lasts less than a minute or two; to moderate — a warm feeling lasting from one to five minutes accompanied by sweating or flushing; to severe — extreme feelings of heat for one to twelve minutes or longer accompanied by sweating. Sometimes feelings of dizziness, chills, or chest pain may accompany severe flashes. Fortunately, most hot flashes are not severe.[29]

While between 16 and 38 percent of all menopausal women are symptom-free, among women who do have symptoms, hot flashes are the most commonly cited symptom; between 43 and 93 percent of women reported hot flashes during menopause or during the year or two after the last menstrual period.[30]

The exact cause of the hot flash is not known, although it is hypothesized that the ovary, pituitary, and hypothalamus are involved. The hypothalamus in the brain not only controls the sex hormones but also regulates the body's temperature through the vasomotor center. Hot flashes and night sweats get their technical name, **vasomotor instability**, from the hypothalamus' vasomotor center. The search for an explanation for hot flashes and night sweats has generated many theories — some more believable than others. For example, one theory suggests that vasomotor instability represents withdrawal symptoms from years of addiction to estrogen.

We can cope with hot flashes in a variety of ways. Vasomotor symptoms respond to estrogen therapy, and so provide an immediate reason for hormone therapy. Other medical alternatives may sometimes also be used. Some doctors may prescribe bellergal tablets, which contain phenobarbital, ergotamine tartarate, and a belladonna-like substance. But contraindications to their use, including any history of cardiovascular problems, liver or kidney disease, or glaucoma, limit their value. Clonidene, an antihypertensive medication, is a medical remedy occasionally prescribed in Canada for the treatment of hot flashes; in the United States, it is used only as a medication for hypertension. Its side effects include constipation, dizziness, and headaches.

Nonmedical methods of dealing with symptoms include techniques that are much more under our control. Practical suggestions such as using a fan, sucking on ice or drinking cold liquids, using less bedding and fewer or lighter night clothes are often helpful. Some women use imagery — imagining themselves walking through the snow or swimming in a clear icy lake. Other women turn to herbal therapy and/or vitamin supplements. The supposition underlying nutritional approaches is that both the ovaries and adrenal glands (which also produce estrogen) need to be nourished, and herbs and vitamins can do that. Some of the items used include: Dong Quai (a Chinese herb associated with healing female complaints); wild yam root and ginseng (both reputed to have estrogen-like properties); unicorn root (reputed to nourish the ovaries, and for women without ovaries, reportedly causes healthful changes in the body); peppermint tea (reputed to lower body temperature); pantothenic acid (one of the B vitamins); Vitamin C; and Vitamin E. Be aware that some herbs in large amounts can be harmful. If you plan to use herbs and supplements, it would be a good idea either to discuss this with an herbalist or a holistic practitioner, or to consult several books to become better informed.

Cognitive Function · The effect of HRT on cognitive function is less clear. In a presentation at the third annual meeting of the North American Menopause Society in 1992, Barbara Sherwin reported on a study of women who had surgically induced menopause. She found that women who were treated with estrogen postoperatively performed better on several tasks of cognitive functioning than those given a placebo.[31]

On the other hand, direct contradiction comes from a study by Barrett-Conner and Kritz-Silverstein.[32] Their 15-year study found there was "no compelling or internally consistent evidence for an effect of estrogen on cognitive function. . . ."[33] An earlier study also found no effect on memory and cognitive function, but did find increased optimism or confidence.[34]

One additional benefit pointed to recently by researchers is estrogen's possible connection with preventing or reducing the severity of Alzheimer's disease (see Chapter Two, p. 20).

Urinary Tract Infections · About 15 percent of women over age 60 get frequent infections of the urinary tract; that is, the bladder and urethra.[36] The increased vulnerability to these infections may be due in part to the vagina's new hospitality to microorganisms after menopause. This occurs because of the drop in estrogen and the subsequent loss of Doderlein's bacilli — making the vagina conducive to opportunistic microbes. The traditional method of treatment — long-term, low-dose antibiotics — can cause allergic reactions and other side effects and lead to drug-resistant bacteria. An alternative method, estrogen cream, has now been suggested by a recent study.[36] Doctors Raz and Stamm showed that applying estrogen cream to the vagina inhibited the growth of infection-causing organisms.

OTHER REASONS NOT TO USE HRT

Many gynecological textbooks warn physicians not to prescribe estrogen therapy for women with diabetes, significant liver or gallbladder disease, large uterine myomas, or history of cancer or blood clots.

Estrogen may increase the degree of concentration of cholesterol in the gallbladder, thus raising the possibility of cholesterol gallstone formation. However, a study published in the *American Journal of Public Health* in 1988 reported that if indeed it is a risk factor, the effect is very small.[37]

If you are naturally past menopause and have been told that you might need a hysterectomy because of fibroids, but you have not yet had the surgery, the use of HRT is a judgment call. Estrogen has the potential to continue fibroid enlargement; however, the amount in current HRT is so small that it does not usually encourage fibroid growth. If you decide to try HRT, monitor the effect on your fibroids with your doctor; and if growth continues, discontinue use.

A survey of Los Angeles gynecologists revealed that almost all of them routinely used hormone supplements for recently menopausal patients.[38] Those asking for a reconsideration see "the tendency to count potential benefits as real benefits; to discount potential risks and to prematurely extend use from high-risk to lower-risk women despite inadequate knowledge of the benefits and risks."[39]

Dr. L. Rosenberg, a member of the Slone Epidemiology Unit of the Boston University School of Medicine, points out that HRT is being used as a preventive of conditions for which alternative methods are known and feasible.[40] She gives as examples: hypertension, which can be treated with diet, weight control, exercise, and antihypertensives; and unfavorable cholesterol levels, which can be treated with diet, exercise, and cholesterol-lowering drugs. However, her recommendations, while eschewing hormones, involve the possible use of other powerful drugs. How and when drugs should be used among healthy people to prevent illnesses that may or may not ever occur is not an easy question to answer. Few can argue with Rosenberg's recommendation that elevated heart disease risk can be reduced by changing lifestyle habits such as smoking, diet, and sedentary behavior.

You may be apprehensive about using any drug. Women for centuries have been postmenopausal without the benefit of HRT. It is a natural phenomenon, so why intervene now? If you share these feelings, psychological resistance to HRT is a serious obstacle and treatment benefits might not be worth the anxiety. For a list of questions to consider before making a decision about hormone replacement therapy for yourself, see Table 11 – 3.

TABLE 11 – 3

QUESTIONS TO CONSIDER IN MAKING A DECISION ABOUT HRT

- Am I at risk for heart disease with a personal or family history of problems such as high blood pressure (140/90 or higher), high cholesterol (above 200 mg/dl), low HDLs (below 45 mg/dl), or high LDLs (above 160 mg/dl)? If yes, then HRT may be especially helpful.
- Am I at risk for osteoporosis with a personal or family history of low bone density, thin body mass, early menopause (before age 40)? If yes, then HRT may be especially helpful.
- Do I smoke, have high alcohol use, lack exercise, have a low dietary intake of calcium and Vitamin D, and have a high coffee consumption (more than four cups daily)? If yes, then I might want to consider lifestyle changes.
- Are my menopausal symptoms impacting my quality of life? If yes, then HRT may be helpful.
- Do I get recurrent urinary tract infections? If yes, then HRT may be helpful.
- Do I have active liver, gallbladder, or thromboembolic disease? If yes, HRT is contraindicated.
- Do I have a personal or family history of breast cancer? If yes, then discuss this with your physician, since HRT may be contraindicated.
- Have I had a recent uterine or ovarian cancer? If yes, then HRT is contraindicated.

A decision regarding hormone replacement therapy is not chiseled in stone. Once you decide, you can still start or stop therapy whenever you choose.

ENDNOTES

1. Bush, T. L. Feminine forever revisited: menopausal hormone therapy in the 1990s. *Journal of Women's Health*, 1992, 1(1), 1 – 4.

2. Smith, D. C., Prentice, R., Thompson, D. J., et al. Association of exogenous estrogen and endometrial carcinoma. *New England Journal of Medicine*, 1975, 293, 1164 – 1167.

Ziel, H. K., & Finkle, W. D. Increased risk of endometrial carcinoma among users of conjugated estrogens. *New England Journal of Medicine*, 1975, 293, 1167–1170.

3. Bush, T. L. Feminine forever revisited: menopausal hormone therapy in the 1990s. *Journal of Women's Health*, 1992, 1(1), 1 – 4.

4. Gambrell, R. D. Jr. *Hormone Replacement Therapy*, 3rd ed. Durant, OK: Essential Medical Information Systems, Inc., 1992.

5. Gambrell, R. D. Jr., Maier, R. C., & Sanders, B. I. Decreased incidence of breast cancer in postmenopausal estrogen-progestogen users. *Obstetrics and Gynecology*, 1983, 62, p. 435.

Nachtigall, L., & Heilman, J. R. *Estrogen: The Facts Can Change Your Life.* New York: Price, Stern, 1987.

6. Bergkvist, L., Adami, H. O., Persson, I., et al. The risk of breast cancer after estrogen and estrogen-progestin replacement. *New England Journal of Medicine*, 1989, 64, 293 – 297.

Ewertz, M. Influence of non-contraceptive exogenous and endogenous sex hormones on breast cancer risk in Denmark. *International Journal of Cancer*, 1988, 42, 832 – 838.

Kaufman, D. W., Palmer, J. R., deMouzon, J., et al. Estrogen replacement therapy and risk of breast cancer: results from the Case-Control Surveillance Study. *American Journal of Epidemiology*, 1991, 134, 1375 – 1385.

7. Gambrell, R. D., Jr. *Hormone Replacement Therapy*, 3rd ed. Durant, OK: Essential Medical Information Systems, Inc., 1992.

8. Pick, R., Stamler, J., Rodbard, S. et al. The inhibition of coronary atherosclerosis by estrogen in cholesterol-fed chicks. *Circulation*, 1952, 6, 276 – 280.

9. Barr, D.P., Ross, E. M., & Eder, H. A. Influence of estrogens on lipoproteins in atherosclerosis. *Transactions of the Association of American Physicians*, 1952, 65, 102 – 113.

10. Bush, T. L., Barrett-Connor, E., & Cowan, L. D., et al. Cardiovascular mortality and non-contraceptive estrogen use in women: results from the Lipid Research Clinics' Program Follow-up Study. *Circulation*, 1987, 75, 1102 – 1109.

Stampfer, M. J., Willett, W. C., Colditz, G. A., et al. A prospective study of postmenopausal estrogen therapy and coronary heart disease. *New England Journal of Medicine*, 1985, 313, 1044 – 1049.

11. Henderson, B. E., Paganinni-Hill, A., & Ross, R. K. Decreased mortality in users of estrogen replacement therapy. *Archives of Internal Medicine*, 1991, 151(1), 75 – 78.

12. Barrett-Connor, E., & Bush, T. L. Estrogen and coronary heart disease in women. *Journal of the American Medical Association*, April 10, 1991, 265(14), 1861 – 1867.

13. Barrett-Connor, E., & Bush, T. L. Estrogen and coronary heart disease in women. *Journal of the American Medical Association*, April 10, 1991, 265(14), p. 1866.

14. Barzal, V. S. Estrogens in the prevention and treatment of postmenopausal osteoporosis: a review. *American Journal of Medicine,* 1988, 85, 847 – 849.

15. Horowitz, M. C. Cytokines and estrogen in bone: anti-osteoporotic effects. *Science*, 1993, 260, 626 – 627.

16. Gambrell, R. D., Jr. *Hormone Replacement Therapy*, 3rd ed. Durant, OK: Essential Medical Information Systems, Inc., 1992.

17. Nachtigall, L. A clinician's dilemma: HRT and breast cancer risk. *Menopause Management*, 1992, 1(1), 12 – 24.

18. Henrich, J. B. The postmenopausal estrogen/breast cancer controversy. *Journal of the American Medical Association*, 1992, 268(14), 1900 – 1902.

19. Skolnick, A. At third meeting, menopause experts make the most of insufficient data. *Journal of the American Medical Association*, 1992, 268(18), 2483 – 2485.

20. Skolnick, A. At third meeting, menopause experts make the most of insufficient data. *Journal of the American Medical Association*, 1992, 268(18), p. 2484.

21. Barrett-Connor, E., & Bush, T. L. Estrogen and coronary heart disease in women. *Journal of the American Medical Association*, April 10, 1991, 265(14), 1861 – 1867.

22. Barrett-Connor, E., & Bush, T. L. Estrogen and coronary heart disease in women. *Journal of the American Medical Association*, April 10, 1991, 265(14), p. 1866.

23. Nachtigall, L. & Heilman, J. R. *Estrogen: The Facts Can Change Your Life.* New York: Price, Stern, 1987.

24. Henderson, B.E., Ross, R.K., & Pike, M. C. Hormonal chemoprevention of cancer in women. *Science*, 1993, 259, 633 – 638.

25. Henderson, B.E., Ross, R.K., & Pike, M. C. Hormonal chemoprevention of cancer in women. *Science*, 1993, 259, 633 – 638.

26. Henderson, B.E., Ross, R.K., & Pike, M. C. Hormonal chemoprevention of cancer in women. *Science*, 1993, 259, 633 – 638.

27. Skolnick, A. At third meeting, menopause experts make the most of insufficient data. *Journal of the American Medical Association*, 1992, 268(18), p. 2483.

28. Brody, J. Personal health. *New York Times*, February 24, 1993, c12.

29. Voda, A. M. Menopausal hot flash. In A. M. Voda, M. Dinnerstein, & S. R. O'Donnell, eds. *Changing Perspectives on Menopause*. Austin: University of Texas Press, 1982, (pp. 136 – 159).

30. Woods, N. F. Menopausal distress: a model for epidemiologic investigation. In A. M. Voda, M. Dinnerstein, & S. R. O'Donnell (Eds), *Changing Perspectives on Menopause*. Austin: University of Texas Press, 1982, (pp. 220 – 238).

31. Phillips, S. M. & Sherwin, B. B. Effects of estrogen on memory function in surgically menopausal women. *Psychoneuroendocrinology*, 1992, 17(5), 485 – 495.

Skolnick, A. At third meeting, menopause experts make the most of insufficient data. *Journal of the American Medical Association*, 1992, 268(18), 2483 – 2485.

32. Barrett-Connor, E. & Kritz-Silverstein, D. Estrogen replacement therapy and cognitive function in older women. *Journal of the American Medical Association*, 1993, 269(20), 2637 – 2641.

33. Barrett-Connor, E. & Kritz-Silverstein, D. Estrogen replacement therapy and cognitive function in older women. *Journal of the American Medical Association*, 1993, 269(20), p. 2637.

34. Ditkoff, E. C., Crary, W. G., Cristo, M., et al. Estrogen improves psychological function in asymptomatic postmenopausal women. *Obstetrics and Gynecology*, 1991, 78(6), 991 – 995.

35. Rubin, R., Silver, M., & Wright, A. Urinary infection rejection. *U.S.News & World Report*, September 20, 1993, 83.

36. Raz, R., & Stamm, W. E. A controlled trial of intravaginal estriol in postmenopausal women with recurrent urinary tract infections. *New England Journal of Medicine*, 1993, 329(11), 753 – 756.

37. Kakar, F., Weiss, N. S., & Strite, S. Non-contraceptive estrogen use and the risk of gallstone disease in women. *American Journal of Public Health*, 1988, 78(5), 564 – 566.

38. Ross, R. K., Paganini-Hill, A., & Roy, S. Past and present preferred prescribing practices of hormone replacement therapy among Los Angeles gynecologists:

possible implications for public health. *American Journal of Public Health*, 1988, 78(5), 516–519.

39. Rosenberg, L. Hormone replacement therapy: the need for reconsideration. *American Journal of Public Health*, 1993, 83(12), p. 1672.

40. Rosenberg, L. Hormone replacement therapy: the need for reconsideration. *American Journal of Public Health*, 1993, 83(12), 1670–1673.

SUGGESTED READING

Gambrell, R. Don, Jr. *Hormone Replacement Therapy*. 3rd edition, Durant, OK: Essential Medical Information Systems, 1992.

Dranov, Paula. *Is Estrogen Right for You?: A Thorough Factual Guide to Help You Decide*. New York: Simon & Schuster, 1993.

Henkel, Gretchen. *Making the Estrogen Decision*. Greenwich, Conn.: Fawcett Book Group, 1993.

Kamen, Betty. *Hormone Replacement Therapy, Yes or No?: How to Make an Informed Decision*. Novato, CA: Nutrition Encounter, Inc., 1993.

Mann, Ronald D. *Hormone Replacement Therapy and Breast Cancer Risk*. Pearl River, NY: Parthenon Publishing Company, 1992.

Notelovitz, Morris. *Estrogen: Yes or No?*. New York: St. Martin's Press, 1993.

Rinzler, Carol A. *Estrogen and Breast Cancer: A Warning to Women*. New York: Macmillan Publishing Company, 1993.

Sitruk-Ware, Regine, ed. *The Menopause & Hormonal Replacement Therapy: Facts & Controversies*. New York: Marcel Dekker, Inc., 1991.

Swartz, Donald P. *Hormone Replacement Therapy*. Baltimore, Md: Williams & Wilkins, 1992.

Whitehead, Malcolm, & Val Godfree. *Hormone Replacement Therapy: Your Questions Answered*. New York: Churchill Livingston, 1992.

Wolfe, Honora L. *Menopause, A Second Spring: Making a Smooth Transition with Traditional Chinese Medicine*. Boulder, CO: Blue Poppy Enterprises Press, 1993.

Chapter 12

LIFE AFTER HYSTERECTOMY: YOUR PHYSICAL & EMOTIONAL HEALTH

"The surgery definitely relieved the pain from menstruation, but I'm still struggling with the effects of menopause and have had so many other problems since surgery : breast cysts, allergies, condyloma, headaches, weight gain, always tired, constant muscle aches and pains, stressed out, can't sleep, dizziness, nausea, and on and on." — Susan, age 52

"The hysterectomy was the best thing that could have happened to me. I have been anemic my entire life — with all the problems that accompany anemia. I had the severe pain of the fibroids and PMS. After surgery I was a new person — the anemia, the pain, and the PMS were gone. I was able to function at a higher level than I could remember." — Bonnie, age 49

There are a number of physical problems, some that are precipitated by hysterectomy and some that occur, unfortunately, naturally. To be forewarned is to be forearmed.

OSTEOPOROSIS

Scientific consensus is in agreement that after menopause, natural or surgical, lack of estrogen can lead to osteoporosis. Osteoporosis is one of the most important health issues women face as we age. The hyperbole of that statement is based on its complications — fractures of sites such as the spine, hip, and arm — which account for an enormous toll in quality of life. About one-third of all postmenopausal Caucasian women will experience at least one osteoporotic fracture during their lives, and 300,000 new cases of osteoporotic hip fractures are reported annually in the United States.[1] It is estimated that postmenopausal osteoporosis affects 1.5 million women each year.[2]

Although we think of osteoporosis as a "women's disease," it strikes men too, and the consequences for them are just as serious. The difference is that it is more common among women, for whom there is a marked link to the depletion of estrogen after menopause. (Men produce small amounts of estrogen for their entire lives.) As a result of the significant drop in estrogen at menopause, women lose bone much faster than men. Our bones are also initially about 30 percent less massive than men's. Those factors combine to make women about eight times more likely than men to suffer from osteoporosis and its fractures.

Contrary to popular belief, bone is not inert material like a steel beam. Bone is living, growing tissue, constantly being broken down, resorbed, and rebuilt. Peak bone mass is achieved in the third decade of life; thereafter, there is a slow but steady loss of bone as a function of aging in both sexes. In menopausal women, a major new stimulus to bone loss, estrogen deficiency, is superimposed on the much slower age-related phenomenon. One particularly vulnerable site is trabecular bone, described in Chapter Eleven. Trabecular bone is found to a large degree in the back, in intermediate amounts in the hip, and in relatively small amounts in the arms and legs (the limbs are composed more of dense and compact bone). Thus, the hip, to a lesser extent than the spine but to greater extent than the arms and legs, is subject to bone loss when estrogen deficiency occurs. The frequency of serious fractures is in that order: spine, hip, limbs.

RISK FACTORS

Researchers have identified genetic, endocrine, and environmental factors associated with increased risk of developing osteoporosis. Genetic factors include a positive family history and being of either Caucasian or Asian race. Endocrine risk factors include late puberty, early menopause (surgical or natural), no children, and small body build. Environmental factors include lifelong low calcium intake, sedentary lifestyle, alcohol abuse, and cigarette smoking. Estrogen replacement should be considered to prevent osteoporotic fractures if you had early surgical or nonsurgical menopause, or relatively few reproductive years, despite your level of bone density (see Table 12 – 1 for a summary of risk factors).[3]

TABLE 12 – 1

SUMMARY OF RISK FACTORS FOR OSTEOPOROSIS

Genetic or Medical Factors	Lifestyle Factors
Female relatives with osteoporosis	High alcohol use
Caucasian or Asian	Smoking
Early menopause (natural or surgical)	Lack of exercise
Late puberty	Low dietary intake of calcium and Vitamin D
Small body build	
Recent fractures not due to major trauma	High caffeine use (more than four cups of coffee daily)
Chronic kidney problems	

Assessing Your Bone's Health · If you are in a high-risk group or if your doctor wants baseline data, it makes sense to be evaluated for osteoporosis. At one time that meant having X-rays of your spine and hips. They were routinely ordered to measure bone density. No longer. Skeletal X-rays have been found to be relatively insensitive, so marked bone loss must occur before it can be detected by conventional X-rays.[4] Unless you already have symptoms of osteoporosis, your X-rays would most probably not detect loss of minerals.

Bone densitometers, a new technology now available, provides doctors with a tool for evaluating women at risk who are symptom-free. Bone densitometers detect with accuracy and precision the actual content of calcium in bone.[5] The method is called **dual photon absorptiometry**. The machine most in use is the **dual energy X-ray absorptiometer (DEXA)**. It gives very little radiation exposure, takes about five minutes, and costs less than $100 (it is covered by many insurance plans). Test results are compared to a set of normal values of healthy young women as well as to age-matched women who do not have osteoporosis or other bone diseases.

Another accurate machine, the CT scanner (discussed in Chapter Four, page 67), has higher amounts of radiation, which might be a problem if used repeatedly over a period of time to monitor changes in bone density.

If the decision is made for an evaluation using either the CT scanner or DEXA, the two major sites of greatest interest are the spine and hip. If, however, you are not at high risk and are having the test done to establish baseline data, then sometimes monitoring of the forearm bone or heel to reflect bone mineral density of the spine and the hip is done. The use of bone densitometry as a mass screening device for asymptomatic women is still controversial, mainly because of quality control in the operation and maintenance of these sophisticated machines.[6] Here again, as in mammography screening for women 40 to 49, the question of cost/benefit to society versus cost/benefit to you as an individual is an issue.

PREVENTION

The best approach to the problem of osteoporosis is prevention. Once you have identified your risk factors, you may need to make changes in your lifestyle so as to preclude the development of osteoporosis. These involve attention to three elements: calcium, exercise, and estrogen. Calcium and exercise are covered in Chapter Thirteen.

The Estrogen Question · Estrogen is important in helping your bones retain calcium and in keeping them thick and strong.[7] Some experts think that estrogen is the only important factor in osteoporosis prevention. This is based on the recognition that deficiency of estrogen, caused by either menopause or surgical removal of the ovaries, results in accelerated bone loss.[8]

The mechanism by which estrogens exert their bone-strengthening effect is beginning to be understood. Recent research points to estrogen's ability to interact with bone cells and regulate the circuitry that controls bone remodeling — the process by which bone resorption is balanced by bone formation.[9]

If you are unsure about starting HRT, you need not rush to make a decision; estrogens' benefits can begin even after 10 to 15 years of postmenopausal life without estrogens.[10] Further, within two years of treatment, a 1 to 2 percent bone gain is possible.[11]

Decisions and Risks · To decide to increase your calcium intake and/or your exercise involves no risk, only a benefit. This may not be the case with estrogen replacement. To reach an informed judgment on the desirability of hormone replacement therapy, a full appraisal of the state of your bone's health as well as your osteoporosis risk profile is necessary.

As discussed in Chapter Eleven, the benefits of estrogen replacement include: additional protection against cardiovascular disease; positive effects on skin and mucous membranes; relief from menopausal symptoms; and osteoporosis protection. These considerations should be balanced against factors that might argue against the use of estrogens, such as the potential side effects also explained in Chapter Eleven.

In all probability, the higher your osteoporotic risk, the more your doctor will encourage you to use HRT. However, whether or not you choose to, you should still increase both your calcium intake and exercise levels.

THE TWO Cs

In the United States, the two major health problems confronting women as we age are cardiovascular disease and cancer. Women seem to be somewhat protected from cardiovascular disease until menopause, provided we do not smoke or take birth control pills. From that time, on heart disease is an equal-opportunity killer. One in nine women between the ages of 45 and 64 — and one in three women over 65 — have cardiovascular disease. When a woman has a heart attack, she is more likely than a man to die in the first few weeks; if she lives, she is more likely to suffer a second heart attack within four years. Bypass surgery, a common surgical remedy, is generally not as successful for women as it is for men.

After cardiovascular disease, cancer is the second leading cause of death and illness in the United States. Breast cancer and lung cancer are the leading lethal malignancies among women, with 150,900 new breast cancer cases a year.

Although researchers have identified many causative factors in the etiology of cancer and cardiovascular disease, some may be self-controllable because they are related to behaviors such as eating, drinking, smoking, and exercising. Since the 1956 Surgeon General's Report, cigarette smoking has been implicated as increasing our risk of both cardiovascular disease and cancer. Research also suggests that a diet high in fat and low in fiber (with few fruits, vegetables, whole grains, and bread) increases the risk of both diseases. Exercise, on the other hand, seems to provide protection against cardiovascular disease and may also protect against some cancers. The type and amount of food we eat and our exercise proclivities will, for the most part, influence whether we become obese. Obesity is a risk factor not only for cardiovascular disease and cancer but also for diabetes and hypertension.

By changing the things we can control such as diet, smoking, and exercise, we can reduce our risk of dying prematurely from either of the two "Cs".

CARDIOVASCULAR DISEASE

The two most common forms of cardiovascular disease in the United States are high blood pressure (hypertension) and coronary artery disease (the gradual narrowing of the blood vessels of the heart). Often these two problems go together and either of them can cause a heart attack (or coronary), which is medically called a **myocardial infarction.** (Infarction means "death of," and the myocardium is the muscular layer of the wall of the heart.) The myocardium receives its blood supply, containing oxygen and nutrients, from the coronary arteries.

Coronary Artery Disease · While **arteriosclerosis** is the general term used to describe any impairment of blood flow through the arteries, the most common form is known as **atherosclerosis.** Atherosclerosis refers to the buildup on the artery wall of plaque — deposits of fat, fibrin (a clotting material), cholesterol, and calcium. An artery that has become occluded by plaque is a likely candidate for a clot (**thrombus**) to form which can block the channel and deprive vital organs of their necessary blood supply. If the blockage is in a coronary artery, it is termed a **coronary thrombosis**; if it occurs in the brain it is a **cerebral thrombosis.**

Hypertension · **Hypertension** is the medical term for high blood pressure. In order to pump blood throughout the body, your heart muscle contracts. Blood pressure is a measure of the force of the contraction and the resistance of the walls of the vessels through which blood flows. Your blood pressure is highest when the heart contracts (called **systolic blood pressure**) and lowest between contractions (called **diastolic blood pressure**). The pressure is expressed as a ratio (systolic over diastolic) of millimeters of mercury (mmHg).

High blood pressure occurs when the artery walls harden due to their narrowing in diameter or losing elasticity. This causes the heart to work harder to send out the same amount of blood. Normal blood pressure is less than 130/85; high normal is 130/85 to 139/89.

Prevention and Treatment · While family history and cholesterol level are taken into account in counseling individuals on their risk of developing cardiovascular disease, much of the thrust of prevention is on lifestyle changes. Lifestyle factors make a difference in both prevention and treatment. The most effective measures for prevention and treatment involve losing weight, a low-fat diet, and exercise.[12]

CANCER

All of us have tumors on and in our body. A tumor is a group of abnormal cells that serve no physiological purpose. As discussed in Chapter Five, tumors can either be benign, self-contained, and not considered to be life-threatening; or malignant, able to spread to other parts of the body, and dangerous. Cancer is the term used to describe a disease characterized by malignant tumors; a particular cancer refers to the malignant tumor itself. Cancer is characterized by its ability to metastasize; that is, to spread to other parts of the body.

No one is immune from cancer, but many factors can influence an individual's risk. Chief among them and the easiest to control is the use of tobacco products. **Cigarette smoking will increase your risk of developing lung cancer by a factor of nine or ten.** Unfortunately, in recent years, the incidence of lung cancer in women has increased dramatically, paralleling increased cigarette usage. It is currently the leading cause of cancer deaths in women.

Breast Cancer · Breast cancer is the second biggest cancer killer. Although it is diagnosed almost three times as often as lung cancer, more breast cancers are curable. Some breast cancer activists say that we are in the midst of an epidemic because incidence rates for breast cancer increased by 21 percent between 1973 and 1989. However, statisticians at the National Cancer Institute (NCI) say that the term epidemic is incorrect because most of the sharp increase in the 1980s was due to increased detection of cancers while they were "in situ" (before they invaded other breast tissue), or at "Stage I."[13] NCI analysts say that the national incidence trends indicate a return to a 1 percent annual increase by the mid 1990s.

In trying to understand even the 1 percent annual increase, the hunt for causes of breast cancer has kept scientists busy. One hypothesis centered on the high-fat diet consumed by most Americans. While circumstantial evidence caused much media hype on the possible association, a recent study using data from the Harvard Nurses Health Study concluded that the evidence for the high-fat diet hypothesis just isn't there.[14] Women on a high-fat diet were at little or no more risk than those on an extremely lean diet. However, there was a clear association between fatty diets and colon cancer. The Nurses Health study results do not rule out a possible role for other dietary factors, such as alcohol.

Researchers have also refocused on estrogen and progesterone as high-risk factors. Recent studies reported that young overweight women have a slightly lower risk of breast cancer, but postmenopausal women who are overweight have a slightly higher risk. This prompted some conjecture of the link between diet and hormones. The possible answer is that young obese women tend to ovulate less frequently and thus have lower estrogen levels and lower risk, whereas overweight menopausal women might have higher levels of estrogen than normal-weight women because body fat itself produces estrogen through conversion of androgens.[15]

What is the likelihood of getting breast cancer? Among naturally postmenopausal women who don't take HRT, breast cancer incidence increases with age by approximately 2.1 percent per year, so that by age 85 you have a one in nine risk of developing this disease.[16] The cause for this rise is probably the small amount of estrogens still produced by the body.[17] Interestingly, when women take ERT, the statistical risk of developing breast cancer is slightly less than 2 percent per year.[18] Comparing these figures suggests that whether or not you take estrogen does not noticeably change your breast cancer risk.

NOTE: The important question — will the risk change with the addition of progesterone — is yet unanswered. Recently, studies have been undertaken to find out.

Breast cancer is believed to take 3 to 30 years to develop, and researchers think that during this time, there are at least three opportunities to interrupt its natural history.[19] Studies currently underway under the auspices of the Women's Health Initiative are designed to test the success of preventive interventions at each of those three stages. Stage one is to prevent or limit cancer-causing exposures; stage two is to reverse, or at least contain the growth of cells that have not yet reached a diagnosable precancerous state; stage three is to remove or kill recognizable precancerous lesions before they cause clinical symptoms.

One trial of interest is hormonal chemoprevention, with the use of **tamoxifen**, of breast cancer in healthy postmenopausal women who are at high risk. Tamoxifen, an anti-estrogenic drug, has been used since the mid-1970s as a mainstay of breast cancer therapy. The use of tamoxifen arose out of observations that primary breast cancer patients treated with the drug appeared to have a lower risk of developing a new cancer in the opposite breast. Because of its toxic side effects, the trial is limited to only those women who because of their high risk are theorized as having ongoing, albeit invisible, carcinogenic activity somewhere in their breast cells.[20]

NOTE: Concerns have been raised by some researchers that the risks of using tamoxifen as a preventative in healthy but at-risk women are sufficient to halt the testing procedure; however, officials at the NCI are not persuaded and are continuing the experiment.[21]

SEXUALLY TRANSMITTED DISEASES

You may think that once you have had a hysterectomy, your sexual activity will diminish, and sexually transmitted diseases (STDs) will not be of personal concern. The authors' research shows neither to be true.

> Mary S. telephoned one night, quite upset. She had a thick, white, curd-like vaginal discharge and was worried that it signaled the reoccurrence of the cervical cancer that had precipitated her hysterectomy two years earlier. She was also entertaining the possibility that her husband had been fooling around, since she hadn't had sex with anyone but her husband. We suggested that it was most likely a yeast infection known as monilia, possibly due to antibiotics she had been taking for a "strep" infection, but that she should see a physician. A checkup with her doctor showed this to be true.

The Centers for Disease Control (CDC) has identified almost 30 sexually transmitted diseases (STDs). Most of us have heard about **AIDS**, **syphilis**, and **gonorrhea**; however, the most ubiquitous one, **chlamydia** (which is responsible for an estimated 4 million cases yearly), is often unknown. All STDs have experienced a resurgence in the late 80s and early 90s. This has occurred because of a confluence of factors: the size of the population at risk for STDs has increased, laboratory diagnostic techniques for detecting STDs have improved, a higher portion of infections with multiple modes of transmission are now being acquired sexually, and many STDs appear to facilitate the acquisition of other STDs.

Three major microbes (bacteria, protozoa, and viruses) are responsible for most STDs. Bacterial and protozoal STDs, such as chlamydia, gonorrhea, syphilis, and trichomoniasis, usually cause either a discharge from the lower genital tract (vagina, cervix, or urethra) or genital ulcers. Specific diagnostic tests are available, and treatment is usually curative.

Viral STDs, such as genital herpes, genital warts (human papillomavirus), or AIDS, have more varied and changeable symptoms and usually cannot be cured. The only STD for which an effective vaccine is presently available is the hepatitis B virus. Many viral STDs become latent in the sense that the infection is still in the body but there are no overt manifestations. Individuals who are infected usually remain so. Prevention of initial infection is particularly important for the currently incurable viral STDs such as AIDS.

While as a woman with a hysterectomy, you do not have a uterus, your vagina and urinary tract are still sites for entrance and infection. Further, some of the STD infections which start genitally can spread systemically or through **autoinoculation** to other parts of the body. For example, in chlamydia, ocular infections can be the result of touching the eye with infected genital secretions. Similarly, the herpes simplex Type 2 virus, which causes genital herpes, can cause cold sores on the lip through autoinoculation or vice versa.

One major risk factor for almost every one of the STDs is multiple sex partners. Because many STDs do not cause any symptoms, you may engage in sexual activity without realizing that you are jeopardizing others or are being endangered. A way to reduce the likelihood of acquiring an STD is to:

1. Maintain a mutually faithful sexual relationship with just one partner. Avoid sexual contact with individuals who have had multiple or anonymous sexual partners, and/or
2. *Always* follow safer-sex practices such as using a latex condom along with a spermicide.

Several common urinary and reproductive tract infections, although included as STDs, are not spread exclusively by sexual contact. The most common of these infections are **trichomoniasis** and **candidiasis**.

Trichomoniasis is a protozoan-caused infection. Its symptoms may include itching, burning, and a white or yellow frothy discharge with an unpleasant odor. Treatment involves taking metronidazole tablets. Since it can be infectious, your partner(s) should also be treated.

Candida (also known as **monilia**) is a yeast infection that produces a thick white curdlike discharge. **Candida Albicans**, the organism responsible for monilia, is a normal inhabitant of the vagina and mouth but is usually held in check by the natural vaginal or oral environment. Old myths claimed that moist, tight, synthetic underwear made women more susceptible to developing monilia. There is no scientific evidence, however, to support that claim. A recent study reported in the *American Journal of Public Health* found that the frequency of sexual intercourse (seven or more times a week) was the strongest risk factor.[22] Other known causative factors include taking antibiotics or birth control pills, both of which alter the vaginal environment. As explained in Chapter Two, estrogen and Doderlein's bacilli help protect the vagina by maintaining its acidity, and both are affected by antibiotics and birth control pills.

If your hysterectomy included removal of your ovaries, and if you are not on hormone replacement therapy, you may find that you are more prone to develop monilia. If so, discuss this with your doctor. Candida can be transmitted sexually but rarely is; however, it is advisable for your partner(s) to wear condoms during an outbreak of the infection.

To be informed is to be prepared. Strategies for change can be used to forestall or prevent osteoporosis, cardiovascular disease, and cancer. Strategies for prevention of STDs can reduce risks of acquisition. The rest is up to you.

EMOTIONAL HEALTH

"When we focus upon what we haven't done, we usually fail to see our accomplishments." — Rita Linda, age 54

MENTAL PROBLEMS

The Myth · Hysterectomy, with or without oophorectomy, has acquired a reputation for causing emotional distress and possible psychiatric problems. This is based on old studies which reported high rates of psychiatric morbidity following surgery.[23] A useful review of this early work can be found in Gath and Cooper.[24] However, most of that research had major methodological flaws. For example, psychopathologies were included which were not reliably defined, and subjects with a varied mix of gynecological problems ranging from cancers to fibroids to sterilizations were treated as if they were one group. However, the major flaw of those older studies is that researchers interviewed subjects who were preselected — that is, they looked at women with known emotional problems who also happened to have had a prior hysterectomy. A causal relationship was assumed between hysterectomy and psychiatric disorder.

In order to scientifically establish cause and effect, a study must be conducted in which psychological status is compared before and after surgery, so as to control for preexisting psychopathology.

The Reality · Two recent reviews have synthesized the substantial available research in this area and concluded that the more scientific the study, the more it discredits the old myth of psychiatric difficulties following hysterectomy.[25] What the authors point to are well-designed studies which include standardized measures of psychiatric status and homogeneous samples of surgical conditions. These studies indicate that hysterectomy for benign pathology does not lead to postoperative psychopathology or depression.[26]

That is not to say that some women do not experience psychological problems after surgery; but if they do, most times they had a preoperative psychopathology. This finding is consistent with the conclusions from the general literature that the best predictor of the future course for any psychiatric illness may be the person's past history.

One interesting side finding of two studies was that women who did have elevated levels of psychiatric problems had fewer symptoms *after* their hysterectomies.[27]

That people experience anxiety prior to major surgery is not unusual. Depending upon the type of surgery, the apprehension relates to issues of surgery survival, recovery, and return to normal functioning. In the case of hysterectomy, there is an additional issue — preoccupation and concern related to postoperative sexual life.[28] Open, informed discussion with your doctor prior to surgery should help alleviate preoperative anxiety and help postoperative adjustment.

In a recent book, guidelines were given to help gynecologists assess and deal with psychological problems before and after surgery.[29] The authors stress the necessity for clear explanations of the surgical procedure by the physician to the patient, and highlight the additional benefits of the doctor's reassurances that sexual functioning need not be affected by the surgery. In the first two weeks after hysterectomy it is not uncommon for patients to feel tired, lethargic, emotionally turbulent, over-sensitive, and occasionally weepy. The researchers emphasize that it is important for the doctor to alert both patients and their caretakers to this occurrence and its essentially benign nature.

STRESS

Surgery is a stressor and may increase or compound other pressures. After surgery, we don't really need more stress, since the body is trying to heal itself and since we may (despite reassurances to the contrary) be having doubts about our sexuality, future athletic ability, and so on.

The word **stress** conjures up negative connotations; yet it is a natural bodily response that has evolved from prehistoric times. In those days the drives of hunger, thirst, and safety were the primary stimuli (called **stressors**) which motivated actions directed towards reducing those needs. Basic physiological responses (the **stress response**) evolved in order to mobilize the body and enable it to satisfy the need to eat, drink, and be secure and safe. Those physiological responses basic to stressor situations have survived intact into modern times, although the external threats — for example, to personal safety — don't always exist. However, internally generated threats still plague us. These mental stressors are the results of thoughts, emotions, and attitudes. The body's response to stressors do not differentiate between ones that are external or internal, positive or negative, real or imagined. A stressor is anything that causes the stress response. It can be mental, emotional, or physical; and include external threats, bereavement, bodily pain, and exercise. Stressors always precede the development of stress. Stressors are the cause; stress is the effect.

The Stress Response · Hans Selye, the father of stress theory, conducted extensive research on stress and described responses of the nervous and endocrine systems.[30] The stress response is complex and varied, but the major effects include an increase in heart rate, blood pressure, breathing, muscle tension, and blood glucose.

Selye created a model, the **General Adaptation Syndrome** (**GAS**), which describes three stages the body passes through when confronted by stressors. In the **Alarm Reaction Stage**, the hormonal and nervous system responses quickly prepare for fight-or-flight. We are now physiologically ready, in a primitive sense, to handle the stressor. However, the high level of preparedness occasioned in this first stage can not be maintained for an extended period. During the **Resistance Stage**, an attempt is made by the body to redirect the generalized response from the first stage to a more manageable level. In this second stage, specific organs and body systems become the focus of the body's response as it allows us to continue to operate under the stress. In the third and final stage, the **Exhaustion Stage**, the specific organs and body systems can not continue to resist the stressor and exhaustion results. In extreme or chronic cases, exhaustion can be so pronounced that physiological functioning is impaired.

The universality of Selye's GAS is remarkable. It describes the response to stressors that originate from physical, psychosocial, or environmental sources. The same physiological responses are produced whether we have lost a friend or started a romance, done poorly at work or received a promotion, had a hysterectomy or had a baby.

Depending upon the severity of the stressor and our resistance, exhaustion may occur quickly or after many years. Prolonged exposure to a low-level stressor, such as a bad work situation, might not cause a breakdown to occur for many years — whereas short exposure to a high-level stressor, such as intense cold, might result in rapid exhaustion. The impact of prolonged and unresolved exposure to a low-level stressor manifests itself in the development of stress-related diseases and disorders. Signs of stress may include insomnia, headaches, backaches, inability to cope, lack of concentration, anxiety, and irritability.

LIVING WITH STRESS

"One of the patterns I have with my workaholism is that before I finish one project, I'm ready to start several others." — Brenda, age 53

The key to living with stress is to understand that stress is neither bad nor good. Selye has compared our stress level to a string on a violin. The string should be tight enough so as to play well but not so tight that it will snap.

Because the results of stress are cumulative, we should take steps to intervene early enough to be able to cope effectively. Traditional and common methods of handling stress have included negative dependency behaviors such as smoking, excessive drinking, pill popping, and overeating; withdrawing from the stressor; or attacking it by direct confrontation. While these methods may provide short-term effectiveness, they are also likely to generate additional stress. Further, most of those methods — escape through negative dependency behavior, withdrawal, and aggressiveness — are not personally rewarding in the long run, nor are they socially acceptable.

Stress Management · Nowadays, the emphasis in stress control is through lifestyle management techniques. One set of mind-altering suggestions comes from the work of cardiologist Dr. Meyer Friedman. In the now classic book, *Type A Behavior and Your Health*, a Type A personality is described and linked to premature heart disease.[31] In a follow-up book, techniques are described which should enable the frenetic, time-conscious, impatient Type A personality "to slow down and smell the roses."[32] They include things such as:

- Reduce your sense of time urgency. Constantly remind yourself that there will always be some unfinished business on your agenda.
- Listen quietly when others are talking. Do not try to finish the sentences of others or interrupt with such speed-up phrases as "Yes, yes."
- Try not to think of more than one thing at a time.
- Move more slowly. Walk at a slower pace and drive with less aggressiveness.
- Expand your vocabulary, use longer sentences, and speak more slowly; all of these reduce the sense of "being in a hurry" that can make you impatient with others.
- Seek time for yourself. This means not just being alone, but searching your "inner self" for understanding and insight.

Another approach to stress management is to use techniques which include exercise, self-hypnosis, relaxation, meditation, biofeedback, and yoga. (For further information on these methods, see the suggested readings at the chapter's end.)

A good time to begin to experiment with these techniques is while you are slowly recovering from surgery and you are confined to the house. However, it might be argued that you should have mastered these tools before surgery so as to enhance recovery. The important point is not when to start but rather that you do begin to use these stress management skills.

Remember, although it might be nice to have a stress-free life, that is an impossibility. Many of us may need a new perspective towards living in today's fast-paced demanding mode. We can begin by taking control of our own future and not viewing ourselves as victims. We can strive to move away from negative thought patterns and not generalize difficulties from one area to another. We need to learn to accept the unchangeable, and cope as effectively as possible with the events over which we have no control. And finally, let us determine to live each day well and fully.

ENDNOTES

1. Favus, M. J., ed. *Primer on the Metabolic Bone Diseases and Disorders of Mineral Metabolism.* Kelseyville, CA: American Society of Bone and Mineral Research, 1990.

2. Horowitz, M. C. Cytokines and estrogen in bone: anti-osteoporotic effects. *Science*, 1993 (April), 260, 626 – 627.

3. Kritz-Silverstein, D., & Barrett-Conner, E. Early menopause, number of reproductive years, and bone mineral density in postmenopausal women. *American Journal of Public Health*, 1993, 83(7), 983 – 988.

4. Bilezikian, J. P., & Silverberg, S. J. Osteoporosis: A practical approach to the perimenopausal woman. *Journal of Women's Health*, 1992, 1(1), 21–27.

5. Johnston, C. C., Siemenda, S. W., & Melton, L. J. Clinical use of bone densitometry. *New England Journal of Medicine*, 1991, 324, p. 1105.

6. Melton, L. J., Eddy, D. M., & Johnston, C. C. Screening for osteoporosis. *Annals of Internal Medicine*, 1990, 112, 516.

7. Richelson, L. S., Wahner, H. W., Melton, L. J.III., et al. Relative contributions of aging and estrogen deficiency to postmenopausal bone loss. *New England Journal of Medicine*, 1984, 311, 1273 – 1275.

8. Kritz-Silverstein, D., & Barrett-Conner, E. Early menopause, number of reproductive years, and bone mineral density in postmenopausal women. *American Journal of Public Health*, 1993, 83(7), 983 – 988.

9. Horowitz, M. C. Cytokines and estrogen in bone: anti-osteoporotic effects. *Science*, 1993 (April), 260, 626–627.

10. Christiansen, C., & K. Overgaard, eds. *Proceeding of the Third International Congress on Osteoporosis*, Copenhagen: Osteopress ApS, 1990; 2; 508.

11. Greenspan, S. L., Myers, E. R., Maitland, L. A. et al. Fall severity and bone mineral density as risk factors for hip fracture in ambulatory elderly. *Journal of the American Medical Association*, 1994, 271, 128 – 133.

12. The Trials of Hypertension Prevention Collaborate Research Group. The effects of nonpharmacological interventions on blood pressure of persons with high normal levels. *Journal of the American Medical Association*, 1992, 267(9), 1213 – 1220.

13. Marshall, E. Search for a killer: focus shifts from fat to hormones. *Science*, 1993 (January 29), 259, 618 – 621.

14. Harris, J. R., Lippman, M. E., Veronesi, U., et al. Breast cancer. *New England Journal of Medicine*, 1992, 327(5), 319 – 328; 327(6), 390 – 398; 327(7), 473 – 480.

15. Henderson, B. E., Ross, R. K., & Bernstein, L. Estrogens as a cause of human cancer: the Richard and Hinda Rosenthal Foundation award lecture. *Cancer Research*, 1988, 48(2), 246 – 253.

16. Marshall, E. Search for a killer: focus shifts from fat to hormones. *Science*, 1993 (January 29), 259, 618 – 621.

17. Henderson, B. E., Ross, R. K., & Pike, M. C. Hormonal chemoprevention of cancer in women. *Science*, 1993(January 29), 259, 633 – 638.

18. Pike, M. C., Bernstein, L., & Spicer, D. V. Exogenous hormones and breast cancer. In D. E. Niederhuber, ed. *Current Therapy in Oncology*. St. Louis, MO: Dekker, Mosby-Yearbook, 1993, (pp 292 – 303).

19. Henderson, M. Current approaches to breast cancer prevention. *Science*, 1993 (January 29), 259, 630 – 631.

20. Henderson, M. Current approaches to breast cancer prevention. *Science*, 1993 (January 29), 259, 630 – 631.

21. Kolata, G. Data on risks create debate about drug to prevent breast cancer. *New York Times*, March 16, 1994.

22. Foxman, B. The epidemiology of vulvovaginal candidiasis: risk factors. *American Journal of Public Health*, 1990, 80(3), 329 – 331.

23. Lindemann, E. Observations on psychiatric sequelae to surgical operations in women. *American Journal of Psychiatry*, 1941, 98, 132 – 137.

24. Gath, D., & Cooper, P. J. Psychiatric aspects of hysterectomy and female sterilization. In Granville-Grossman, K., ed. *Recent Advances in Clinical Psychiatry.* London: Churchill, 1982, (pp. 75 – 100).

25. Gitlin, M. J., & Pasnau, R. O. Psychiatric syndromes linked to reproductive function in women: a review of current knowledge. *American Journal of Psychiatry*, 1989, 146(11), 1413 – 1422.

Oates, M., & Gath, D. Psychological aspects of gynaecological surgery. *Bailliere's Clinical Obstetrics and Gynaecology*, 1989, 3(4), 729 – 749.

26. Coopen, A., Bishop, M., Beard, R. J., et al. Hysterectomy, hormones and behavior: a prospective study. *Lancet*, 1981, 1, 126 – 128.

Gath, D., Cooper, P., Bond, A., et al. Hysterectomy and psychiatric disorder: II. demographic, psychiatric and physical factors in relation to psychiatric outcome. *British Journal of Psychiatry*, 1982, 140, 343–350.

Gath, D., Cooper, P., Day, A. Hysterectomy and psychiatric disorder: I. levels of psychiatric morbidity before and after hysterectomy. *British Journal of Psychiatry*, 1982, 140, 335 – 342.

Martin, R. L., Roberts, W. V., Clayton, P. J. Psychiatric status after hysterectomy—a one-year prospective follow-up. *Journal of the American Medical Association*, 1980, 244, 350 – 353.

Meikle, S., Brody, H., & Pysh, F. An investigation into the psychological effects of hysterectomy. *Journal of Nervous and Mental Disease*, 1977, 164(1), 36 – 41.

27. Gath, D., Cooper, P., Bond, A., et al. Hysterectomy and psychiatric disorder: II. demographic, psychiatric and physical factors in relation to psychiatric outcome. *British Journal of Psychiatry*, 1982, 140, 343 – 350.

Martin, R. L., Roberts, W. V., Clayton, P. J., et al. Psychiatric illness and noncancer hysterectomy. *Diseases of the Nervous System*, 1977, 38, 974 – 980.

28. Lalinec-Michaud, M., & Engelsmann, F. Anxiety, fears and depression related to hysterectomy. *Canadian Journal of Psychiatry*, 1985, 30, (1), 44 – 47.

29. Oates, M., & Gath, D. Psychological aspects of gynaecological surgery. *Bailliere's Clinical Obstetrics and Gynaecology*, 1989, 3(4), 729 – 749.

30. Selye, H. *Stress in Health and Disease*. Boston: Butterworth Publishing, 1976.

31. Friedman, M., & Rosenman, R. *Type A Behavior and Your Health*. New York: Fawcett Group, 1981.

32. Friedman, M., & Ulmer, D. *Treating Type A Behavior and Your Heart*. New York: Alfred A. Knopf, 1984.

SUGGESTED READING

DeGregorio, Michael W., & Valerie J. Wiebe. *Tamoxifen and Breast Cancer*. New Haven, Conn: Yale University Press, 1994.

Douglas, Pamela S., ed. *Cardiovascular Health and Disease in Women*. Philadelphia, PA: W. B. Saunders, 1993.

Gaby, Alan. *Preventing and Reversing Osteoporosis: Every Woman's Essential Guide*. Roseville, CA: Prima Publishing, 1993.

Hirshaut, Yashar. *Breast Cancer: The Complete Guide*. New York: Bantam Books, 1993.

LaTour, Kathy. *The Breast Cancer Companion: From Diagnosis, Through Treatment, to Recovery, Everything You Need to Know for Every Step Along the Way*. New York: William Morrow & Company, 1993.

Legato, Marianne, & Carol Colman. *The Female Heart: The Truth About Women and Heart Disease*. New York: Avon Books, 1993.

McIlwain, Harris H., and others. *Winning with Osteoporosis*. New York: Wiley, 1993.

Notelovitz, Morris, Diana L. Tonnessen, & Marsha Ware. *Stand Tall!: The Informed Woman's Guide to Preventing Osteoporosis*. Gainesville, Fl: Triad Publishing, 1994.

Novotny, Pamela P. *What Women Should Know About Chronic Infections and Sexually Transmitted Diseases*. New York: Dell, 1991.

Rinzler, Carol A. *Estrogen and Breast Cancer: A Warning to Women*. New York: Macmillan, 1993.

Royak-Schaler, Renee, & Beryl Lieff-Benderly. *Challenging the Breast Cancer Legacy: A Program of Emotional Support and Medical Care for Women at Risk*. New York: Harper Collins, 1992.

Stevenson, John, & Michael C. Ellerington. *Osteoporosis — Questions and Answers*. Santa Monica, CA: Merrit Communications, 1993.

Vierck, Elizabeth. *Special Report: Osteoporosis: How to Stop It, How to Prevent It, How to Reverse It*. Englewood Cliffs, NJ: Prentice Hall, 1993.

Padus, Emrika, ed. *The Complete Guide to Your Emotions and Your Health: Hundreds of Proven Techniques to Harmonize Mind and Body for Happy, Healthy Living*. Emmaus, PA: Rodale Press, 1992.

Peterson, Christopher. *Health and Optimism*. New York: Macmillan, 1991.

Chapter 13

EAT RIGHT AND GET FIT

"I did not exercise 15 years ago. I do now, and love it!" — Jane, age 51

"I do aerobics with a Jane Fonda video about three times a week. I especially enjoy watching the gray-haired woman in the video class. I've set her up to be my model." — Lucille, age 58

NUTRITIONAL CONCERNS: RETHINKING YOUR DIET

If you are like most Americans and have poor eating habits, your surgery can be used as an opportunity to rethink and if necessary reform a faulty diet. A good diet, appropriate weight, and a regular exercise program can contribute to a healthier, and often happier, life. One important reason to actively attend to food intake is that as we age, our bodies are not as forgiving. We can't eat as we did as teenagers and expect it not to show. Two important considerations regarding diet and weight are total caloric consumption and dietary fat/cholesterol intake.

TOTAL CALORIC CONSUMPTION

While the recommendation is to monitor and control our food intake on a daily basis, few Americans do so and consequently are prone to excess weight gain. These gains are followed frequently by strict diets which aim to remove the fat that has accumulated as a result of indulgence and lack of exercise. Unfortunately, although successful in losing weight when we follow one of the fad diets, our weight loss is usually temporary. Once we resume old eating patterns, which initially caused the weight problem, weight gain is inevitable.

For those of us who have gained weight because we enjoy indulging in food, there is no psychologically pain-free way of losing weight. However, in theory it is quite simple to lose excess poundage with a combination of restricting caloric intake and/or increasing caloric expenditure.

While there are many ways of cutting one's calories, a no-frills, basic, balanced low-calorie diet makes the most sense. That type of diet causes weight loss by stressing awareness of eating patterns, and therefore has a stronger possibility of keeping excess pounds from reaccumulating.

THE BASICS OF LOSING WEIGHT

In order to satisfy our body's metabolic needs, we eat food. Food can be evaluated in terms of the energy it provides in the form of calories. There are technical definitions for the terms *calorie* or *Calorie* when used to describe the energy value of a food by scientists. However, most of us use the terms interchangeably. We will use Calorie with a capital C to refer to food values.

Gaining or losing weight can be viewed as a mathematical game involving balancing a Calorie equation. If we take in more Calories than we expend, we gain weight. If we expend more than we take in, we lose weight. One pound of weight equals approximately 3,600 Calories. In order to lose one pound, we have to consume or use about 3,600 Calories less than usual. In a typical day, the average woman needs approximately 1,800 – 2,400 Calories. If intake is cut by 500 Calories per day, at the end of one week she has lost one pound ($500 \times 7 = 3{,}500$ Calories).

Obviously, this is a simplified rule of thumb, but it is based upon our body's energy needs, also known as **metabolism.**

Metabolism · Metabolism represents the sum total of all physical and chemical changes that take place within the body, and reflects how the body is using its energy stores. Metabolism can be thought of as having two components: basal metabolism and our activity requirements.

Basal metabolic rate (BMR) represents the energy necessary to carry on basic life functions (such as circulation, respiration, body temperature maintenance, and brain activity), and accounts for about 60 to 70 percent of the body's total daily energy expenditure.

Activity requirements include the energy expenditures for everyday activities such as sitting, reading, standing, brushing our teeth, and working, as well as the energy expended during recreational physical activity.

As we age, our body's requirements for energy decrease. This change reflects the loss of muscle tissue with age and the concomitant alteration of the ratio of lean body tissue to fat. As the proportion of fat increases, our energy needs decrease, because fat cells have a lower metabolic need. Unfortunately, that negative change in our body's requirement for energy is usually accompanied by a reduction in activity — which makes our energy needs even lower.

Thus, while a typical college-age female (with a median height of 5′4″ and a weight of 130 pounds) needs approximately 2,500 Calories per day, by the time she is menopausal she might only require 1,900 – 2,200 Calories.

THE ROLE OF EXERCISE

Weight loss occurs when the energy demand of the body exceeds the food energy consumed. A diet that reduces the Calories (energy) entering the body is one way to accomplish weight loss. The other way is to increase the need for energy. Since we can't change our basal metabolism (without medical intervention), it makes sense to increase what we can change — our voluntary activity. By increasing our physical endeavors we increase the number of Calories our body requires. That increase allows us to eat more and not gain weight or eat the same and lose weight. For example, if our metabolic need is usually for 2,000 Calories and we increase our activity, we might raise our energy need by 500 Calories. By eating our usual 2,000 Calories per day, by week's end we will have lost one pound because of our increased physical activity. Compare that with the example earlier in this chapter, where the hypothetical woman, in order to lose one pound, had to cut back food intake by 500 Calories per day.

Additional benefits derive from increasing our physical activity. Proportionately more fat is lost through exercise than through dieting. We also gain psychological and physiological benefits. There are some things to note. First, if we increase our activity and also increase our food intake, we will not lose weight! Second, it takes the addition of a significant amount of activity to burn up calories. We need to generate a lot of calories through exercise to have the luxury of indulging in food. For example, a 130-pound female uses only approximately 200 Calories per hour when walking 2 to 2.5 miles. (If she increases or decreases her distance in that hour, she will use more or fewer Calories.) That hour of exercising to accumulate the 200-Calorie deficit will be negated if she eats approximately what is found in four granola cookies, or ½ cup dried peaches, or 2 tablespoons of peanut butter. Moral: exercise helps, but don't count on it as the sole focus for weight reduction.

The best approach to weight reduction is one which combines Calorie reduction and increased exercise along with conscious behavioral and attitudinal changes regarding food and eating. Set a realistic, long-term goal; the chances of keeping weight off are better if you lose one pound rather than five pounds per week. Total deprivation of enjoyable foods is neither wise nor necessary. Some practical suggestions include: stop eating after one serving; try not to snack between meals, but if you must, choose small, nutritious low-Calorie snacks; and substitute carbohydrates for fats — for example, jam for butter, pasta for meat.

Exercise and Osteoporosis · Exercise works to maintain healthy bones in a positive way — by increasing bone mass — rather than by retarding the process of bone thinning. However, not all kinds of exercise are equally beneficial to bone strength, and some types do little good. Further, some researchers report that exercise without adequate intake of calcium and estrogen replacement therapy is not effective.

Muscle-joint stress-producing exercise makes bones stronger in two ways. First, it causes an acceleration of blood flow within the bone's Haversian canals, thereby increasing the nutrients carried to bone-building cells. Second, by creating an electrical charge (piezoelectricity) when the bone is stressed, exercise stimulates the bone-building cells.

Bones are stressed when the muscles attached to them are contracted and strengthened. Strength training, which involves lifting weights or working out on resistance machines, has recently emerged as one of the best ways to strengthen bones.

The benefits of exercise seem to be specific to the activity. Runners and cyclists have denser bones in their legs and hips but not their arms or spines, while swimmers tend to have denser bones in their arms and shoulders. It would make sense, therefore, for you to use a variety of activities to make sure that bones are strengthened bodywide.

A recent study indicated that hip fractures are related not only to bone mass but also to the characteristics of the fall and the individual's body structure (height, weight, and body mass index — weight divided by the square of height).[1] The investigators concluded that in addition to the maintenance of bone density, preventive strategies should also include enhancement of muscle strength and neuromuscular function through exercise.

In addition to buildup of bone, another benefit of exercise is the possible increase in stability and development of quicker reaction time — which have the effect of decreasing the likelihood of a bone-breaking fall. However, if you fall, your exercise program may still have served you well. Exercise not only has made your bones denser and your muscles stronger, but you also may have developed faster reflexes which allow you to break the force of the fall with an outstretched arm. A broken wrist is a lot less debilitating than a fractured hip.

DIETARY FATS

Fat is one kind of nutrient (carbohydrate, protein, vitamins, minerals, and water are the others) which is an essential component of daily dietary needs. Fat serves as the most concentrated source of energy and as a body insulator. It also provides a vehicle for the fat-soluble vitamins (A, D, E, and K); is a structural component of cell membranes; and is the only source of linoleic acid — an essential fatty acid required by the body.

If you are like most Americans, your current diet will consist of approximately 46 percent carbohydrates, 12 percent proteins, and 42 percent fats. According to the federal government's recently released recommended dietary goals, the healthiest diet should be 58 to 60 percent carbohydrate, 12 percent protein, and no more (and hopefully less) than 30 percent fat.[2] Fat intake should break down to roughly 10 percent saturated, 10 percent polyunsaturated, and 10 percent monounsaturated fats.

Fat-Cholesterol Connection · All fats in our diet are technically known as **lipids,** a general term for a number of different water-insoluble compounds found in the body. Lipids are composed chiefly of fatty acids (known as **triglycerides**) and **phospholipids** (which include **cholesterol**). Triglycerides represent about 95 percent of the fat we eat; the phospholipids (cholesterol and lecithin) represent the other 5 percent of our dietary fat intake.

Triglycerides are fats which are composed of glycerol (an alcohol) attached to fatty-acid molecules. Triglycerides are found in both plant and animal foods, and can be considered either saturated or unsaturated. **Unsaturated triglycerides (fats)**, generally liquid at room temperature, are derived primarily from plant sources such as corn, soybeans, and peanuts. Unsaturated fats are further divided into monounsaturated and polyunsaturated, depending on their molecular composition. **Saturated fats** are derived mainly from animal sources, and include the fat in meats as well as the fat in egg yolks and dairy products.

As with any rule, there are exceptions. For example, coconut and palm oil, which are from plant sources, are highly saturated. Vegetable oils are initially polyunsaturated, but through processing to convert them to margarine they become partially saturated. This process of adding hydrogen atoms to produce a solid oil is known as **hydrogenation.** Although margarine might be considered to be a healthy fat, it is more saturated than the oil from which it is made. Additionally, questions have been raised recently about possible harmful health effects that might occur from the process of hydrogenation.

The difference between fat and cholesterol, although simple, causes much confusion. Cholesterol is a waxy, soapy-looking, yellowish substance which is normal and useful to the body. It is an essential component in the formation of the cell membrane and in several hormones, such as testosterone and prostaglandin. Cholesterol is manufactured by the body and is also found in the animal foods we eat. It is not found in fruits, vegetables, nuts, grains, or other plant sources. So, all margarines are automatically cholesterol-free if they are made from a vegetable oil, but they can contain saturated fats. Diets which are high in saturated fats, such as meat and dairy products, usually are high in cholesterol. Accordingly, people with elevated blood cholesterol levels are often advised to reduce their intake of saturated fats and increase their intake of polyunsaturated fats. Although fat is necessary to maintain bodily functions, the body can manufacture the cholesterol it needs from any of the three basic foodstuffs (fat, protein, and carbohydrate). A diet with fat intake as low as 5 to 10 percent is sufficient to provide the necessary substances for the body to manufacture cholesterol.

Cholesterol is transported through the cardiovascular system in the form of lipoproteins (lipids covered by a protein coat). The **lipoproteins** can be either of high-density (**HDL**) or low-density (**LDL** or **VLDL**) varieties. The HDLs are "the good guys," because higher concentrations of them are associated with a lessened risk of coronary heart disease; presumably because they remove cholesterol from blood vessel walls and transport it to the liver for disposal. Higher levels of LDL are associated with increased cardiovascular risk because of their propensity to deposit any excess amount of cholesterol on the walls of the arteries. This deposition contributes to the buildup of atherosclerotic plaque, which progressively blocks the arteries and effectively narrows the blood vessels' diameter.

Fat/Cholesterol and Disease Connection · Researchers have known for some time that populations with diets high in saturated fat tend to have elevated blood cholesterol levels and increased heart disease rates. However, the critical question of whether altering one's diet reduces coronary risk has not yet been adequately answered. Certain drug studies indicate that diet can reduce heart problems, but dietary studies have not been as conclusive.

Nevertheless, an offensive against high fat and cholesterol has been launched in the United States. The National Cholesterol Education Program (NCEP) campaign has defined elevated cholesterol as 200 milligrams per deciliter of blood or more. Officials of NCEP estimate that about one in three adults will require a doctor's care to achieve that target. Diet usually is the first weapon in cholesterol reduction; this is followed by exercise and cholesterol-lowering drugs if necessary.

While health officials in the United States have taken an activist role, other countries, reviewing the same body of evidence of the link between cholesterol level and heart attack, have opted for a more conservative approach. According to *Consumer Reports,* these countries "consider it unreasonable to test huge numbers of seemingly healthy people, then medically supervise major dietary changes — and, in many cases, provide lifetime treatment with costly drugs — in order to prevent a possibly modest number of heart attacks."[3]

The issue for women who are postmenopausal (either naturally or because of surgery) is more complicated. After menopause, HDL falls and both LDL and total cholesterol rise. Coronary risk rises as well with the result that nearly half of all heart attacks that are fatal occur in postmenopausal women. Yet surprisingly, the question as to whether postmenopausal women with elevated cholesterol levels can benefit from cholesterol-reducing measures has not been addressed until recently.

Conservative advice would probably stress that postmenopausal women with moderate or high cholesterol levels and elevated LDLs should strongly consider hormone replacement therapy and the adoption of the American Heart Association's prudent diet. In that diet, fat intake is limited to 30 percent of total calories, with saturated fat 10 percent of that; dietary cholesterol is limited to 250 – 300 milligrams or less a day (slightly more than the amount in one large egg) rather than the current daily 400 – 600 mg.

Even if the American Heart Association's diet does not lower coronary risk through cholesterol and fat reduction, it would probably lower caloric intake and so aid in weight control. Obesity is a risk factor not only in cardiovascular disease but for some cancers as well, so weight loss would only enhance health.

GOOD NUTRITION

Good nutrition means eating for variety, balance, and moderation. Seven basic elements should be kept in mind when planning a diet. They are:

1. Eat a variety of foods.
2. Maintain ideal weight.
3. Avoid too much fat, saturated fat, and cholesterol.
4. Eat foods with adequate starch and fiber.
5. Avoid too much sugar.
6. Avoid too much sodium.
7. If you drink alcohol, do so in moderation.

Fiber · **Dietary fiber** is a collective term used for the indigestible residue of the structural components of plants. The different types of dietary fiber can be divided into two main categories: those that are soluble in water and those that are not. During digestion, while water-soluble fibers become gel-like or viscous and are partially digested by bacteria in the colon, water-insoluble fibers remain essentially unchanged.

Fiber in the diet exerts a variety of physiologic and metabolic effects. Based on their physiological effects, some benefits which have been attributed to both soluble and insoluble fiber include: increased satisfaction after eating; rapid passage of food through the intestines and out of the body (because of increased fecal bulk due to their absorption of water); and greater frequency of bowel movements. While both types of fibers provide those benefits, soluble fibers have been shown to have additional beneficial metabolic effects, including: delaying glucose absorption, lowering insulin requirements, decreasing serum cholesterol and triglycerides, and lowering blood pressure.

Because it is important to get both soluble and insoluble fiber, it makes sense to get dietary fiber from more than one source. Fruits, vegetables, and grains contain varying amounts of soluble and insoluble fibers. The amounts and types of fiber differ from one food to another. For example, while carrots and celery are much higher in total fiber than tomatoes, carrots provide 50 percent more soluble fiber than celery. And while bran is one of the best sources of total fiber, it has a low percentage of soluble fiber. In general, fruits and vegetables (rather than grains) are among the best sources of soluble fiber. When you select a wide variety of fiber-rich foods daily, it maximizes the benefits of fiber to the body by ensuring that you get a mix of the necessary soluble and insoluble fibers.

The majority of Americans eat only about 15 to 20 grams of dietary fiber each day. The National Cancer Institute recommends that most of us should increase our daily fiber intake to 25 to 35 grams per day. To do that, we should eat approximately six servings of whole grain breads and cereals and four servings of fruits and vegetables. Cooking, canning, freezing, and freeze-drying do not appear to significantly decrease the fiber content of most foods. Peeling fruits and vegetables, however, will decrease their fiber content; making fruits and vegetables into juices also causes much of the fiber content to be lost.

Note: When you increase fiber intake,

1. you should increase it gradually to the optimal amount to avoid distention, excessive gas, and flatulence
2. you should drink plenty of water and other liquids, and
3. you should spread your intake throughout the day.

CALCIUM AND OSTEOPOROSIS

Calcium, the most abundant mineral in the body, is necessary for strong bones and teeth as well as for muscular contractions, blood coagulation, and nerve membrane stability. While the Food and Drug Administration recommends a daily intake of 800 milligrams for adults over age 24, some researchers recommend that premenopausal women should increase that to 1,000 milligrams. After your menopause, the recommendation is that you increase the amount to 1,500 milligrams of calcium a day if you are considered to be at high risk of developing osteoporosis. However, a recent study in the *New England Journal of Medicine* found that calcium supplementation of only 1,000 mg per day significantly slowed bone loss in the spine and legs of normal postmenopausal women.[4]

Realistically, it is hard to achieve that goal through normal dietary sources of calcium. Ingestion of the required amount of dairy products presents problems because of high calories, fat content, and lactose intolerance.

It would mean consuming, for example, six 8-ounce glasses of milk or the equivalent in other dairy products high in calcium. (See Table 13–1 for other good sources of calcium). Even if you decide to meet your daily calcium requirement of 1,000 – 1,500 mg by consuming two glasses of skim milk, two containers of yogurt, and two ounces of cheddar cheese, you'll have taken in 900 Calories. Since you need only approximately 2,000 Calories per day, you would have only a little more than one-half of your calories still available to allot to meeting your other nutritional requirements.

TABLE 13 – 1

GOOD SOURCES OF CALCIUM

	Portion Size	Calcium* (mg)	Calories*
Skim milk	8 oz.	300	90
Whole milk	8 oz.	285	160
Yogurt (lowfat, plain)	8 oz.	295	125
Cheddar cheese	1 oz.	225	120
American cheese	1 oz.	210	110
Cottage cheese (uncreamed)	8 oz.	200	200
Sardines (unboned, drained)	3 oz.	370	175
Salmon (canned)	3 oz.	170	120
Broccoli (medium stalk)		205	50
Spinach	4 oz.	84	84

* Approximate figures

A way around this problem is through supplemental calcium. Because of increased media coverage of women's health issues, calcium-containing supplements have flooded the over-the-counter market and are available as calcium carbonate, calcium lactate, or calcium gluconate tablets. Calcium carbonate tablets have the highest percentage of calcium per tablet (40 percent); the others contain approximately 13 percent and 9 percent, respectively. Because of those percentage differences, to get 1,000 milligrams you would need to take 4 tablets of carbonate; whereas to get the equivalent with the other calcium salts, you would need 12 tablets of lactate and 18 tablets of gluconate. *Tums,* although sold as an antacid, is a calcium carbonate tablet which *Consumer Reports* recommends as an inexpensive way to take calcium.[5]

Although taking excessive amounts of most vitamins and minerals can be harmful to your body, this is rarely true with calcium. As much as 2,500 milligrams daily, for example, rarely cause problems in healthy people. The exception is for women who have previously had calcium-containing kidney stones; if this is your case, you need to discuss this problem with your doctor.

Coffee or caffeine consumption has been identified in some studies (and contradicted in others) as a potential risk factor for osteoporosis and hip fractures because it decreases bone density. A recent study that supports the negative impact of coffee found that there was a significant association between lifetime intake of two cups per day of caffeinated coffee and decreased bone mineral density.[6] The good news from that study was that in the subjects who drank 8 ounces of milk on a daily basis, bone mineral density did not change. This study reinforces the need for adequate calcium intake throughout a woman's life.

Calcium and Vitamin D. Nutritionists point out that in order for the small intestines to absorb adequate calcium — no matter how much is available — Vitamin D must be present. In most seasons, the majority of people get adequate amounts of Vitamin D through exposure to sunlight for at least 20 to 30 minutes daily, during which time the skin synthesizes Vitamin D. However, both winter and aging present problems.

Since most people are not outdoors much in winter, the recommendation for those in that category is to take daily supplements of 400 IU of Vitamin D — which is usually the standard amount in a multi-vitamin tablet — one pint of whole, fresh enriched milk contains 200 IUs. Scientists have evidence that aging reduces the skin's capacity to produce Vitamin D. It is therefore recommended that the daily supplement should be increased to 800 IU year-round for those over 50. Amounts over 800 IUs are not recommended because they may be toxic.[7]

TABLE 13 – 2

CALCIUM HINTS

- When you eat dairy products, choose those that are nonfat wherever possible.
- Choose other calcium-rich alternatives such as sardines (packed in water), other canned fish, tofu, spinach, broccoli, and greens. A six-ounce stalk of broccoli supplies about a quarter of the RDA for calcium.
- Use an acid dressing, made with citrus juices or vinegar, to enhance calcium absorption from salad greens.
- Be aware that some experts claim that high-fiber diets can impair the absorption of calcium from the intestines.
- Lifetime coffee or caffeine intake of two cups per day is reported to lower calcium in bone. This can be offset by drinking at least one glass of milk per day during most of your adult life.
- More than two or three alcoholic beverages a day impairs intestinal calcium absorption.

Vitamins · Prevailing dogma would have us follow a daily diet chosen from the FDA food pyramid recommendations. Presumably, we would then consume enough vitamins and minerals to satisfy our recommended daily allowance (RDA). However, if because of work or lifestyles, a nutritious daily diet is not always possible, then vitamin supplements should be considered. Ordinary multiple vitamin pills — not therapeutic or mega-vitamin doses — are all that are necessary as a supplement. They should be taken either daily or three to four times per week.

Since all vitamins are chemically the same, our recommendation is to buy a generic vitamin pill and not spend (waste) extra money on brand-name vitamins. Check ingredients and dosage levels before buying.

EXERCISE AND FITNESS

Exercise should have been a normal part of your life prior to your surgery. If it was not, the advent of your operation marks an opportune time to refocus on both exercise and nutrition in a way that they will become intrinsic to your lifestyle. You might ask, Why should I start to exercise now if I've never done it before and didn't miss it? In answer, there are some exercise advocates who go so far as to say that exercise can "profoundly affect this period of transition [menopause] by enhancing quality of life."[8] In a recent article in *The Physician and Sportsmedicine,* Dr. K. M. Hartgarten cites studies showing that postmenopausal women participating in an exercise program can improve their cardiorespiratory fitness, reduce their risk of coronary artery disease, prevent osteoporosis, and experience psychological benefits.[9]

The types of physical activity which we can incorporate into our life are endless and range from the exotic, like rock climbing, to the mundane, like walking. Each has its attractions, benefits, and liabilities.

In choosing an activity to pursue, consider at least one which will help protect you from osteoporosis. As we discussed in Chapter Twelve, osteoporosis can be forestalled with a combination of hormone replacement therapy, calcium, vitamin D, and muscle-joint-bone stress producing exercise.

Ideally we should have a mix of activities that we do over a week's period so that we work the bones throughout our body. Swimming/bicycling/running could be juxtaposed with weight resistance activities. Women who are not exercise-oriented should not be intimidated by these suggestions. Don't get discouraged if you don't have the time or inclination to do as much as is recommended. Do as much as you feel comfortable. Every little bit will help enhance both body and health.

DEVELOPING PHYSICAL FITNESS

Depending upon the specific activity program you choose, you will be improving your performance to varying degrees in each of the five components of fitness: cardiovascular endurance, muscular strength, muscular endurance, flexibility, and body composition. See Table 13 – 3 for a list of physical activities broken down by fitness components.

TABLE 13 – 3

ACTIVITIES FOR PHYSICAL FITNESS DEVELOPMENT

High	Moderate
Cardiorespiratory Endurance	
Aerobic dancing	Basketball
Aerobic walking	Calisthenics
Backpacking	Downhill skiing
Bicycling	Field hockey
Cross-country skiing	Handball
Hiking	Racquetball
Jogging	Squash
Running	Tennis (singles)
Skating	
Stair climbing	
Swimming	
Muscular Strength	
Backpacking	Aerobic dancing
Bicycling	Calisthenics
Gymnastics	
Swimming	
Weight training	
Muscular Endurance	
Jogging	Calisthenics
Running	Fencing
Swimming	Handball
Weight training	
Body Composition (body mass)	
Aerobic exercise	
Cross-country skiing	
Jogging	
Running	
Swimming	
Flexibility	
Calisthenics	Aerobic dancing
Gymnastics	
Karate	
Modern dance	
Stretching	

The Overload Principle · The golden rule for developing overall physical fitness involves attention to the *overload principle,* which states that our bodies must be stressed beyond their normal levels of activity if they are to improve. To increase the overload and consequently your level of physical conditioning, you must gradually increase the *intensity, duration,* or *frequency* of your activity.

Intensity. Intensity is the rate you do an exercise, or, for weight training, the amount of resistance that you work against. Heart rate is usually used as a measure of intensity in aerobic activities such as walking, running, and swimming. The amount of weight lifted is the intensity measurement used in weight training activities.

Using heart rate as a measure of intensity for achieving a training effect involves knowing your **Target Heart Rate (THR).** To get that figure we need the following. First, calculate your **Maximal Heart Rate (Max HR).** An easy approximation of that rate is achieved by subtracting your age from 220. Second, calculate your **Resting Heart Rate (RHR)** — simply count your pulse rate for six seconds and add a zero or count your pulse rate for ten seconds and multiply by six. Third, you have to arbitrarily choose a **Range Percentage (RP).** Traditionally, a RP was 60 to 90 percent of the difference between your resting heart rate and your maximum heart rate. Recent research has revealed that lower levels (40 – 45 percent) may also be effective, especially in individuals with low levels of physical fitness.

All three of these figures then get entered into the formula for Target Heart Rate, which is: THR = [RP (MaxHR – RHR) + RHR]. That sounds daunting, but if put into everyday numbers it means that if you choose a 60 percent range level and your RHR is 70 and your MaxHR is 180, then your THR is 136 [.6 (180 – 70) + 70].

Using those same figures, in order for you to achieve a conditioning level from the aerobic activity you have chosen, you need to get your heart rate to 136 beats per minute during the exercise period. A simple way of checking whether you have achieved this is to immediately monitor your pulse rate when you have stopped the activity. To increase the intensity goal, raise your range percentage (for example, to 65 percent instead of 60 percent) which means that you will need to exercise more vigorously to get to your new targeted heart rate.

The same principle of increasing the intensity applies to weightlifting, but in this case it means increasing either the amount of weight lifted or the number of repetitions done at each of the weights.

If you plan to start either a weightlifting or aerobic activity program, you should consult one of the many available books on the subject which will provide you with more detailed descriptions (see "Suggested Readings in Fitness" at the end of this chapter).

Duration. This term is used to describe the length of time of an exercise period. By increasing the amount of time we exercise, we can contribute to the overload principle. Be aware that in general, the intensity of an exercise is inversely related to the duration — that is, as one increases, the other usually decreases. As we age, it is often advised to increase duration rather than focus on intensity.

Frequency. Frequency refers to the number of days per week that an exercise program is pursued. Three to four days per week is generally believed to be sufficient to maintain a beneficial effect. The other days could be used as "rest" days. Recuperation time between exercise days is important in order for our body systems to adapt to and recover from the stress placed on them during exercise.

HOW TO BEGIN

Note: Before engaging in an exercise program, get your doctor's okay. This is especially important if you are at risk for coronary artery disease or osteoporosis.

Putting the above into practical terms, and using aerobic walking as an example, we might decide to aim at walking one mile in 20 minutes, three times a week by the end of one month.

A one-month long "phase in" to reach the goal is necessary when planing to begin an exercise regimen. This helps to prevent the "drop-out" syndrome, which occurs when we enthusiastically begin a program at too high a level for untrained muscles and abruptly end the program due to muscle strain. Remember, surgery contributes to muscle atrophy and weakness due to disuse while you are recuperating for at least four weeks after your hysterectomy. During that time most of us can do only minimal exercise. Thus, even if prior to surgery you could run two miles nonstop, don't attempt to start your program at that level after your operation. The severe muscle soreness that you will develop may cause you to abandon your exercise program.

For the former nonexerciser — remember, don't get discouraged. It's better to do some exercise, even if it's not as much as recommended, than to do nothing. (See Table 13 – 3 for a list of activities that you might consider.)

Start at a reasonable level for whatever activity you pursue, and as your body begins to adapt, slowly increase intensity, duration, or frequency.

If you were involved in some type of physical activity before surgery and now wish to try something new, be aware of a phenomenon known as **mus-**

cle specificity. Despite your previous level of conditioning, your new activity may use different muscle groups and it will be as if you are starting from scratch. Do not be surprised if you develop soreness in those newly used muscle groups.

When planning an exercise program, try to think of each session as a unit consisting of a warm-up, the specific exercise, and a cool-down. Warm-up describes the activities done to prepare our body for the more strenuous physical requirements of the exercise, while cool-down immediately follows the exercise and allows the various body systems to return to pre-exercise levels. Exercise physiologists have identified the warm-up and cool-down as important in the possible prevention of muscle soreness, injury, and also in alleviating excessive heart strain which may result from sudden engagement in strenuous exercise.

Warm-ups and cool-downs will vary depending upon the specific activity, but in general, warm-ups might include some type of calisthenics or stretching, and/or be specific to your activity but at a lower level of intensity. Warm-downs are usually a graduated tapering of exercise intensity and perhaps some gentle stretching as well.

KEEPING FIT

If you are already involved in an activity program or if you are about to start one, there is one more thing to consider — a supplementary exercise program to strengthen your abdominals and improve the flexibility of your lumbar, or lower back, region.

Lower (Lumbar) Back Muscles · You might have been lucky so far and have avoided an affliction common to many Americans — lower back problems. Over 80 percent of the population will experience low back pain at some time in their lives; it accounts for over 25 percent of all injuries, and nearly 40 percent of all worker's compensation claims. It is important to note that most cases of back pain resolve in one to two weeks by themselves; however, some linger or become chronic and require medical intervention.

Low back pain occurs more frequently as we get older. Back pain can often be prevented or an existing problem helped by following two guidelines. First, avoid behaviors that may increase the risk of back injury or reinjury, and second, develop muscular strength and flexibility.

The usual causes of low back injury are mechanical harm due to improper lifting techniques, lifting too heavy a load, or improper posture. Avoiding or correcting problems involves using proper lifting techniques, improving posture, and gaining greater flexibility.

Lifting techniques. To lift properly, keep your back relatively straight rather than stooped over. You should use your leg rather than back muscles as the main source of power; that is, bend at the knees when lifting. Avoid lifting objects that are too heavy for you; and keep objects being lifted as close to your body as possible. Further, when you pick up objects (or touch your toes), slowly bend over and remember to bend your knees at the same time.

Posture. The major cause of poor posture is inadequate muscle tone with an accompanying shortening and tightening of certain muscles and a concurrent lengthening and weakening of the opposite set of muscles. For example, in round shoulders caused by habitual slouching of the shoulders, muscles in the chest are shortened and tightened, while those in the upper back are lengthened. In the lower body, poor posture contributes to lengthening and weakening of the abdominal muscles and a concomitant tightening of the lower back muscles. Tightening of lower spinal muscles may cause the development of lumbar lordosis, or hollow back, in which there is an exaggeration of the natural curve of the lower back. In addition to avoiding movements which increase this curvature of the lumbar spine (for example, slouching while standing, or sleeping on your stomach), you should consciously work to increase both the strength of your abdominals and the flexibility of your lower spine.

Flexibility. For flexibility of the lower spine, include exercises that flatten out the curve of the lumbar spine. For example, while sitting with your legs extended straight in front, reach as far towards your toes as possible; hold that position for 15 to 60 seconds, then relax and repeat three times. Consult an exercise manual for other suggestions (see "Suggested Readings in Fitness" at the end of this chapter).

Abdominals. Weak abdominals often contribute to weak backs. The abdominals are comprised of three major muscle groups: the internal obliques, external obliques, and the rectus abdominus. The rectus abdominus serves the upper and lower abdominal areas. The upper rectus abdominals draw the rib cage toward the pelvis, while the lower ones draw the pelvis toward the rib cage. Together they also help to hold the internal organs in place. The internal and external obliques are the muscles that form the waist and act as the rotational muscles of the abdomen — twisting the trunk and bending to the side and forward.

Before beginning an abdominal strengthening regimen, you might want to assess your abdominal strength using the one-minute curl-up test described on the next page. An exercise program to achieve abdominal strength includes using sit-ups or curl-ups with your knees bent and feet flat on the floor. Other abdominal exercises include variations which aim at the specific abdominal muscle group you want to strengthen. (For specific exercises, consult one of the books recommended at the end of this chapter in "Suggested Readings for Fitness.") Two precautions to keep in mind when doing abdominal exercises: don't hook your feet under an object, and don't perform straight-leg exercises where both legs are lifted or lowered simultaneously. In both movements, the hip flexors are the main muscles used, and not the abdominals. Any straining can cause excessive and possibly painful arching of the lower back — the condition these exercises are designed to help prevent or cure!

Remember: Strong abdominals, good posture, flexibility, and care in lifting help keep backs from causing problems.

ONE-MINUTE CURL-UP TEST

Purpose: To measure the muscular strength and endurance of the abdominal muscles.

Equipment: Watch with second hand

Procedure: A curl-up is a sit-up in which you only come up less than halfway (about 30 degrees).

Lie on your back with your knees bent and your shoulders touching the floor. Your arms are completely extended by your sides, with palms facing down. It is helpful if you have someone hold your feet to the floor and do the timing.

With your arms fully extended, lift your head and shoulders off the floor and slide your hands forward. Then return to the lying position — it is not necessary to return your head to the floor with each curl-up. Do as many as you can for one minute.

Evaluate your score against the standards listed below.

Age	Beginner	Intermediate	Advanced
30 – 39	<20	20 – 40	>40
40 – 49	<18	18 – 35	>35
50 – 59	<12	12 – 30	>30
60 +	<11	11 – 25	>25

< means less than

> means more than

Hints:

1. Exhale as you curl up — don't hold your breath.
2. Rest at any time, but don't stop the clock.
3. If you don't have a partner to hold your feet, try not to slide back during the test.

Putting It All Together · Workaholics trying to reform their compulsive behavior have been heard to say "I need to work on my working too much." The great majority of us need to work on our poor eating habits and infrequent exercise regimens. Don't wait until next January 1st to start changes. Let your operation serve as the impetus to change things — you owe it to yourself.

ENDNOTES

1. Greenspan, S. L., Myers, E. R., Maitland, L. A. et al. Fall severity and bone mineral density as risk factors for hip fracture in ambulatory elderly. *Journal of the American Medical Association,* 1994, 271, 128 – 133.

2. Human Nutrition Information Service. *USDA's Food Guide Pyramid.* Hyattsville, MD: United States Department of Agriculture, 1992.

Nutrition and Your Health: Dietary Guidelines for Americans, 3rd ed. U. S. Department of Agriculture and U. S. Department of Health and Human Services. Washington, D.C.: Government Printing Office, 1990.

3. *Consumer Reports.* Forget about cholesterol. 1990, 55(3), p.154.

4. Reid, I. R., Ames, R. W., Evans, M. C., et. al. Effects of calcium supplementation on bone loss in postmenopausal women. *New England Journal of Medicine,* 1993, 328(7), 460 – 464.

5. *Consumer Reports.* The truth about calcium. May 1988, 53, 288 – 291.

6. Barrett-Conner, E., Chang, J. C., & Edelstein, S. L. Coffee-associated osteoporosis offset by daily milk consumption: the Rancho Bernardo study. *Journal of the American Medical Association,* 1994, 271(4), 280 – 283.

7. Wymelenberg, S. Osteoporosis: alternatives to estrogen. *Harvard Health Letter,* 1994, 19(5), 6 – 8.

8. Hargarten, K. M. Menopause: how exercise mitigates symptoms. *The Physician and Sportsmedicine,* 1994, 22(1), p. 49.

9. Hargarten, K. M. Menopause: how exercise mitigates symptoms. *The Physician and Sportsmedicine,* 1994, 22(1), 49 – 57.

SUGGESTED READINGS

General

Barnard, Neal. *Food for Life: How the New Four Food Groups Can Save Your Life.* New York: Crown Publishing, 1993.

David, Marc. *Nourishing Wisdom: A Mind — Body Approach to Nutrition and Well-Being.* New York: Crown Publishing, 1994.

Foreyt, John P., & G. Ken Goodrick. *Living Without Dieting.* New York: Warner Books, 1994.

Everson, Cory, & Carole Jacobs. *Cory Everson's Fat-Free & Fit: A Complete Program for Fitness, Exercise & Health Living.* New York: Putnam Publishing Group, 1994.

Goldberg, Linn, & Dianne L. Elliot, eds. *Exercise for the Prevention and Treatment of Medical Illness.* Philadelphia, PA: Davis Company, 1994.

Hoffer, Abram & Morton Walker. *Smart Nutrients: A Guide to Nutrients That Can Prevent and Reverse Senility.* Garden City Park, NY: Avery Publishing Group, 1994.

Janklowicz, Gilad & Ann M. Brown. *Bodies in Motion: Discovering Joy in Fitness.* San Francisco, CA: Foghorn Press, 1993.

Moog, Shirleigh. *A Guide to the Food Pyramid: Recipes and Information.* Watsonville, CA: The Crossing Press, 1993.

Ornish, Dean. *Eat More, Weigh Less: Dr. Dean Ornish's Life Choice Program for Losing Weight Safely While Eating Abundantly.* New York: HarperCollins, 1993.

University of California at Berkeley Wellness Letter Editors. *The Wellness Guide to Lifelong Fitness.* New York: Rebus, Inc., 1993.

Vertinsky, Patricia A. *The Eternally Wounded Woman: Women, Exercise, and Doctors in the Late Nineteenth Century.* Urbana, Il: University of Illinois Press, 1994.

FITNESS

Anderson, B. *Stretching.* Bolinas, CA: Shelter Publications, 1980.

Cooper, K. *The Aerobics Program for Total Well-Being.* New York: Bantam Books, 1983.

Fahey, T. *Basic Weight Training.* Mountain View, CA: Mayfield Publishers, 1989.

Hales, D., & R. Hales. *The U.S. Army Total Fitness Program for Men and Women.* New York: Ballantine Books, 1985.

Kusinitz, I., & M. Fine. *Your Guide to Getting Fit.* Mountain View, CA: Mayfield Publishers, 1987.

Lederach, N., N. Kauffmann, & B. Lederach. *Exercise As You Grow Older.* Intercourse, PA: Good Books, 1986.

Maglischo, E. W., & C. F. Brennan. *Swim for the Health of It.* Mountain View, CA: Mayfield Publishing, 1984.

Noakes, T. *Lore of Running*. 3rd ed. Champaign, IL: Human Kinetics Press, 1991.

Prentice, W. *Fitness for College and Life.* 3rd ed. St. Louis: Mosby-Yearbook, 1991.

Riley, D. *Maximum Muscular Fitness.* Champaign, IL: Leisure Press, 1982.

Chapter 14

THE CHOICES ARE YOURS: THE TIME IS NOW

CONGRATULATE YOURSELF

By reading this book, you have demonstrated that you care enough about yourself to put forth some effort. You are well on your way to becoming an informed consumer of health care. Everything you read, every action you take, puts you further ahead in accepting rightful responsibility for your own life and welfare.

NO MORE A PATIENT

Susan Sherwin, in her powerful work *No Longer Patient: Feminist Ethics and Health Care,* admonishes women to give up passivity, especially in matters of health.[1] Decisions regarding contraception, abortion, birth, surgery, and hormone replacement therapy must not be made by others. It is up to each of us to choose or refuse specific medical or surgical intervention. Sherwin observes that medical practice of the past was largely paternalistic. Physicians gave the "orders," and "patients" (of both sexes) were expected to be "compliant." Sherwin calls for a change in the current health care model. She recommends a system which is concerned with "empowering consumers in their own health by providing them with the relevant information and the means necessary to bring about the changes that would contribute to their health."[2] Together, through this book, we have embarked on contributing to these changes.

Dr. Paul Arnston, professor of Communication at Northwestern University, takes this concept of "consumer" a step further. He writes that people must act as "citizens" in regard to health care. What he means is that we should not let ourselves be persuaded to make health decisions based on "advertising," as we might choose a brand of breakfast cereal. As citizens, we assume responsibility for our own well-being. We *actively* seek information from others. We consider and evaluate health prevention and treatment options recognizing that the choices are ours. It is up to each individual to develop health competencies so as to act wisely.[3]

For years the medical literature and physicians were concerned with "patient **compliance**," which actually means "bending to the will of another."[4] Doctors would order medication or treatment only to find that it was not taken or followed. For any number of reasons, "patients" did not do as they were told. In many cases this was to the consumers' detriment, since physicians had information which could contribute to "patients'" welfare.

As we move toward shared responsibility for individual health, the term **adherence** has been proposed instead of compliance.[5] Adherence suggests that the procedure leading to a medical decision includes active patient involvement. In other words, rather than bending to follow the doctor's orders, a patient thoughtfully adheres to a plan of treatment because it has been agreed upon mutually.

Becoming more and more involved in your own medical status has clear benefits. You likely will find, as many researchers have demonstrated, that you achieve greater health and experience more satisfaction with health-related decisions.[6]

TAKE STOCK

This is the time to review where you are medically. If hysterectomy or other gynecological surgery has been prescribed for you, a number of informed decisions need to be made. If you already have had surgery, different options exist.

Gynecological Problems Awaiting Solution

If you have problems such as those described in Chapter Four, you should be busy evaluating your condition and actively selecting the best solutions available. Some guidelines may be helpful.

DON'T RUSH

Unless you have had a Pap smear or other test which shows invasive cancer, the best thing that you can do is slow down. Do not let a gynecologist or surgeon rush you into an operation. If you have fibroids, they grow slowly. Endometriosis and uterine prolapse are also not emergency procedures. Be sure to have the appropriate medical tests, then take your time in investigating your options and making your decisions.

DO YOUR HOMEWORK

Prepare Your Medical History · The Appendix contains an example of a medical history that you should have ready to show every time you see a new health care provider. Doctors sometimes hurry you as they take information. This can have serious consequences. Did someone in your family have ovarian cancer? Your physician may not ask this question, but a "yes" answer will put you at greater risk for this disease, and so special tests may be appropriate. *You* need to provide the information, and having it in writing assures that it won't be overlooked.

What's the Problem? · It is remarkable how often our symptoms seem to disappear as soon as we enter a health care practitioner's office. We sometimes even forget what brought us there. As you begin to think about consulting a physician, write down a description of your ailments and concerns. What's wrong? Why are you seeking help at this time? The Appendix outlines the type of information you should record prior to each visit to your health specialist.

Do Some Reading · In earlier chapters, we suggested books that describe medical tests, give advice on selecting doctors and hospitals, and generally help you become more knowledgeable about your health options. Many can be purchased at reasonable cost and should become part of your personal reference library. Read what pertains to you and apply what is appropriate.

Popular magazines often contain helpful articles on health. Check to make sure that these are well researched. A responsible article will refer to scientific studies by respected researchers at known institutions. Be aware of what authorities conclude based on their investigations, and then make your decisions wisely.

Talk and Listen · While many of us tend to just listen to a doctor we trust or base our decisions on what we read, others explore a variety of avenues for becoming more educated about health concerns. Dr. Paul Arnston notes that family, peer, school, work, mass media, self-help groups, and community action groups are all potential sources of information.[7]

Talking to people, being careful not to bore them with your medical problems, may turn up friends, relatives, or coworkers who have symptoms similar to your own. While each encounter will not be productive, and some may be of questionable reliability, none should be disregarded without fair consideration.

Seek Several Medical Opinions · The first physician you consult may not be as current or sensitive as you would wish, or he or she may appear to be wise and understanding. Whatever the situation, especially if surgery or any other major procedure is recommended, seek at least one other opinion. If these disagree, talk to a third, and perhaps a fourth physician. Chapters Three and Eight offer guidelines in selecting a doctor. The major suggestions include choosing a physician who is board certified in the relevant specialty (gynecology and perhaps oncology or endocrinology) and, where possible, has been recommended by a consumer group or trusted friends or relatives. A family practitoner can also be a source of valuable information.

After Hysterectomy

If you have already had a hysterectomy, you still need to take stock of your health and life and make some decisions.

MEDICAL CHECKUPS

Health maintenance is important throughout life. While some women visit their health care provider only when they have a problem, it is far wiser to have regular medical checkups. For those over age 50, it is generally acknowledged that an annual medical checkup is appropriate. When you go for this, you can expect your height, weight, blood pressure, and pulse to be measured and recorded. Your skin will be looked over for skin cancers or other lesions, and your lymph glands will be palpated. Other assessments will be made which may or may not require that you go for other tests. As you enter your 60s, you may expect your vision and hearing to also be tested.[8]

Many illnesses, such as heart problems, breast cancer, and osteoporosis, are associated with older ages. Some serious problems may be symptom-free in the early stages, but can be identified through medical tests. As you recall, early diagnosis and treatment permit better outcomes.

TABLE 14 – 1

BLOOD PRESSURE READINGS AND RECOMMENDED FOLLOW-UP

Category	Systolic	Diastolic	Follow-up•
Normal	<130	<85	Recheck in 2 years
High Normal	130 – 139	85 – 89	Recheck in 1 year
Hypertension**			
Mild	140 – 159	90 – 99	Confirm within 2 months
Moderate	160 – 179	100 – 109	Evaluate or refer within 1 month
Severe	180 – 209	110 – 119	Evaluate or refer within 1 week
Very Severe	210 +	120 +	Evaluate or refer immediately

*When the systolic and diastolic readings are in different severity categories, the higher level is considered more indicative.

**Blood pressure readings taken on three separate occasions are required to make a diagnosis of hypertension.

Source: Tierney, et al., 1994.

Heart Disease and Stroke · Elevated cholesterol and LDL levels are associated with a greater risk of heart disease, yet it is impossible to know your cholesterol and LDL levels without blood tests. While diet and exercise can help reduce these blood components, you would be prudent to stay informed regarding your current condition. The National Institutes of Health suggest that for people over age 40, a cholesterol reading of more than 240 mg/dL or more than 260 mg/dL is a sign of moderate or high risk, respectively, although the National Cholesterol Program considers any cholesterol level over 200 mg/dL too high.[9] (See Chapter Thirteen.)

An electrocardiogram provides baseline information in case of later emergencies, and many health care professionals recommend this be taken at about age 40.[10]

Blood pressure also cannot be known without testing. At every adult age, individuals with high blood pressure (hypertension) are at greater risk than normal for stroke and heart failure. If your reading is high normal or mild, you may be able to bring it down to normal by reducing the amount of salt in your diet, losing weight, exercising regularly, and/or engaging in relaxation techniques.[11] Table 14 – 1 indicates categories and appropriate follow-up for different readings.

Cancer · Cancer has sometimes been called a silent killer. Symptoms may not appear until the disease is well advanced. The American Cancer Society provides guidelines for when and how often you should be tested for cancer if you have no symptoms. These are summarized in Table 14 – 2.

TABLE 14 – 2
RECOMMENDATIONS FOR FREQUENCY AND TYPE OF CANCER TESTING

Procedure	Age	Frequency
Sigmoidoscopy	50 or over	Every 3 – 5 years
Stool test for occult blood	50 or over	Every year
Digital rectal exam	40 or over	Every year
Pap test	20 or over; under 20 if sexually active	Every year until 3 negative exams; then every 3 years, more or less at doctor's discretion
Endometrial tissue sample	If you have not had a hysterectomy, at menopause; earlier, if high risk*	At menopause, then at doctor's discretion
Breast self-exam	20 or over	Every month
Breast exam by physician	20 – 39	Every 3 years
	40 or over	Every year
Mammogram	40 – 49	Every 1 – 2 years
	50 or over	Every year
Health counseling & cancer checkup**	20 – 39	Every 3 years
	40 or over	Every year

*History of infertility, obesity, failure of ovulation, abnormal uterine bleeding, unopposed estrogen or tamoxifen therapy.
**Includes examination for cancers of the thyroid, ovaries, lymph nodes, mouth, and skin.
Source: Tierney, et al., 1994.

TO BE OR NOT TO BE A CRONE

After a hysterectomy you are no longer reproductively capable. You are now in the third stage of your biological life. The first was childhood; the second was your reproductively possible period, and now you are post-menopause.

Susun Weed has a provocative plan to welcome the third stage of life. She advises that within a year after your last menstrual period, you engage in a ritual of "Crone's Crowning." [12] This can be performed either alone or with similarly minded women. You are no longer a "'bleeding woman',… you are now free from worry about conception, pregnancy, or mothering." You should celebrate your new position as "crone."

The word "crone" used to be synonymous with witch. The classic fairy-tales show old women as ugly, mean, and clever. But Webster's definition for crone includes the words "elder" and "matriarch." As a woman who is past menopause, you can choose to enact the definition that appeals to you. You can stop caring about your physical appearance and permit yourself to be irritable and cross. Or, you can opt for the role of experienced older person, someone whose judgment and understanding are valued.

REDEFINING BEAUTY

> Her old friends had trouble not commenting when Karen walked into the room. Karen, age 62, tall, elegant, and divorced, just had a face lift. Hair dyed the shade of strawberry blond she once was, Karen was dressed in a short skirt and low-cut blouse. One acquaintance whispered that Karen resembled "a dead teenager." Another said that "Karen looked fantastic."

As we age, we have the opportunity to reevaluate our personal appearance. One option is Karen's way, to do what we can to look young. Cosmetic surgery is often effective, although expensive. Wrinkles and jowls can temporarily be lessened. (In several years, the skin is likely to sag again.) How do you evaluate the cost/benefit ratio? All operations carry the risks associated with anesthesia and medical mishap. Insurance is not likely to pay the fees, which are certain to be high. On the other hand, you may wipe years off your appearance, which can do wonders for your self-esteem. The decision is yours.

> Nadine had a hysterectomy at 36 and had started to gray in her twenties. Now aged 38, Nadine was a fourth grade teacher and had just returned to her home after a summer of "trail work" in the Rockies. She and her husband had volunteered to help maintain hiking trails in the high mountains.
>
> Upon seeing her again after several months, some friends were startled by Nadine's appearance. Her flowing tresses were white; she

had stopped dyeing her hair. During the summer out-of-doors, Nadine had determined to let her appearance return to its natural state. She was motivated in part by the knowledge that hair-dyeing is considered a risk factor in ovarian cancer. Although she recognized the connection might be minimal, she opted to look older but eliminate a potentially dangerous behavior.

Nadine is an example of someone whose age is hard to judge. Her body is fit from physical work. She glows with enthusiasm from her summer experience, and she is eager to get back to the classroom and share some of her new knowledge with the children. Nadine's hair ages her, but her energy is that of a much younger person.

Diane recently turned 50. She had a hysterectomy at age 46, and her husband died two years later. Diane works as an administrative assistant in a large corporation. She has been with the company for 20 years; she could do her job in her sleep. Twenty years of sedentary work have taken their toll. Diane is clearly overweight, and she no longer invests in her appearance. Her hair is salt-and-pepper, shoulder-length, but lacking in style. She generally wears pants suits with oversized jackets to cover her girth. Although always friendly, Diane gives the impression of having given up on life.

Karen, Nadine, and Diane offer three contrasting approaches to personal appearance. Karen and Nadine, although very different in style, care about how they look and it shows. Diane has let go, perhaps as part of a general retreat from life.

Naomi Wolf, in her book *The Beauty Myth,* talks about how women's beauty has been marketed, packaged, and sold.[13] As we grow older, none of us look as we did in our teens or early 20s. Our body weight is harder to control. Our faces have developed lines (some say character). Our hair may not have the color or texture it had. Our decision is not to forego beauty, but to redefine it in keeping with the options we now have.

A NEW BEGINNING

Increasing interest is currently being paid to the third phase of women's lives. Gail Sheehy, in her best-selling book *The Silent Passage,* claims that at last women are breaking the silence and speaking out on "the last taboo" — menopause and the years beyond.[14] Whether you had a hysterectomy at a relatively young age or lost your uterus closer to the time of natural menopause, the chances are that you do not want to live your postmenopausal years in the same way as your mother. Women today are often more active and more liberated. Most of us do not intend to settle into back-seat roles as grandmothers. And, if grandparenthood has been achieved, many of us do it very differently from our predecessors.

Lottie, a smartly-dressed retired businesswoman in her 70s, described the older women she knew when she was growing up in Europe:

> "After 50 women only wore black. They were always in mourning. First their parents had died, then their husband, perhaps a brother, maybe even a child. What was the point in having colorful clothing? As for me, although my parents are long gone and I lost my first husband to the second world war, I'll only wear black to a funeral."

> Mary, now 53, had a hysterectomy at age 48. She has four grandchildren. When Mary's not working in her important government position, she can generally be found in running clothes or chic casual wear. Mary has successfully run a marathon four times since turning 50. Her trim body, stylish blond hair, and vibrant personality define a new image of the postmenopausal woman.

Perhaps surprisingly, once over the hill of going through menopause, many women feel a new energy and clarity in their lives. Gail Sheehy received responses to a detailed questionnaire on personal life history from almost 700 women, with an average age of 50. They were from all over the country and were in lower middle and upper middle income brackets. The vast majority reported that the most critical factor in their happiness was not wealth or marital status, but age — and older is better! Ninety percent of Sheehy's respondents reported that 50 is "an optimistic, can-do stage of life."[15]

Postmenopause often means that children are grown, and domestic responsibilities have lessened. Some women become depressed at their "empty nest"; others take the opportunity to find new personal fulfillment. You may choose to take the time to think about those things which are truly most important to you as an individual. Your life may no longer be dictated by the needs of others. As such, it is up to you to make plans and define meaning for this "second adulthood."[16]

SET GOALS

Your hysterectomy may be the occasion to recognize that to a large extent you have control over your well-being. What do you want? Who do you want to be?

YOUR PHYSICAL SELF

Chapter Twelve discussed in detail physical problems which are associated with the post-hysterectomy/postmenopausal years. Chapter Thirteen considered ways of staying fit and healthy. What plans should you make to improve your physical well-being?

Smoking · If you smoke, we join the chorus of voices urging you to stop. Smoking is the single most important cause of preventable illness and premature death. Smokers suffer twice as many fatal heart attacks and are much more likely to get cancer than nonsmokers.[17] The current outcry against the dangers of cigarette smoking (and secondhand smoke) should be an inducement. You can no longer light up on domestic airplane flights, most places of business, some restaurants, and other public places. Cigarette smoking is no longer fashionable — in fact, it is often an embarrassment.

While smoking is an addiction that is often hard to break, it is well worth your while to make the effort. If you can't stop on your own, consider consulting your physician or a hypnotist, or working with a self-help group. The reward may be a longer and healthier life.

Diet · Your options are whether to continue in your eating patterns of the past, or to invest energy in changing them for a more healthful diet. Remember the suggestions made in Chapter Thirteen:

1. Eat a variety of foods.
2. Maintain ideal weight.
3. Avoid too much fat, saturated fat, and cholesterol.
4. Eat foods with adequate starch and fiber.
5. Avoid too much sugar.
6. Avoid too much sodium.
7. If you drink alcohol, do so in moderation.

Examine your food habits. Do you routinely eat lunch out with coworkers and feast on high-calorie fast food? Many chains now offer salads and other nutritious dishes. Think about what you order.

Do you prepare meals to please the tastes of others? If they can't be persuaded to join you in the guidelines noted above, consider preparing separate items or encouraging each person to cook their own food.

Do you nibble on leftovers? Is it better to throw some food away or eat more than you need? Can you plan to cook a little less? Or a little more — so that you can make extras into "planned-overs" for a later meal?

Can't resist the ice cream always kept on hand in your freezer? Switch to light ice cream or frozen yogurt, which are lower in fat (but high in sugar, so don't overdo it!). Look for the no-fat cookies at the grocery, and substitute them for richer cakes and cookies. The ways of eating better are numerous; the hardest part is making the decision to do so.

Exercise · Cleaning house, preparing meals, tending a garden, and taking care of children all provide a modicum of exercise. These activities are more beneficial physically than sitting at a desk all day. However, optimum fitness can only be obtained through following a carefully thought-out regimen. As discussed in Chapter Thirteen, attention needs to be paid to five components of physical fitness:

1. cardiovascular endurance
2. muscular strength
3. muscular endurance
4. flexibility
5. body composition

Reasons not to exercise are plentiful: time, money, boredom, difficulty. But solutions to these potential problems also exist.

Time. Your days may be filled to capacity. Job responsibilities, home duties.... Where can the hour be found to work out? If you have not exercised before, walking as much as possible, instead of riding, is an excellent way to begin. Walking contributes to four of the five fitness components listed before. Instead of the elevator, take the stairs. If you drive to work, park a little further away than usual. If you take public transportation, get off a stop ahead of the one you need. The extra time this takes will be minimal and you will have made a start.

If you are already walking and want to do more, you will need to set aside a time that is just for you. This may require some effort. Many women get up an hour earlier than normal to permit a "workout" period. Others convince their families to have the evening meal later so they can exercise prior to dinner. So as not to delay the meal too much, you might consider preparing food the evening before and/or using some (nutritious) convenience items so that the time needed before dinner is minimal. Another exercise period might be noon. Some employers are sympathetic to the importance of exercise in maintaining health and will permit a flexible lunch hour. It's worth inquiring.

Money. You may complain that exercise is expensive if you base your opinion on advertisements for joining health clubs. It's true that many gyms and even "Y's" charge $500 or more a year. If funds are not a problem, and you actually *use* the facilities, this is money well spent. However, you can work out much less expensively.

To start, walking can be free. Of course, once you get going, you may want to invest in special walking shoes. We recommend these for the support that they provide. But you do not need a special outfit, old comfortable clothing will certainly do. If you've moved to jogging, the expense can be limited to running shoes and a good "jog-bra."

Exercise/aerobic classes may cost $10 per session. But for $10 – $15 you can purchase an exercise tape to play on your VCR and use repeatedly when convenient. As you progress you can purchase additional tapes so as to vary your routines. These tapes also have the advantage of taking less time, since you can work out at home. However, if you are just starting, you may want to take a class or two with a knowledgeable instructor to make sure that you do not hurt yourself. Also, some people require the motivation of a class to keep going. Again, the choice is yours.

Boredom. Vary your exercise. This is important not only to keep you interested, but also to stretch and strengthen different muscle groups as explained in Chapter Thirteen. You might choose to walk or jog three days a week and work out with an exercise tape on alternate days (allowing for one or two days a week off). If you are walking, jogging, or biking, find different routes. If you are using a stationary bike or treadmill at home, play music, watch television, or read while you exercise. As you become familiar with your exercise videotapes, you might try turning off the sound and simply following the picture while you listen to something else on the radio.

Difficulty. Some women stop exercising because working out can be hard work. If you push to your limits for maximum benefits, you may find that you are straining, sweating, and watching the clock hoping that it will be over soon. Don't overdo — increase your activity gradually. Expecting to make improvements too quickly can cause bodily injury, thereby negating the beneficial effects.

But exercise does require effort. Few things that are truly worthwhile are easy. Once you have made exercise a part of your life, you will miss it on days that you can not work out. Aerobic exercise increases our bodies' production of adrenaline and endorphins and provides us with a good feeling; some call this "an exercise high." It is work to get there, but the rewards are great.

Hormones · Will you take hormone replacement therapy? This is another decision which you must make. Chapter Eleven provided details of the arguments for and against hormone replacement.

In making your decision, weigh the advantages and drawbacks to HRT.

Advantages:

Reduces or eliminates hot flashes
May reduce insomnia if due to night sweats
Reduces or eliminates vaginal dryness
Reduces risk of osteoporosis
May reduce risk of heart disease
May prevent or reduce severity of Alzheimer's disease

Drawbacks:

May increase risk of breast cancer (although this conclusion is controversial)

May increase risk of gallbladder problems

Expense of prescription and medical follow-up

Whatever you decide, remember that your position is reversible. HRT is helpful even if started several years after menopause. You may also stop at any time, although you should taper down your dosage under your doctor's care. If you have opted for HRT, it is essential to have your health monitored by a physician at least once a year.

Alternatives:

The benefits of HRT can often be derived in other ways.

To reduce or eliminate hot flashes

- Dress in layers, so you can peel as necessary
- Adjust the heat in your home to suit you
- Drink lots of room-temperature liquid
- Carry and use an old-fashioned hand fan

To reduce insomnia due to night sweats

- Be ready to adjust your bedding
- If you are awake, get up and use the time to read or watch television — consider this your "bonus" time

To reduce or eliminate vaginal dryness

- Use vaginal moisturizers or gels

To reduce risk of osteoporosis

- Engage in weight-bearing and aerobic exercise
- Take extra calcium and eat food high in calcium (broccoli, dairy products, sardines with bones)

To reduce risk of heart disease

- Eat a diet that is varied and low in fat
- Stop smoking
- Take one low-dose aspirin a day

FEELINGS AND RELATIONSHIPS

Menopause is reputed to be a time of emotional swings. Whether it is due to hysterectomy or natural processes, tradition forecasts that you may expect to experience angry outbursts or weepy periods for no good reason. Your psyche is supposedly hooked up to the change in hormones and you are at their mercy. While recent research questions the inevitability of psychological problems at this time, recognizing that you *may* be a little more on edge than before can help you set goals to achieve more emotional comfort.

Moods · Have you developed a way for dealing with "the blues?" If when you are feeling fine you think of things that tend to cheer you up, you may have ammunition for when you need it.

> Delores often came home from work feeling stressed and angry. Unfair pressures from her boss, ridiculous deadlines, traffic, and a husband who expected her to be cheerful and chatty at day's end frequently made Delores feel that she was at the breaking point. Following her hysterectomy, the situation appeared to be even worse and she would end up yelling at her spouse and then crying inconsolably. Several drinks at day's end did not help her situation. Finally, after much thought and discussion, Delores determined that every day following work, she would quickly go in her house, change her clothes and go for a bike ride in a nearby park. Biking was something she and her husband had occasionally enjoyed on weekends. Since her husband wanted to go with her, at least some of the time, they set up a rule: no talking until they got back to the house. This new routine helped!

The method for getting through testy periods is up to you. Exercise in some form is often helpful. Some women find a short walk by themselves a real mood lifter. Others feel better after a swim, aerobics class, yoga, or meditation. Still others find comfort in cooking, baking, or even cleaning out a closet. The trick is to indulge in some activity that will transport you to a more peaceful state of mind.

Friends · Good friends and companions to talk to and do things with are precious. In this age, when people move frequently, it is often difficult to maintain long-term relationships. But as we age, those with whom we have shared histories through the years are sometimes especially treasured. Older friends perhaps knew us when we were students together. They may have been our confidants as marriage thoughts approached and as children enriched and complicated our lives. A continued investment in these old relationships is often fruitful.

Newer friends with more immediate interests in common are also vital. Susan McDaniel and Allison McKinnon, Canadian researchers, observe that "it is well known that contacts with people are important to well-being."[18] So, it may be beneficial to welcome new associations with those with whom we feel a bond.

But family and friendships do not come without a price. As we age, we are more likely to assume responsibilities for the welfare of others. McDaniel and McKinnon note that "the informal support that women provide as spouses, daughters, daughters-in-law, sisters, nieces, friends, and volunteers, can leave women with little time, energy or resources to care for themselves and to work outside the home and family."[19]

We need to choose on an individual basis whether to initiate, maintain, or discontinue our connections with others. These are difficult decisions, and usually best done thoughtfully rather than by simply letting things happen.

Partners · Experiencing a hysterectomy or natural menopause can tax the best of relationships. You will need extra support and understanding. Try to prepare your partner to know what to expect.

A few women find this a time to end a relationship which is no longer vital. Others opt to reinvigorate and perhaps redefine their relationship. Rather than continuing as things were, this new stage of life calls for a fresh examination of your most intimate partnership.

Solo · Life as a single older woman has many advantages. Gail Sheehy observes that alone, many women can pursue the dreams of their youth — or later years — unfettered by rigorously accommodating to another.[20]

> Barbara had a hysterectomy at age 36 and was divorced at 38. Today, at age 50, she has not remarried. Her life is full, and for now, she does not want the constraints of a full-time relationship. In addition to running a successful private preschool, Barbara teaches "Euro-dancing" primarily to older women three evenings a week. She travels during the summer, when her school is not in session, and is active in a local political organization. Although she has dated from time to time, she can't visualize herself "tied down" at least at this point in her life.

Sex · After menopause, our sexual rhythms may change. We may not desire sexual activity as frequently, and orgasm may occur less readily. Lonnie Barbach observes that many couples engage in less intercourse but more "touching, self-pleasuring and oral sex."[21] Chapter Ten provides suggestions for enhancing sexual satisfaction.

ON THE JOB — IN THE COMMUNITY

For some women, the years past 40 contain extra financial and emotional pressures. Children may be in college, getting married, and/or starting their careers. Parents of mid-life adults may be aged and require special attention. You may feel squeezed in the middle — caring for needy parents (or in-laws) and still providing for your children who are struggling to establish themselves. If this is your situation, you need to be sure to allow time for yourself.

For other women, middle and later adulthood permit more personal time. Either never married, or single again, work patterns may be more flexible and the competence which comes from experience may be strengthening. Gail Sheehy observes that "the Woman of the 90s is in her 50s — enjoying power, glory, and life."[22]

What Do You Want? · Whether you are caught in the middle of two needy generations or are feeling relatively free, this is a good time to pause to consider your personal desires. Reexamine your career aspirations and think about the things you like to do. Are there courses you'd like to take? Job changes you are tempted to make? Have you always wanted to contribute more to your community but lacked the time? Obviously you can't do everything, but you should give it some thought. Sit down and make a list. Permit yourself stream of consciousness. Write down every activity that you truly enjoy, every ambition which you have harbored. If you don't plan your life, the days will go by and be out of your control.

Hillary Rodham Clinton observed that many of us "lack at some core level, meaning in our individual lives and meaning collectively."[23] Attempt to identify what is personally important and fulfilling. Unforeseen events, illness, financial concern, and responsibilities to others all influence what finally occurs — but each of us has a hand in our destiny, if we choose to play it.

TAKE ACTION

Drawing up a plan to eat better, exercise more, and identify the components of personal satisfaction is perhaps half the work. The remainder is to actually follow through. This requires determination and a measure of fearlessness.

> At age 49, Barbara was tired of driving a school bus. Her hysterectomy the previous year gave her a forced vacation and time to reflect on what she really wanted to do. Barbara was good at her job; she took pride in that. The children respected her and she loved them.... But Barbara felt that she could do more; she'd been a secretary for many years and knew that was no longer for her. Taking courage in hand, Barbara enrolled as a nonmatriculated student at the local community college. Many mornings she literally had diarrhea before taking her seat among the mostly younger students. Her brain often felt rigid — how could she learn so much new information? But finally, at 58, a Bachelor's degree in hand, Barbara found a satisfying professional-level position as a hospital dietician. This was accomplished despite personal doubts and anxiety, and excessive questioning and some derision by her husband. Tremendous support from her grown son and daughter, however, helped her through some of the more trying periods.

KEEP INFORMED

The work of a thoughtful life is never over. Recognizing that you are largely responsible for your health and happiness means that you must keep reading, talking, and listening.

Dr. Gary L. Kreps, a professor at Northern Illinois University, in writing about cancer, insists that "consumers should be in charge of their own treatment."[24] But whatever your diagnosis, whether you are healthy or ill, you need to know enough to make intelligent choices.

Several newsletters are available which highlight important recent medical information in a readable fashion. You might consider subscribing to one or more of these:

Consumer's Report on Health
Harvard Women's Health Watch
The Johns Hopkins Medical Letter – Health After 50
The Harvard Medical School Health Letter
Tufts University Diet and Nurtition Letter
University of California at Berkeley Wellness Letter

If you have been diagnosed with cancer, you should know about and use the following toll-free resources:

American Cancer Society 1-800-ACS-2345
National Cancer Institute's Cancer Information Service (CIS)
1-800-FOR-CANCER

Read health articles as they appear in your local newspaper, and clip and file those which may be relevant to you. Become familiar with the medical/health section of your local library. In this way you will know where to find information, should the need arise.

Go to lectures, watch health shows on television, join a support group. Your personal physician is only one source of health information. The broader and more complete your own knowledge, the better able you will be to contribute wisely to health decisions which concern you.

FIND THE JOY

No matter what health condition or procedure you have experienced or anticipate, you can strive to make the most of the situation.

> Ellen, age 48, had ovarian cancer. She had a hysterectomy and bilateral salpingo-oophorectomy. This was followed by rounds of radiation and chemotherapy. However, the cancer had spread and these treatments were only buying time. Ellen, with support of family and friends, was determined to use her remaining days as fully as she could. Ellen had been a high school French teacher and had lived in France for several years. She was fascinated by the nuances of differences in meaning provided by the French and English languages. She chose to embark on a project to translate and write commentaries on the works of some relatively obscure French philosophers whom she believed were not well understood by Americans. During the hours in

which she felt reasonably well, Ellen rejoiced in her task. She told friends that her illness relieved her from mundane chores and provided her with the gift of time to do work which intrigued her.

Ellen found happiness where others would have suffered only despair. Each life is filled with struggle and hardship that often seem overwhelming. The challenge is to find the joy; the options are yours.

ENDNOTES

1. Sherwin, S. *No Longer Patient: Feminist Ethics and Health Care.* Philadelphia: Temple University Press, 1992.

2. Sherwin, S. *No Longer Patient: Feminist Ethics and Health Care.* Philadelphia: Temple University Press, 1992, p. 239.

3. Arnston, P. Improving citizens' health competencies. *Health Communication,* 1989, 1 (1), 29-34.

4. Sharf, B. F. Physician-patient communication as interpersonal rhetoric: a narrative approach. *Health Communication,* 1990, 2 (4), p. 218.

5. Sharf, B. F. Physician-patient communication as interpersonal rhetoric: a narrative approach. *Health Communication,* 1990, 2 (4), 217 – 231.

6. Ballard-Reisch, D. S. A model of participative decision making for physician-patient interaction. *Health Communication,* 1990, 2 (2), 91 – 104.

7. Arnston, P. Improving citizens' health competencies. *Health Communication,* 1989, 1 (1), 29 – 34.

8. Branch, Jr., W. T. *Office Practice of Medicine,* 3rd ed. Philadelphia: W. B. Saunders, 1994.

9. Tierney, Jr., L. M., McPhee, S. J., & Papadakis, M. A., eds. *Current Medical Diagnosis & Treatment 1994.* Los Altos, CA: Appleton & Lange, 1994.

10. Branch, Jr., W. T. *Office Practice of Medicine,* 3rd ed. Philadelphia: W. B. Saunders, 1994.

11. Tierney, Jr., L. M., McPhee, S. J., & Papadakis, M. A., eds. *Current Medical Diagnosis & Treatment 1994.* Los Altos, CA: Appleton & Lange, 1994.

12. Weed, S. S. *Menopausal Years: The Wise Woman Way — Alternative Approaches for Women 30 – 90.* Woodstock, NY: Ash Tree Publishing, 1992.

13. Wolf, N. *The Beauty Myth.* New York: Doubleday, 1991.

14. Sheehy, G. *The Silent Passage.* New York: Random House, 1991.

15. Sheehy, G. The flaming fifties. *Vanity Fair,* October 1993, p. 272.

16. Sheehy, G. The flaming fifties. *Vanity Fair,* October 1993, 270 – 273, 302, 304 – 311.

17. Tierney, Jr., L. M., McPhee, S. J., & Papadakis, M. A., eds. *Current Medical Diagnosis & Treatment 1994.* Los Altos, CA: Appleton & Lange, 1994.

18. McDaniel, S. A., & McKinnon, A. L. Gender differences in informal support

and coping among elders: findings from Canada's 1985 and 1990 General Social Surveys. *Journal of Women and Aging,* 1993, 5 (2), p. 95.

19. McDaniel, S. A., & McKinnon, A. L. Gender differences in informal support and coping among elders: findings from Canada's 1985 and 1990 General Social Surveys. *Journal of Women and Aging,* 1993, 5 (2), p. 95.

20. Sheehy, G. The flaming fifties. *Vanity Fair,* October 1993, 270 – 273, 302, 304-311.

21. Barbach, L. *The Pause: Positive Approaches to Menopause.* New York: Signet, 1993, p. 248.

22. Sheehy, G. The flaming fifties. *Vanity Fair,* October 1993, 270 – 273, 302, 304 – 311.

23. Sheehy, G. The flaming fifties. *Vanity Fair,* October 1993, p. 305.

24. Kreps, G. L. Refusing to be a victim: rhetorical strategies for confronting cancer. In Thornton, B. C., & Kreps, G. L., *Perspectives on Health Communication,* Prospect Heights, IL: Waveland Press, 1993, p. 45.

SUGGESTED READING

Barbach, Lonnie. *The Pause: Positive Approaches to Menopause.* New York: Signet, 1994.

Barbach, Lonnie, & David L. Geisinger. *Going the Distance: Finding and Keeping Lifelong Love.* New York: Plume, 1993.

Cobb, Janine O'Leary. *Understanding Menopause.* New York: Plume, 1993.

Doress-Worters, Paula B., & Diana Laskin Siegal. *The New Ourselves, Growing Older: Women Aging with Knowledge and Power.* New York: Simon & Schuster, 1994.

Friedan, Betty. *The Fountain of Age.* New York: Simon & Schuster, 1993.

Greer, Germaine. *The Change: Women, Aging, and the Menopause.* New York: Knopf (distributed by Random House), 1992.

Jones, A., Kreps, G.L., & G. M. Phillips. *Communicating with Your Doctor: Getting the Most Out of Health Care.* Cresskill, NJ: Hampton Press, 1995.

Sheehy, Gail. *The Silent Passage: Menopause.* New York: Random House, 1992.

Sherwin, Susan. *No Longer Patient: Feminist Ethics and Health Care.* Philadelphia: Temple University Press, 1992.

Weed, Susun S. *Menopausal Years: The Wise Woman Way — Alternative Approaches for Women 30 – 90.* Woodstock, NY: Ash Tree Publishing, 1992.

Wolf, Naomi. *The Beauty Myth.* New York: Doubleday, 1991.

APPENDIX

SPECIAL INTEREST GROUPS THAT MAINTAIN LISTS OF OBSTETRICIANS/GYNECOLOGISTS

Boston Women's Health Collective
465 Mt. Auburn Street
Watertown, MA 02172
(617) 924-0271

The Institute for Reproductive Health
8721 Beverly Boulevard
Los Angeles, CA 90048
(213) 854-6375 or 6483

HERS (Hysterectomy Educational Resources and Services)
501 Woodbrook Avenue
Philadelphia, PA 19119

(for doctors who specialize in cancer of the female organs)

The Resource Center
American College of Obstetricians and Gynecologists
600 Maryland Avenue SW
Washington, DC 20024-2588
(202) 863-2518

NATIONAL CANCER INSTITUTE (NCI) DESIGNATED CANCER CENTERS

The following list is not inclusive, nor is it an endorsement; it is provided as a starting place in your search for an outstanding facility to treat your medical problem. Included in this list are comprehensive care cancer centers as well as clinical cancer centers that focus on both treatment and research (basic and clinical). For additional NCI-designated cancer centers, call 1-800/4-CANCER.

California
University of California at San Diego
225 Dickinson Street
San Diego, CA 92103

University of California at Los Angeles (Jonsson Comprehensive Cancer Center)
10833 Le Conte Avenue
Los Angeles, CA 90024

Colorado
University of Colorado Cancer Center
4200 East 9th Avenue
Denver, CO 80262

Connecticut
Yale University Comprehensive Cancer Center
333 Cedar Street
New Haven, CT 06510

Illinois
University of Chicago Cancer Research Center
5841 South Maryland Avenue
Chicago, IL 60637

Massachusetts
Dana Farber Cancer Institute
44 Binney Street
Boston, MA 02115

New York
Albert Einstein College of Medicine
1300 Morris Park Avenue
Bronx, NY 10461

Memorial Sloan-Kettering Cancer Center
1275 York Avenue
New York, NY 10021

University of Rochester Cancer Center
601 Elmwood Avenue
Rochester, NY 14642

Ohio
Case Western Reserve University
University Hospitals of Cleveland
Ireland Cancer Center
2074 Abington Road
Cleveland, OH 44106

Rhode Island
Roger Williams General Hospital
825 Chalkstone Avenue
Providence, RI 02908

Tennessee
St Jude Children's Research Hospital
332 North Lauderdale Street
Memphis, TN 38101

Texas
Institute for Cancer Research and Care
8122 Datapoint Drive
San Antonio, TX 78229

Utah
Utah Regional Cancer Center
University of Utah Medical Center
50 North Medical Drive
Salt Lake City, UT 84132

Virginia
Massey Cancer Center
Medical College of Virginia
Virginia Commonwealth University
1200 East Broad Street
Richmond, VA 23298

Washington
Fred Hutchinson Cancer Research Center
1124 Columbia Street
Seattle, WA 98104

Wisconsin
University of Wisconsin
Wisconsin Clinical Cancer Center
600 Highland Avenue
Madison, WI 53792

Adapted from Robert Arnot, M.D. *The Best Medicine: How to Choose the Top Doctors, the Top Hospitals, and the Top Treatments*. Reading, MA: Addison-Wesley, 1992.

HEALTH & MEDICAL HISTORY

IDENTIFICATION

Your name ____________________ Date of completing this form ____________

(You should update this form following each medical checkup, illness, and personal or family life change.)

Home address ____

Work address ____

Home phone ____________________ Work phone ____________________

Who should be notified in case of emergency?

Name ____________________ Phone number(s) ____________________

Name ____________________ Phone number(s) ____________________

Marital status ____________________ Spouse/partner's name ____________________

CHILDREN

Name ____________________ Birth date ____________________

Address ____

Name ____________________ Birth date ____________________

Address ____

Name ____________________ Birth date ____________________

Address ____

Name ____________________ Birth date ____________________

Address ____

FAMILY HISTORY

Mother ____________________ Present age ____________________

Current health condition ____

Past health problems & surgeries ____

____

If applicable: date of death ____________ Age at death ____________________

Father ____________________ Present age ____________________

Cause of death ____

Current health condition ____

Past health problems & surgeries ____

____

If applicable: date of death ____________ Age at death ____________________

Cause of death ____

Number of brothers ________ sisters ________

What health problems and surgeries have they had?________________________________

____

What do you know about health problems and surgeries of your maternal and paternal grandparents?____

____

Aunts? ____

Uncles?____

BIRTH HISTORY

Date of birth ____

Place of birth ____

Conditions of birth (such as Caesarian, premature, mother had problems during pregnancy, used DES; mother had previous miscarriages, etc.) ______________________________

____

VACCINATIONS

(note approximate dates)

Polio: injection ________ oral ________; Smallpox ________; Mumps ________;

measles (year is important) ________; German measles (rubella) ________;

diphtheria/pertussis/tetanus (DPT) ________;

DT booster ________, ________, ________; Influenza ________, ________;

Chicken pox (varicella) ________; Hepatitis B ________; Other ________________

CHILDHOOD ILLNESSES, ACCIDENTS & SURGERIES

Age____________ Illness, accident, or surgery ______________________________

Age____________ Illness, accident, or surgery ______________________________

Age____________ Illness, accident, or surgery ______________________________

OTHER PAST SERIOUS ILLNESSES FROM WHICH YOU HAVE RECOVERED

(Include sexually transmitted disease, drug reactions, etc.)

Illness	Date	Your age then	Symptoms & treatment

PREVIOUS ACCIDENTS, SURGERIES AND HOSPITALIZATIONS

Date	Your age then	Nature of operation or circumstances (be as specific as possible)
____________	____________	____
____________	____________	____
____________	____________	____

CURRENT CHRONIC CONDITIONS

Disease	Date diagnosed	What are you doing for it?
____________	____________	____
____________	____________	____
____________	____________	____

FOOD, DRINK, SMOKE, ALLERGIES

List the foods which you commonly eat ____

____

____

Foods which you avoid ____

Food allergies ____

Other allergies (include pollen, medicines) ___________________________

How often do you drink alcohol? ____________________________________

How much each time? ____

How often do you drink caffeinated beverages? _________________________

How much each time and what form (e.g. coffee, tea, hot chocolate)? _________

Do you currently smoke? ____________ What do you smoke? ____________

How much per day? ________________

Did you ever smoke? ______________ How much per day? ______________

Years in which you smoked, from ________ to ________

Reason for stopping ____

Do you use any recreational drugs? ________ Specify ____________________

History of recreational drug use ____________________________________

____

____

OCCUPATIONS & OTHER ACTIVITIES

(List your current job and all previous jobs. For each, describe the nature of your work. Your specific tasks and your employment environment can provide important clues to diseases you may acquire later in life. Use as many pages as necessary for this section.)

Domestic chores

Hobbies

Favorite activities

Exercise patterns (include walking and sports)

HEIGHT & WEIGHT

(You should note this about once a year)

Date Height Weight

(Note special conditions such as pregnancy, surgery, illness.)

DOCTORS and OTHER HEALTH CARE PROVIDERS YOU HAVE SEEN

(Begin with the most recent. Try to repeat this as far back as possible for each medical provider and visit.)

Doctor's name ______________________________

Location ______________________________

Specialty ______________________________

Date of visit ________ Your symptoms/reasons for visit ______________________________

Diagnosis ______________________________

Treatment ______________________________

Outcome ______________________________

Reason you stopped seeing doctor ______________________________

(Repeat as necessary)

Doctor's name ______________________________

Location ______________________________

Specialty ______________________________

Date of visit ________ Your symptoms/reasons for visit ______________________________

Diagnosis ______________________________

Treatment ______________________________

Outcome ______________________________

Reason you stopped seeing doctor ______________________________

Doctor's name ______________________________

Location ______________________________

Specialty ______________________________

Date of visit ________ Your symptoms/reasons for visit ______________________________

Diagnosis ______________________________

Treatment ______________________________

Outcome ______________________________

Reason you stopped seeing doctor ______________________________

Adapted from J. Alfred Jones, Gary L. Kreps, & Gerald M. Phillips. *Communicating with Your Doctor: Getting the Most out of Health Care.* Cresskill, NJ: Hampton Press, 1995.

CURRENT HEALTH PROBLEMS

(Fill this out before each medical visit, and bring it with you.)

What are your symptoms? ______________________________

When did they start? ______________

Do you feel pain? ______________ Where? ______________

Can you point to it? ______________

What kind of pain is it? (Sharp, piercing, dull, throbbing, steady, intermittent, shooting—describe its pattern) ______________________________

____

When do you feel it? (After meals? When you wake up? When you exercise? All the time? Other? Describe in detail.) ______________________________

____

Write down details similar to above for each of the following possibilities that might be relevant in your case.

Heavy, irregular, or postmenopausal bleeding ______________________________

Sexual difficulties, including lack of interest, vaginal dryness, inability to orgasm, pain with intercourse ______________________________

Nausea ______________________________

Vomiting ______________________________

Loss of appetite ______________________________

Fatigue ______________________________

Sleep problems ______________________________

General feeling of uneasiness or anxiety ______________________________

Lack of interest in things ______________________________

Depression ______________________________

Feelings of hopelessness ______________________________

Diarrhea ______________________________

Constipation ______________________________

Itching, rash ______________________________

Feeling faint or dizzy ______________________________

Vision problems ______________________________

Hearing problems ____________________

Balance — falling problems ____________________

Sneezing, coughing, wheezing ____________________

Other (describe in detail) ____________________

Was there some event that set it off? ____________________

Did it come on suddenly or gradually? ____________________

Has it gotten worse? ____________________

Did you ever have it before? ____________________

When and under what circumstances? ____________________

PREVIOUS MEDICAL CONSULTATION

Have you spoken to a medical person previously about this? ________

Who? ____________________ When? ____________________

What was the diagnosis? ____________________

What physical, laboratory, or X-ray findings were there? ____________________

____

What treatment was recommended? ____________________

____

What did you do? ____________________

What were the results? ____________________

Bring in all prescription bottles which you have for medicines you are currently taking.

What over-the-counter medicines are you taking? ____________________

____

List all health problems for which you are currently being treated. ____________________

____

____

____

____

____

____

Adapted from J. Alfred Jones, Gary L. Kreps, & Gerald M. Phillips. *Communicating with Your Doctor: Getting the Most out of Health Care*. Cresskill, NJ: Hampton Press, 1995.

GLOSSARY

abdominal endoscopy — use of the laparoscope to examine the interior of the abdomen.

ablate — to remove or destroy.

acupressure — the use of pressure to various body parts to relieve aches and pains.

adenomyoma — see also *adenomyosis;* a benign, tumorlike nodule in the uterine wall.

adenomyomata — plural of *adenomyoma.*

adenomyosis — benign growth of the endometrium into the uterine musculature.

adhesions — the abnormal formation of internal scar tissue sometimes following surgery or D&C.

AIDS — (acquired immunodeficiency syndrome) a disease that breaks down the body's immune systems to the extent that it cannot fight off infections.

Alarm Reaction Stage — the first stage of Selye's General Syndrome where the hormonal and nervous system responses quickly prepare for a fight-or-flight response.

ampulla — the part of the fallopian tubes nearest the ovary.

analog — a chemical which has similar properties as another; for example, GnRH analogs are manufactured preparations which have similar effects as GnRH.

antineoplastic — anti-cancer.

antiprostaglandins — drugs which counter the effect of the prostaglandin hormones; prostaglandins encourage uterine contractions and may account for painful menstrual periods; antiprostaglandins include ibuprofens (Motrin, Advil, Nuprin) and aspirin.

anus — the external opening of the large intestine.

areola — the wrinkled dark skin around the nipple.

arteriosclerosis — the general term used to describe any impairment of blood flow through the arteries.

atherosclerosis — the buildup on the artery wall of plaque (deposits of fat, fibrin, cholesterol, and calcium) which increase the risk of a heart attack.

atrophic vaginitis — thinning of the vaginal walls and related problems caused by the loss of estrogen.

autoinoculation — spreading an infection from one body area to another.

autologous blood donation — the process of donating your own blood which is then kept available for your use in case it is needed during a surgical procedure.

Bartholin's ducts — passageways which are situated on each side of the vestibule in the groove between the hymen and the labia minora which pass inward to the Bartholin's glands.

Bartholin's glands — an aggregate of cells which secrete a small amount of lubricating fluid during sexual excitement.

basal metabolic rate (BMR) — represents the energy necessary to carry on basic life functions (such as circulation, respiration, body temperature maintenance, and brain activity).

benign — a noncancerous condition; a situation with a favorable outcome.

benign cervical dysplasia — abnormal cells in the cervix that are not cancerous.

bikini cut — see *Pfannestiel incision.*

biofeedback — a technique for teaching people to become aware of and gain control over involuntary body functions.

biopsy — the removal and microscopic examination of body tissue for diagnostic purposes.

bisexual — interested in sexual interactions with both women and men.

BMR — see *basal metabolic rate.*

board certified — a physician who has passed licensing requirements in a particular medical specialty.

bone densitometers — a technology which detects with accuracy and precision the actual calcium content in bone.

bony pelvis — the bowl-like structure formed by the two hip bones and the bottom of the spinal column.

breakthrough bleeding — irregularly occurring small endometrial discharges not associated with the menses; spotting.

Caesarean section — see *Cesarean section.*

cancer — a tumor which has the property of spreading and invading neighboring tissue as well as metastasizing to more remote tissue.

cancer in situ — a malignancy that is localized, not invasive.

Candida — see *monilia.*

Candida Albicans — the organism responsible for monilia.

cannula — a tube through which material may be inserted into a cavity such as the vagina and cervix.

carcinogenic — producing or causing cancer.

carcinoma — a malignant, cancerous tumor.

carcinoma in situ — a malignant tumor that is not invasive and confined to the epithelium tissue in which it originated.

castration — see *oopherectomy*; also refers to removal of male gonads (testes).

CAT scan — see *computerized axial tomography.*

catheter — a tube inserted through the urethra into the bladder to withdraw urine.

CBC — see *complete blood count.*

cell cycle nonspecific agents — used in chemotherapy for cancer; chemicals which are most effective against "solid" tumors which grow relatively slowly.

cell cycle specific agents — used in chemotherapy treatment for cancer; chemicals which are most effective against rapidly growing tumors.

cerebral thrombosis — a blockage that occurs in any brain vessel such as an artery.

cervical biopsy — the microscopic examination of suspicious cells taken from the cervix.

cervical cone biopsy — also *cone biopsy;* also *conization;* a method of removing a "cone" of tissue from the cervix for microscopic evaluation to detect the possible presence of cancer cells.

cervical intraepithelial neoplasia — new growth in the epithelial cells of the cervix, the quantity and nature of which is used in classifying tissue taken during a Pap test as indication of cervical cancer.

cervical stenosis — the narrowing of the cervical canal.

cervix — the lower portion of the uterus.

Cesarean section — also *Caesarean* or *C-section;* the delivery of a child through a cut in the abdomen.

chemotherapy — the use of drugs or chemicals to treat disease, specifically cancer.

chlamydia — a common sexually transmitted disease.

cholesterol — a waxy, soapy-looking, yellowish substance which is normal and useful to the body. It is an essential component in the formation of the cell membrane and in several hormones, such as testosterone and prostaglandin. Cholesterol is manufactured by the body and is also found in the animal foods we eat.

chronic — a disease or disorder which continues over an extended period of time.

cilia — hairlike projections.

CIN — see *cervical intraepithelial neoplasia.*

Class — a traditional method for categorizing cervical tissue removed during a Pap smear.

climacteric — the lead-up time to menopause during which a woman adjusts to a diminishing and then ceased menstrual flow, and the physiologic changes that may be associated.

clitoris — the erogenous small cylindrical erectile structure situated at the top of the vestibule and at the lower border of the pubic symphysis.

cobalt-60 gamma rays — a type of radiation used in cancer treatment.

coinsurance (or co-payment) — the requirement by your insurance company that you pay a certain percentage of your medical costs.

coitus — sexual intercourse.

colonoscopy — viewing the interior of the colon through a special scope.

colpohysterectomy — also *vaginal hysterectomy;* removal of the uterus through the vagina.

colposcopy — examining the cervix through a scope placed at the opening of the vagina.

combined opposed regimen — a hormone replacement protocol where progestogen is taken with estrogen.

comfrey — an herb that was believed to be helpful against cancer, but is actually ineffective.

complete blood count (CBC) — one of the most commonly performed blood analyses, consisting of seven different tests that are automatically machine-analyzed.

complete hysterectomy — see *total hysterectomy.*

computerized axial tomography — also called *CT scan* or *CAT scan;* an X-ray procedure in which a dye is injected into the veins, findings are processed by computer, and information about the health of body organs can be obtained.

cone biopsy — see *cervical cone biopsy.*

conization — see *cervical cone biopsy.*

conjugated estrogens — estrogen derived from the urine of pregnant mares.

co-payment — see *coinsurance.*

coronary thrombosis — a blockage in a coronary artery.

corpora cavernosa — the two spongy erectile tissues which make up the clitoris in women and part of the shaft of the penis in men.

corpus — in the uterus, the larger top portion or body.

corpus albicans — or "white body,"develops from the corpus luteum; if fertilization does not occur, corpus luteum regresses, stops hormone production, and turns white.

corpus luteum — the yellow body which forms from the cells of the graffian follicle after ovulation.

corpus spongiosum — the erectile tissue through which the male's urethra passes.

Cowper's glands — the aggregate of cells that provide pre-ejaculatory secretions which serve to cleanse the male urethral canal.

cryosurgery — the use of liquid nitrogen to freeze and kill cancerous cells.

C-section — see *Cesarean section.*

CT scan — see *computerized axial tomography.*

curette — a small spoon-shaped instrument used to scrape tissue; used in a D&C.

cystocele — a hernia, or bulge, of the bladder, intruding it into the vagina.

Danazol — a synthetic steroid that has been used as an anti-estrogen drug.

D&C — see *dilation and curettage.*

deductible — the amount that must be paid by the insured before their medical insurance takes effect.

DES — see *diethylstilbestrol.*

DEXA — see *dual energy X-ray absorptiometer.*

diastolic blood pressure — the lowest blood pressure reading; occurs between the heart's contractions.

dietary fiber — the collective term used for the indigestible residue of the structural components of plants.

diethylstilbestrol — also DES; a synthetic estrogen that was used to treat pregnancy and childbirth problems but may have had deleterious effects on the offspring years later.

differentiated cells — the normal, healthy manner in which body cells resemble others of the same type of tissue.

dilation and curettage — also known as D&C, a method of opening (dilating) the cervix and scraping tissue from the endometrium (with a curette) for diagnostic or treatment purposes.

dildo — an object, usually penis-like in shape, used to sexually stimulate the genitalia.

Doderlein's bacilli — the bacteria which are normal vaginal residents.

dual energy X-ray absorptiometer (DEXA) — a machine most commonly used to measure bone density.

dual photon absorptiometry — a method of measuring bone density.

durable power of attorney for health care — a document which lets you choose a person to make medical or health care decisions for you in case you become incapable of doing so.

dyspareunia — pain in the genital area during sexual intercourse.

dysplasia — abnormal body cells.

ECG — see *electrocardiogram.*

ectopic pregnancy — development of the embryo outside of the uterus.

EKG — see *electrocardiogram.*

electrocardiogram — (also known as EKG and ECG) performed to evaluate heart function.

electron beam — a type of radiation energy used in cancer treatment.

endometrial ablation — a procedure used to therapeutically destroy the inner lining (the endometrium) of the uterus.

endometriosis — the presence of endometrial tissue in places other than the uterus.

endometrium — the inner mucosal lining of the uterus. The endometrium is the tissue that thickens as estrogen causes the uterus to prepare for a fertilized egg's implantation, and then sloughs off as the menstrual period when hormones subside — if no pregnancy has occurred.

enterocele — a bulge, or hernia, of the small intestine, intruding into the vagina.

epidermoid carcinoma — cancer cells which resemble the outermost layer of cells of skin tissue.

ERT — see *estrogen replacement therapy.*

estradiol — one of the members of the hormone group for which the term estrogen is generally used.

estrogen replacement therapy (ERT) — the use of estrogen postmenopausally.

estrogen stimulation hypothesis — the theory that excessive estrogen stimulation may eventually convert normal endometrial tissue to cancer.

estrogenic group — one of the two main groups of female hormones produced primarily in the ovaries (and also by the adrenal glands in both men and women). It is comprised of several compounds, such as estradiol, estrone, and estrol, for which the term estrogen is generally used.

estrol — one of the members of the hormone group for which the term estrogen is generally used.

estrone — one of the members of the hormone group for which the term estrogen is generally used.

estrus — the female animal's sexually receptive time.

excitement — the first stage (or arousal) of the sexual response cycle during which, in women, the uterus pulls upward, while the inner two-thirds of the vagina expands.

exhaustion stage — the last stage of the General Adaptation Syndrome, where the specific organs and body systems cannot continue to resist the stressor.

external os — the opening of the cervix into the vagina.

external radiation — cancer therapy in which radiation is beamed into your body.

fallopian tubes — passageways through which the egg travels from the ovary to the uterus.

false negative — a mistaken clinical diagnosis which indicates that a condition is not present when in fact it is.

false positive — a mistaken clinical diagnosis which indicates that a condition is present when it is not.

fee-for-service insurance — the traditional type of health insurance, where the practitioner is paid for services rendered to the insured person.

ferning — the branching appearance of the vaginal mucous discharge at the time of ovulation.

fibroids — technical term is *leiomyomata uteri;* benign tumors which stem from the smooth muscle of the uterus.

fimbria — the small finger-like extensions that are at the end of the fallopian tube's infundibulum.

flushes — see *hot flashes.*

follicle-stimulating hormone (FSH) — the hormone released by the pituitary which stimulates egg and sperm maturation.

follicular phase — the stage in the ovarian cycle when there is initial follicle growth under the stimulation of FSH.

FSH — see *follicle-stimulating hormone.*

fundus — the upper end of the uterus.

GAS — see *General Adaptation Syndrome.*

General Adaptation Syndrome (GAS) — the model created by Hans Selye which describes three stages the body passes through when confronted by stressors.

GnRH — see *gonadotropin-releasing hormone.*

goal-free pleasuring — sexual stimulation and activity that is not directed at achieving orgasm.

gonadotropin-releasing hormone — also *GnRH;* hormones produced by the hypothalamus which prompt the pituitary to secrete gonadotropins.

gonorrhea — a sexually transmitted disease caused by a bacteria. Untreated gonorrhea can cause infertility in women.

Grafenberg area — also *G-spot;* the front portion of the vagina that is supposed to be especially sensitive to stimulation.

graffian follicle — the housing for an ovum inside the ovary.

group prepaid practice plans — since 1973, known as Health Maintenance Organizations.

G-spot — see *Grafenberg area.*

guided imagery — a technique that uses mental imagery to facilitate the healing process.

gynecologist — a board-certified physician who specializes in the health of the female reproductive/sexual system.

gynecology — the study of female anatomy and physiology, and its health.

hand-over-hand — see *hand-riding.*

hand-riding — also *hand-over-hand;* placing one's hand on top of the hand of another person to guide intimate touch.

HDLs — see *high density lipoproteins.*

health care proxy — a document that lets you choose a person to make medical or health care decisions for you in the event that you become incapable of doing so.

health maintenance organization (HMO) — an organization which delivers medical services for a fixed fee paid by enrollees and/or employers.

hematocrit — a blood test which measures the percentage of the blood volume that is made up of red blood cells.

herbal medicine — the use of balms and medications prepared from flowers, leaves, and other parts of plants.

high density lipoproteins (HDLs) — protein molecules which carry cholesterol from the blood to the liver.

histology — the study of cells and body tissue.

HMO — see *health maintenance organization.*

holistic medicine — an umbrella term for care which considers all aspects of a patient's needs and functioning.

homologous — corresponding in basic type of structure and deriving from a common primitive origin.

hormone replacement therapy (HRT) — used in this book as a general term for any hormonal therapeutic intervention (that is, estrogen replacement with or without progesterone).

hot flashes — also called flushes or, technically, vasomotor instability; temporary rises in body temperature associated with menopause.

HPV — see *human papilloma virus.*

HRT — see *hormone replacement therapy.*

human papilloma virus — also HPV; the virus associated with genital warts.

hydrogenation — the process of adding hydrogen atoms to produce a solid oil.

hymen — a thin, vascularized membrane that partially closes the external opening of the vagina.

hyperfractionated radiation therapy — radiation therapy in which relatively small doses are given several times a day.

hyperplasia — an abnormal increase in the number of cells in a tissue, as in endometrial hyperplasia (the overgrowth of endometrial tissue).

hypertension — the medical term for high blood pressure.

hyperthermia — elevating body temperature in experimental, and ineffective, treatment of cancer.

hypnotherapy — a method of inducing a trancelike state.

hysterectomy — surgical removal of the uterus.

hysterectomy with bilateral salpingo-oopherectomy — surgical removal of the uterus, fallopian tubes, and ovaries.

hysterosalpingogram — an X-ray procedure, using dyes injected through the cervix to detect fibroid tumors and/or blockage in the fallopian tubes.

hysteroscope — an instrument for viewing the interior of the uterus by entering through the vagina and cervix.

iatrogenic — problems "caused" by the medical care system; includes infections or surgical mishaps such as damage to surrounding organs.

immunotherapy — encouraging the body's own immune system to be active in fighting a disease.

implant radiation — see *internal radiation therapy.*

incentive deep breathing exerciser — a device which gets you to activate your lungs in order to keep them from filling with fluid.

incontinence — failure to "hold" one's urine.

informed consent — being fully advised of the procedures and consequences prior to treatment.

infundibulum — the end of the fallopian tubes which extends toward the ovary.

in situ — limited to the tissue of origin (used in reference to cancer that has not spread to other sites in the body).

interferon — a drug with limited effectiveness in the immunotherapy approach to cancer treatment.

interleukin-2 — a protein produced by the body which was considered as immunotherapy for cancer; it has not been found to be effective.

internal os — the opening of the cervix into the corpus of the uterus.

internal radiation therapy — radiation treatment through implanting a radioactive substance into the body; also called *implant radiation.*

intramural — the section of the fallopian tubes that is within the walls of the uterus.

intraoperative radiation — introducing radiation therapy for cancer during a surgical procedure.

intrauterine device (IUD) — a coil, t-shaped, or similar object placed in the uterus which helps prevent conception.

intravenous pyelogram (IVP) — a form of X-ray, using injected dyes, which tests the health of the kidneys.

invasive carcinoma — cancer which has spread beyond its original site.

isthmus — the narrow part of the fallopian tubes adjoining the uterus. Also, a slight constriction which divides the interior of the uterus into two parts — the corpus and the cervix.

IUD — see *intrauterine device.*

IVP — see *intravenous pyelogram.*

Kegel exercises — a series of exercises used to strengthen genital muscles.

keloid — a knotty scar which occasionally forms after surgery.

labia majora — two longitudinal folds of skin that extend from the mons veneris and form the lateral (side) borders of the vulva.

labia minora — (or minor lips) two longitudinal folds of skin located within the labia majora. The minor lips form the lateral and lower borders of the vestibule and fuse at the top to form the clitoral prepuce, which encloses the clitoris.

laetrile — Vitamin B-17, derived from apricot pits, and despite claims, found to be ineffective as a drug against cancer.

laparoscope — an instrument used for viewing the interior of the abdomen.

laparoscopic hysterectomy — a procedure for removing the uterus with the aid of the laparoscope.

laparoscopic tubal ligation — the procedure in which the fallopian tubes are "tied" to prevent conception; a laparoscope is used.

laparoscopy — also known as *peritoneoscopy, pelvic endoscopy,* or *abdominal endoscopy;* viewing the abdominal organs through a special scope placed through a small incision in the abdominal wall.

laparotomy — surgical abdominal incision used for both diagnostic purposes and to remove diseased organs.

large loop excision of the transformation zone — see *loop electrosurgical excision procedure.*

laser — Light Amplification by Stimulated Emissions of Radiation; the use of focused light in surgical procedures.

LDLs — see *low density lipoproteins.*

LEEP — see *loop electrosurgical excision procedure.*

leiomyoma — the singular form of *leiomyomata.*

leiomyomata — benign tumors stemming from smooth muscle (of the uterus); commonly called fibroids.

lesbian — a woman desiring sexual/affectional interactions mainly or exclusively with other women.

leuprolide acetate — a GnRH agonist used to shrink fibroids.

LH — see *lutenizing hormone.*

libido — the desire for sexual activity.

lipids — the fats in our diet; technically, it is a general term for a number of different water-insoluble compounds found in the body.

lipoproteins — molecules covered by a protein coat which transport cholesterol within the bloodstream.

lithotomy position — the gynecological position where the patient is on her back, with knees bent and feet in a pair of stirrups which are attached to the examining table.

living will — (often called a Medical Directive or Directive to Physicians) a document which lets you tell your physician in advance that you do not want your life artificially extended in certain situations.

loop electrosurgical excision procedure (LEEP) — a method for removing precancerous cells of the cervical area.

loop excision of the transformation zone — see *loop electrosurgical excision procedure.*

low density lipoproteins (LDLs) — protein molecules which carry large amounts of cholesterol to the arteries.

Lupron — a synthetic GnRH analog which blocks estrogen production.

luteal phase — the stage in the ovarian cycle in which the corpus luteum reaches full maturity.

luteinizing hormone (LH) — produced by the pituitary, this hormone in females causes ovulation and then helps maintain the corpus luteum.

magnetic resonance imaging (MRI) — also known as *nuclear magnetic resonance, NMR.* A procedure for diagnosing a variety of disorders based on the electrical resonance within the body.

malignant — the tendency to become increasingly worse, even fatal; often used to indicate cancer.

mammogram — a diagnostic X-ray of the breast.

mammography — the process of obtaining a mammogram.

managed care — the term used to describe how medical insurance companies now monitor the quality of medical treatment and determine its appropriateness for the patient's condition.

masturbation — stimulating oneself for sexual pleasure.

maximal heart rate — the theoretical highest rate at which your heart will pump blood.

medical curettage — the use of hormone treatment to stimulate the uterine lining to shed and begin a new cycle.

menarche — the onset of menstruation.

menopause — the final cessation of menstruation, either as a normal part of aging or as a result of surgery. Also the general term for the combination of symptoms associated with that period of a woman's life.

menstrual phase — the stage in the endometrial cycle when, if the egg is not fertilized, progesterone diminishes and the lining of the uterus breaks down. The superficial two-thirds of the endometrium is almost all sloughed off as part of the menstrual flow.

metabolism — represents the sum total of all physical and chemical changes that take place within the body, and reflects how the body is using its energy stores.

metastasis — the process by which abnormal (cancer) cells from one part of the body are spread to other sites not directly connected to the original source.

mittelschmerz — a German term for pain in the middle of the cycle which indicates that ovulation is occurring.

monilia — also known as *candida,* a yeast infection of the vagina.

mons veneris — also known as *mons pubis*, translates as Mountain of Venus. The mons veneris consists of pads of fatty tissue lying below the skin and over the pubic symphysis.

MRI — see *magnetic resonance imaging.*

mucous plug — an additional protection provided by the cervix in the form of thick secretions which separate the uterus from both the vagina and the outside environment, thereby lessening the possibility of infection.

mullerian ducts — embryonic tubes which, if the embryo is to be a female, form the fallopian tubes, the uterus, and the top four-fifths of the vagina.

muscle specificity — refers to the fact that different muscles are used in different activities so that being in good condition in one activity does not necessarily imply that your muscles are ready for a different activity.

myocardial infarction — the technical term for a heart attack. Infarction means "death of"; the myocardium is the muscular layer of the wall of the heart.

myoma — also *fibroid;* a benign tumor made of muscular fiber; plural is myomata.

myomata — plural form of *myoma.*

myomectomy — surgical removal of a myoma or myomata — uterine fibroids.

myometrium — the middle muscular layer of the wall of the uterus.

myotonia — increased bodily muscle tension.

negative — a condition or test result which is normal and shows no pathology.

nerve growth factor (NGF) — a protein produced by the body with hormone-like action that affects the growth and care of nerve cells.

NGF — see *nerve growth factor.*

NMR — see *magnetic resonance imaging.*

nuclear magnetic resonance — see *magnetic resonance imaging.*

nulliparous — never pregnant.

oocyte — an ovum in an early stage of development.

oophorectomy — also *ovariectomy;* also *castration;* the surgical removal of the ovaries.

oophoritis — inflammation of an ovary.

orgasm — sexual climax.

oscilloscope — a TV-like screen on which sound waves, or a sonogram, is viewed.

osteoporosis — thinning, demineralization, and weakening of the bones, making them more vulnerable to breakage; sometimes accompanied by pain or body deformity.

ovariectomy — see *oopherectomy.*

ovaries — the female gonads, which are homologous to the male testicles. The function of the ovary is to store and release eggs and to manufacture hormones.

ovulation — when the follicle ruptures within the ovary, thereby releasing the ovum.

ovum — the egg in the follicle in the ovary.

palpation — touch used during examination.

panhysterectomy — see *hysterectomy with bilateral salpingo-oopherectomy.*

Pap smear — test used as a screening for cervical cancer; can also detect vaginal cancer and chlamydia, a sexually transmitted disease.

partial hysterectomy — also subtotal hysterectomy; the removal of the body of the uterus, leaving the cervix in place.

pelvic endoscopy — examining the interior of the pelvic cavity using a laparascope.

pelvic girdle — the two hip bones, the sacrum and the coccyx.

pelvic inflammatory disease (PID) — infection and/or inflammation of the fallopian tubes, ovaries, and/or uterus.

pelvis — "basin" in Latin, the lower part of the trunk of the body; these bones that provide an attachment for the legs and support the lower spine.

perimetrium — the uterine walls' outer layer of elastic fibrous tissue.

peristalsis — the muscular action which pushes food through the large intestine.

peritoneoscopy — see *laparoscopy.*

peri-urethral glands — the aggregate of cells which surround the urethra; the female equivalent of the prostatic gland in men.

pessary — a device inserted into the vagina which may ease the symptoms of a vaginal hernia.

Pfannestiel incision — also *bikini cut;* a horizontal cut just above the pubic hairline; may be used for abdominal hysterectomy.

phospholipids — compounds such as cholesterol and lecithin.

PID — see *pelvic inflammatory disease.*

pituitary gland — one of the body's endocrine glands, at one time considered to be the master gland of the body.

plateau — according to Masters and Johnson, the second stage in sexual response; it follows arousal and precedes orgasm.

PMS — see *premenstrual syndrome.*

polyp — a protruding benign growth from a mucous membrane; for example, cervical polyps.

positive imagery — see *visualization.*

postmenopausal bleeding — bloody vaginal discharge six months or more after a presumed last menstrual period.

post-operative residual ovary syndrome — when the ovaries have been left in place following hysterectomy, thick adhesions may form on them which prevents the development and release of eggs. Ovarian hormones may also be blocked.

precancerous lesion — a change in cell appearance that suggests a condition which may become malignant.

premenstrual syndrome (PMS) — the diagnostic term used to describe a variety of symptoms occurring prior to menstrual flow.

primary dysmenorrhea — painful menstrual periods caused by uterine contractions.

progesterone — in humans, the naturally occurring progestin. It accomplishes its function of preparing the uterus for implantation of a fertilized ovum and then maintaining it.

progestins — compounds (both natural and synthetic) which produce changes in the uteral endometrium — after it has been previously prepared by estrogen.

progestogen — synthetic progesterone.

progestogen challenge test — a test which assesses potential natural or medicinal estrogenic stimulation of the endometrium which could result in a higher risk for developing hyperplasia or adenocarcinoma.

prolapsed uterus — see *uterine prolapse.*

proliferative phase — the stage in the endometrial cycle when the endometrial wall is very thin but, under the stimulation of estrogen, begins to grow.

prostate — the gland located directly below the male's bladder. Its secretions make up part of the seminal fluid.

pruritis — intense itching.

puberty — the point when males or females are first able to reproduce; that is, to produce viable sperm or eggs.

pubescence — the time period and the physical and biological changes leading to puberty.

pubic — the anterior (front) portion of the hip bone.

pubic symphysis — the joining place of the two pubic bones in the front of the body.

pubococcygeal — the area including the muscles around the pubic bone and the coccyx; associated with Kegel exercises.

pudendum — Latin for *vulva*, or "covering"; refers to the outer genitalia.

radiation therapy — the use of X-ray techniques to destroy cancer cells.

radical hysterectomy — the removal of the cervix and body of the uterus, the fallopian tubes, and often a portion of the vagina.

range percentage (RP) — a target cardiac goal to achieve for physical fitness. RP can be 60 to 90 percent of the difference between your resting heart rate and your maximum heart rate.

rectocele — a hernia, or bulging, of the rectum, intruding into the vagina.

resectoscope — an electrical instrument used for surgical cutting.

resistance stage — the second stage of the General Adaptation Syndrome, in which an attempt is made by the body to redirect the generalized response from the first stage to a more manageable level.

resolution — according to Masters and Johnson, the final stage of sexual response; it follows orgasm and is characterized by the body returning to its prearousal state.

resting heart rate — the number of heartbeats per minute when your body is at rest.

Robinul — an anticholinergic drug which dries up excess secretions during surgery.

RP — see *range percentage.*

salpingitis — inflammation of the fallopian tubes.

salpinx — the Greek word for "trumpet" or "tube"; refers to the fallopian tubes.

same-day admission surgery — the procedure whereby you enter the hospital on the morning of your scheduled surgery.

saturated fats — fats derived mainly from animal sources.

scrotum — the pouch which holds the male's testicles.

second opinions — seeing a second doctor for a consultation and confirmation of an original diagnosis.

secondary dysmenorrhea — painful menstrual periods due to problems associated with an IUD, polyps, fibroids, endometriosis, etc.

secretory phase — the stage in the endometrial cycle when the glands of the endometrium become swollen and fill up with secretions of fat and glycogen in preparation for pregnancy.

sensate focus — massage-like touch used to explore a sexual partner's body.

serology test — laboratory analysis of blood for antibodies, immune complexes, and antigen-antibody reactions.

sexual response cycle — the term used by Masters and Johnson to describe the sexual stages: arousal, plateau, orgasm, and resolution.

sexually transmitted disease (STD) — any disease usually contracted through sexual intimacy. The old term was *venereal disease,* or *VD.*

SIL — see *squamous intraepithelial lesion.*

simulation — a procedure involved in cancer treatment in which the area to be targeted in radiation therapy is marked.

Skene's ducts — serve as large collecting conduits for the female's peri-urethral glands.

smegma — the white cheese-like substance produced by the glands in the penis and the clitoris.

sonogram — ultrasound pictures taken of internal organs that can reveal their condition.

speculum — an instrument used to separate the walls of a body cavity to permit examination; for example, the vaginal speculum.

spinbarkeit — the term for the thick, viscous vaginal discharge which occurs at the time of ovulation.

squamous cell carcinoma — cancer cells which have developed from flat, scalelike epithelial tissue.

squamous intraepithelial lesion — the presence of atypical, possibly cancerous, cells.

stage — a period in the progression of a disease or cancer.

STD — see *sexually transmitted disease.*

stress — in common usage, refers to two different things — the situations that produce physiological changes, and the physiological changes themselves.

stress incontinence — leaking urine when there is increased abdominal pressure, such as while sneezing, laughing, running, or straining.

stress response — the basic physiological responses to a stressor: they mobilize the body and enable it to reduce the stressor.

stressors — any physical or psychological event or condition that produces stress.

subtotal hysterectomy — see *partial hysterectomy.*

surgical menopause — technically, the removal of the ovaries (oopherectomy or castration); but also sometimes used to refer to the removal of the uterus.

Synarel — a GnRH analog which blocks estrogen production.

synthetic estrogen — compounds, like diethylstilbestrol (DES), which have an estrogenic effect.

syphilis — a sexually transmitted disease caused by a bacteria.

systolic blood pressure — a measurement which reflects the heart's force at its maximum contraction.

tamoxifen — a drug used to treat breast cancer but which may contribute to endometrial cancer.

target heart rate (THR) — the use of heart rate as a measure of intensity for achieving a training effect in exercise.

taxol — a drug which has been used in the treatment of ovarian tumors.

testosterone — the hormone associated with males. It is also produced by females, mainly by the adrenal glands and in limited amounts.

THR — see *target heart rate.*

thrombus — a clot.

total blood cholesterol — the sum of cholesterol carried by the several types of lipoproteins.

total hysterectomy — also *complete hysterectomy;* the removal of both the cervix and the body of the uterus.

trabecular bone — the honeycombed network of bone plates that give elasticity and strength to the bones.

transducer — a hand-held, wandlike instrument which is used to send sound waves to internal organs; these are then reflected and viewed on a video monitor.

treatment port — in cancer therapy, the place to which external radiation beams are to be directed.

trichomoniasis — a protozoan-caused infection characterized by genital itching and discharge.

triglycerides — fatty acids, which represent about 95 percent of the fat we eat.

tumor — a swelling or new growth of tissue; may be benign or malignant.

ultrasonography — the use of very high frequency sound waves in the visualization of body organs.

ultrasound — see *ultrasonography*.

unopposed HRT — hormone therapy where progestin is not included.

unsaturated fats — generally liquid at room temperature, they are derived primarily from plant sources.

urethra — the canal through which urine is discharged from the bladder.

urinalysis — a series of tests aimed at studying urine makeup.

urinary incontinence — difficulty in retaining urine.

uterine prolapse — also prolapsed uterus; the abnormal protrusion, or falling, of the uterus through the pelvic floor.

uterus — a hollow, thick-walled muscular organ that houses the developing fetus. It has the ability to grow from a weight of two ounces to two pounds during pregnancy and then shrink back to original size by six weeks after delivery.

vagina — a muscular tube about three inches long connecting the uterine cervix with the external female genitals.

vaginal hernia — any bulge into the vaginal wall; including cystocele (coming from the bladder), rectocele (coming from the rectum), enterocele (coming from the small intestine), and uterine prolapse.

vaginismus — a painful, involuntary contraction of the outer third of the vagina, making it impenetrable.

vasocongestion — increased blood flow to the sexual organs occuring during sexual arousal.

vasomotor instability — see *hot flashes*.

venipuncture — the method by which blood is taken from a vein in the arm.

Versed — a short-acting central nervous system depressant, used as a sedative and to block memory of surgical events.

vestibular bulbs — the female equivalent of the male's corpus spongiosum. They are located internally and laterally alongside the vagina and become engorged with blood during sexual excitement.

vestibule — which means "entry," describes the entire cleft enclosed by the labia minora. It houses the hymen and the openings of the vagina, urethra, Bartholin's ducts, and Skene's ducts.

vibrator — a battery- or electrically-powered device that may be used to massage or stimulate any part of the body, including the genitals.

visualization therapy — imagining or visualizing that medicine, other treatment, or the body itself is curing a disease or disorder.

vulva — the term for the visible female anatomical structures. It includes the structures located in the space between the thighs, bounded in the front by the mons veneris and in the back by the anus.

withdrawal bleeding — menstrual-like bleeding that may accompany hormone replacement therapy when progestins are used.

X-rays — electromagnetic radiation that can be used at high levels to treat cancer and at low levels to diagnose disease.

Index